PROGRESS IN BRAIN RESEARCH

VOLUME 74

TRANSDUCTION AND CELLULAR MECHANISMS
IN SENSORY RECEPTORS

Recent volumes in PROGRESS IN BRAIN RESEARCH

PROGRESS IN BRAIN RESEARCH

VOLUME 74

TRANSDUCTION AND CELLULAR MECHANISMS IN SENSORY RECEPTORS

EDITED BY

W. HAMANN

Faculty of Medicine, The Chinese University of Hong Kong, Shatin, NT, Hong Kong

and

A. IGGO

Department of Preclinical Veterinary Sciences, University of Edinburgh, Edinburgh EH9 1QH, UK

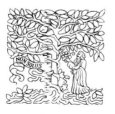

ELSEVIER
AMSTERDAM — NEW YORK — OXFORD
1988

© 1988, Elsevier Science Publishers B.V. (Biomedical Division)

ISBN 0-444-80971-6 (volume)
ISBN 0-444-80104-9 (series)

Published by:
Elsevier Science Publishers B.V. (Biomedical Division)
P.O. Box 211
1000 AE Amsterdam
The Netherlands

Sole distributors for the USA and Canada:
Elsevier Science Publishing Company, Inc.
52 Vanderbilt Avenue
New York, NY 10017
USA

Library of Congress Cataloging-in-Publication Data

Transduction and cellular mechanisms in sensory receptors / edited by
  W. Hamann and A. Iggo.
      p.   cm. -- (Progress in brain research ; v. 74)
    Proceedings of a symposium held in the spring of 1987 at the
Chinese University of Hong Kong.
    Bibliography: p.
    Includes index.
    ISBN 0-444-80971-6
    1. Sensory receptors--Congresses.   I. Hamann, W.   II. Iggo,
Ainsley.   III. Series.
QP376.P7 vol. 74
[QP447]
612'.82 s--dc19
[591.1'82]   88-14689
                                                       CIP

Printed in The Netherlands

List of Contributors

A. Adachi, Department of Physiology, Okayama University Dental School, Shikata-cho, Okayama 700, Japan

A. Anand, DST Centre for Visceral Mechanisms, V.P. Chest Institute, University of Delhi, Delhi-110 007, India

K.H. Andres, Anatomisches Institut, Abteilung Neuroanatomie, Ruhr-Universität Bochum, Postfach 102148, 4630 Bochum, FRG

J.F. Ashmore, Department of Physiology, Medical School, University of Bristol, UK

A.R. Astbury, Department of Anatomy, Guy's Campus, United Medical and Dental Schools of Guy's and St. Thomas's Hospitals, London SE1 9RT, UK

L.H. Bannister, Department of Anatomy, Guy's Campus, United Medical and Dental Schools of Guy's and St. Thomas's Hospitals, London SE1 9RT, UK

K.I. Baumann, Department of Physiology, Faculty of Medicine, The Chinese University of Hong Kong, Shatin, N.T., Hong Kong

L.A.M. Bharali, Department of Physiology, Medical School, University Walk, Bristol BS8 1TD, UK

H.A. Braun, Physiologisches Institut, Universität Marburg, D-3550 Marburg, FRG

R.H. Cohen, Department of Neurosurgery, Johns Hopkins Medical School, 600 N. Wolfe St., Baltimore, MD 21205, USA

J. Diamond, Department of Neurosciences, McMaster University, 1200 Main Street West, Hamilton, Ontario, L8N 3Z5, Canada

B.G. Dinger, Departments of Pharmacology and Toxicology, University of Utah School of Medicine, 410 Chipeta Way, Research Park, Salt Lake City, UT 84108, USA

H.C. Dodson, Department of Anatomy, Guy's Campus, United Medical and Dental Schools of Guy's and St. Thomas's Hospitals, London SE1 9RT, UK

E.E. Douek, E.N.T. Department, Guy's Hospital London SE1 9RT, UK

S.J. Fidone, Department of Physiology, University of Utah School of Medicine, 410 Chipeta Way, Research Park, Salt Lake City, UT 84108, USA

G.S. Findlater, Department of Anatomy, University of Edinburgh Medical School, Teviot Place, Edinburgh, UK

Å. Flock, Department of Physiology, Karolinska Institute, S-104 01 Stockholm, Sweden

C. Gonzalez, Departamento de Fisiología y Bioquímica, Facultad de Medicina, Valladolid, Spain

J.E. Gregory, Department of Physiology, Monash University, Clayton, Victoria, Australia

Z. Halata, Anatomisches Institut der Universität in Hamburg, Abteilung für Funktionelle Anatomie, Martinistrasse 52, D-2000 Hamburg 20, FRG

W. Hamann, Department of Physiology, Faculty of Medicine, The Chinese University of Hong Kong, Shatin, N.T., Hong Kong

G.R. Hanson, Departments of Pharmacology and Toxicology, University of Utah School of Medicine, 410 Chipeta Way, Research Park, Salt Lake City, UT 84108, USA

W. Hartschuh, Dermatological Clinic, University of Heidelberg, 6900 Heidelberg, FRG

T. Hashimoto, Institute for Medical and Dental Engineering, Tokyo Medical and Dental University, Surugadai, Kanda, Chiyoda-ku, Tokyo 101, Japan

T. Horikoshi, Department of Physiology, School of Dental Medicine, Tsurumi University, 2-1-3 Tsurumi, Tsurumi-ku, Yokohama 230, Japan

S.H.S. Hughes, Department of Physiology, Medical School, University of Bristol, Bristol, BS8 1TD, UK

A. Iggo, Department of Preclinical Veterinary Sciences, University of Edinburgh, UK

R.D. Johnson, Department of Physiological Sciences, College of Veterinary Medicine, University of Florida, Gainesville, FL 32610, USA

F. Jørgensen, Physiological Institute, Odense University, Campusvej 55, 5230 Odense M, Denmark

E. Jyväsjärvi, Department of Physiology of the University of Helsinki, Siltavuorenpenger 20 J, SF-00170 Helsinki, Finland

J. Kieschke, Anatomisches Institut III, Universität Heidelberg, Im Neuenheimer Feld 307, D-6900 Heidelberg, FRG

K.-D. Kniffki, Physiologisches Institut der Universität Würzburg, Röntgenring 9, D-8700 Würzburg, FRG

M. Kobashi, Department of Physiology, Okayama University Dental School, Shikata-cho, Okayama 700, Japan

G.-M. Koschorke, II Physiologisches Institut, Universität Heidelberg, Im Neuenheimer Feld, D-6900 Heidelberg, FRG

L. Kruger, Departments of Anatomy and Anesthesiology and Brain Research Institute, UCLA Center for Health Sciences, Los Angeles, CA 90024, USA

T. Kumazawa, Department of Nervous and Sensory Functions, Research Institute of Environmental Medicine, Nagoya University, Nagoya, 464 Japan

R.H. LaMotte, Department of Anesthesiology, Yale University School of Medicine, 333 Cedar Street, New Haven, CT 06510, USA

J. Leah, II Physiologisches Institut, Universität Heidelberg, Im Neuenheimer Feld, D-6900 Heidelberg, FRG

M.S. Leung, Department of Physiology, Faculty of Medicine, The Chinese University of Hong Kong, Shatin, N.T., Hong Kong

R.W.A. Linden, Department of Physiology, King's College London, Strand, London WC2R 2LS, UK

S.J.W. Lisney, Department of Physiology, Medical School, University Walk, Bristol BS8 1TD, UK

B. Matthews, Department of Physiology, Medical School, University of Bristol, Bristol BS8 1TD, UK

A.K. McIntyre, Department of Physiology, Monash University, Clayton, Victoria, Australia

K.M. Mearow, Department of Neurosciences, McMaster University, 1200 Main Street West, Hamilton, Ontario, L8N 3Z5, Canada

M.K.C. Mengel, Physiologisches Institut der Universität Würzburg, Röntgenring 9, D-8700 Würzburg, FRG

S. Mense, Anatomisches Institut III, Universität Heidelberg, Im Neuenheimer Feld 307, D-6900 Heidelberg, FRG

L.R. Mills, Department of Neurosciences, McMaster University, 1200 Main Street West, Hamilton, Ontario, L8N 3Z5, Canada

K. Mizumura, Department of Nervous and Sensory Functions, Research Institute of Environmental Medicine, Nagoya University, Nagoya, 464 Japan

D.L. Morgan, Departments of Physiology and Electrical Engineering, Monash University, Clayton, Victoria, Australia

B.L. Munger, Department of Anatomy, The Milton S. Hershey Medical Center, Pennsylvania State University, P.O. Box 850, Hershey, PA 17033, USA

A. Niijima, Department of Physiology, Niigata University School of Medicine, Niigata 951, Japan

D. Nohr, Anatomical Institute, University of Mainz, 6500 Mainz, FRG

H. Ogawa, Department of Physiology, Kumamoto University Medical School, Honjo 2-2-1, Kumamoto 860, Japan

H. Ohmori, National Institute for Physiological Sciences, Myodaiji, Okazaki 444, Japan

E.G. Pacitti, Department of Preclinical Veterinary Sciences, University of Edinburgh, Edinburgh, UK

A.S. Paintal, DST Centre for Visceral Mechanisms, V.P. Chest Institute, University of Delhi, Delhi 110 007, India

E.R. Perl, Department of Physiology, University of North Carolina, Chapel Hill, NC 27514, USA

N.R. Prabhakar, Department of Medicine, Pulmonary Division, University Hospitals, Abbington Road, Cleveland, OH 44116, USA

U. Proske, Department of Physiology, Monash University, Clayton, Victoria, Australia

B.H. Pubols Jr., Neurological Sciences Institute, Good Samaritan Hospital and Medical Center, 1120 N.W. Twentieth Avenue, Portland, OR 97209, USA

P.W. Reeh, Institut für Physiologie und Biokybernetik, Universitätsstrasse 17, D-8520 Erlangen, FRG

L. Rempe, Institut für Zoophysiologie, Universität Hohenheim, D-7000, Stuttgart 70, FRG

J. Sato, Department of Nervous and Sensory Functions, Research Institute of Environmental Medicine, Nagoya University, Nagoya, 464 Japan

K. Schäfer, Institut für Zoophysiologie, Universität Hohenheim, D-7000 Stuttgart 70, FRG

B.J.J. Scott, Department of Physiology, King's College London, Strand, London WC2R 2LS, UK

J.-X. Shen, Institute of Biophysics, Academia Sinica, Beijing, People's Republic of China

K.-F. So, Department of Anatomy, Faculty of Medicine, University of Hong Kong, Hong Kong

M. Sokabe, Department of Physiology, School of Medicine, Nagoya University, 65 Tsuruma-cho, Showa-ku, Nagoya 466, Japan

I. Taniguchi, Medical Research Institute, Tokyo Medical and Dental University, Yushima, Bunkyo-ku, Tokyo 113, Japan

M. von Düring, Anatomisches Institut, Abteilung Neuroanatomie, Ruhr-Universität Bochum, Postfach 102148, 4630 Bochum, FRG

E. Weihe, Department of Anatomy, Johannes Gutenberg-Universität, 6500 Mainz, FRG

E. Welk, II Physiologisches Institut, Universität Heidelberg, Im Neuenheimer Feld, D-6900 Heidelberg, FRG

H. Wissing, Physiologisches Institut, Universität Marburg, D-3550 Marburg, FRG

Z.-M. Xu, Institute of Biophysics, Academia Sinica, Beijing, People's Republic of China

Y. Yamashita, Department of Physiology, Kumamoto University Medical School, Honjo 2-2-1, Kumamoto 860, Japan

K. Yanagisawa, Department of Physiology, School of Dental Medicine, Tsurumi University, 2-1-3 Tsurumi, Tsurumi-ku, Yokohama 230, Japan

T. Yoshioka, Department of Physiology, School of Medicine, Yokohama City University, 2-33 Urafune-cho, Minami-ku, Yokohama 232, Japan

M. Zimmermann, II Physiologisches Institut, Universität Heidelberg, Im Neuenheimer Feld, D-6900 Heidelberg, FRG

Foreword

In 1983 the first international symposium on sensory receptors was held at the Department of Physiology of the Chinese University of Hong Kong. Around fifty specialists participated, who were working in relevant disciplines. The work presented triggered some very interesting and constructive discussion, so that the symposium ended with a consensus that there should be a follow-up. The second international symposium was held at the same venue with equal success in the spring of 1987 and is reported in this volume.

A number of factors contributed to the success of both events. Firstly, the cost of attending was sufficiently low to enable young scientists to attend. This was achieved by generous financial support from the Chinese University of Hong Kong, the Croucher Foundation, the Wellcome Trust and from local business. Furthermore, the Chinese University provided the conference facilities and administrative support. Secondly, the group of participants was small enough to avoid the anonymity of large conferences. Thirdly, the meetings were held at a place, Hong Kong, that offers considerable touristic attractions. Fourthly the main topic of the second symposium, 'stimulus transduction', is usually overshadowed at large neuroscience meetings by the central nervous sensory neurosciences. Whilst understandable, this is to the detriment of sensory neuroscience. Sensory receptors are, after all, the interface between environment and the nervous system, and the present rapid progress in molecular biology is producing a re-appraisal of transduction mechanisms in sensory receptors.

The initiation and implementation of a successful symposium depend heavily on the whole-hearted support of many people. Though it is invidious to make a special mention we would both like to express our very warm thanks to Miss Dori Yang for her conscientious and courteous help at all stages of the symposium and in the editing of the proceedings. Finally, a word of thanks to the participants who not only contributed fully to the symposium but also, and quite remarkably, made the work of editing a pleasure.

We hope that the two symposia in Hong Kong are the beginning of an informal tradition with further symposia to follow, not necessarily all at the same place.

W. Hamann   A. Iggo
Hong Kong   *Edinburgh*

Preface

Colleagues, Ladies and Gentlemen, it is a pleasure to welcome you to the symposium on Transduction and Cellular Mechanisms in Sensory Receptors here at the Chinese University. Over the course of two and a half days, forty plenary lectures and papers reporting new findings in the area will be given. The topics cover a wide range including the structure and function of sensory receptors. There will be plenty of opportunities for discussion and exchange of views.

During recent years, significant progress has been made in the understanding of transduction mechanisms, so that it seems timely to hold a follow-up to the last symposium held here in 1983. We are pleased that so many distinguished scientists were able to come.

We often take our sensory receptors for granted, and it is only in illness and disease that malfunction teaches us how much we depend on intact sensory detection facilities. As in other specialities of medicine, the neurologist aims to treat the cause of an illness, rather than symptoms only. If in disease, sensory pathology has its origin in the periphery, treatment should aim at the specific cause in the periphery. Unfortunately, this is not always possible, largely because of limited knowledge about mechanisms of sensory transduction, and often the only available course of action is symptom control with drugs aimed at the central nervous system. As an example, pain of clearly peripheral origin often needs to be treated with centrally acting drugs with all the unpleasant side effects which many of these drugs have.

This symposium will be another step towards a better understanding of sensory processes. Its importance will be enhanced by the fact that the proceedings are to be published as a volume of *Progress in Brain Research*. Symposia like the present one depend on outside financial support, particularly to enable young scientists to attend. I should like to thank the Croucher Foundation and the Wellcome Trust for their generous financial assistance.

I wish you success with this symposium, and I believe that your expectations will be met. At the same time, I hope that there will be sufficient time for you to explore Hong Kong and to discover some of its unique features.

G.H. Choa
Department of Administrative Medicine,
Hong Kong University,
Hong Kong

Contents

Section 3 — Visceral Receptors, Chemoreception and Molecular Aspects of Receptor Function

Section 4 — Mechanoreceptors and Structural Aspects of Receptor Function

Section 5 — Modulation and Efferent Control of Transduction

SECTION I

Mechanisms of Transduction I

W. Hamann and A. Iggo (Eds.)
Progress in Brain Research, Vol. 74
© 1988 Elsevier Science Publishers B.V. (Biomedical Division)

CHAPTER 1

Ionic mechanisms in hair cells of the mammalian cochlea

J.F. Ashmore

Department of Physiology, Medical School, Bristol BS8 1TD, UK

Introduction

The sensory element common to all vertebrate inner ear structures is the hair cell. Placed between a K-rich endolymph and a low-K perilymph, it is believed that the hair cell transducer channels gate the K flow into the cell. The recent use of a variety of techniques in hair cell physiology has, however, revealed subtle differences between hair cells from different species. To cover a wide dynamic and frequency range, the mammalian cochlea is organised to separate frequencies mechanically along the basilar membrane. This separation is actively controlled (Davis, 1983), by local feedback from the hair cells themselves. In lower vertebrates, however, hair cells act like individual bandpass filter elements, either by membrane electrical resonance (Crawford and Fettiplace, 1981; Lewis and Hudspeth, 1983; Art et al., 1986) or by control of the micromechanics of the stereocilial hair bundle (Holton and Hudspeth, 1983).

The mammalian cochlea contains two morphologically distinct populations of hair cells, inner and outer hair cells. There is growing support, however, for the idea that outer hair cells are capable of both sensing and generating forces (Brownell et al., 1985; Ashmore, 1987), which may influence the motion of the cochlear partition. Although such 'bidirectionality' is a common principle in physical mechano-transducers (Weiss, 1982), its implementation in the cochlea is indirect. Insights into the mechanisms in mammalian hair cells have been obtained by the introduction of patch recording techniques: these will be described in this paper.

Methods

Solitary hair cells were obtained by microdissection of the organ of Corti in the guinea pig into tissue culture medium (Ashmore and Meech, 1986; Ashmore, 1987). Cells were placed in a 300 μl chamber on the stage of an inverted microscope equipped with Nomarski optics and observed at a magnification of 640×. Cells remained in good condition, judged by morphological criteria, for 4 – 5 h at room temperature (20 – 23°C). Mild enzymatic treatment (trypsin, 0.5 mg/ml, for 30 min) was found useful to prepare cells free of the basal synaptic apparatus and facilitate patching, gigaseals forming virtually instantaneously. No difference was found between cells in which the trypsin was washed out from the medium, probably because the enzyme is inactivated. Simple trituration of the cells was also used for dissociation: in this case, seals formed much more slowly (1 – 2 min). Outer hair cells were obtained more readily than inner hair cells. Cells were identified on the basis of their stereocilial pattern, outer hair cells possessing a distinct V-shaped pattern (e.g., Lim, 1986). Conventional patch recording techniques were used (Hamill et al., 1981), using pipettes with internal diameters of 0.5 – 1 μm to dialyse the cells.

Results

Membrane properties of inner hair cells

Inner hair cells are the primary sensory cells of the cochlea, but remain constant in morphology from the basal to the apical end of the cochlea. A distinct non-linear current – voltage curve was apparent when the cells were recorded in whole-cell configuration (Fig. 1). Cells showed an outward current activating sharply at membrane potentials more positive than about – 60 mV. Near physiological membrane potentials (typically – 50 to – 40 mV (Cody and Russell, 1987)), the current appeared to be fully activated, with a slope conductance of 23 nS (range 5 – 30 nS). Below – 60 mV, the current inactivated, almost completely. Reducing the pipette K concentration 10-fold shifted the I – V curve along the voltage axis by 40 mV and reduced the slope conductance of the outward current. These results indicate that the inner hair cell membrane is K-selective. Assuming that both Na and K can pass through the membrane channel, a shift of 40 mV with low internal K suggests a high selectivity for K, $P_K/P_{Na} = 6.6$.

In some cells, individual channels, which are K-permeable, can also be observed in cell-attached patches, with a typical unit conductance of about 95 pS. Surprisingly, the reversal potential of such single channel currents suggests that the intracellular K in these isolated cells may be below 30 mM. This will be discussed again below.

Membrane properties of outer hair cells

The membrane conductances of outer hair cells differ from those of inner hair cells. The simplest observations suggest that the membrane is also permeable to K but is controlled largely by internal Ca concentrations (Ashmore and Meech, 1986). Buffering intracellular calcium by including chelators in the pipette made the membrane potential more negative and decreased the input conductance. When patched with pipettes containing the Ca buffer BAPTA, the cell resting potential gradually increased over about 2 – 3 min to give values near – 60 mV, comparable to values found in vivo (Cody and Russell, 1987). The simplest interpretation is that removal of calcium from within the cell closes most of the K(Ca) channels, leaving

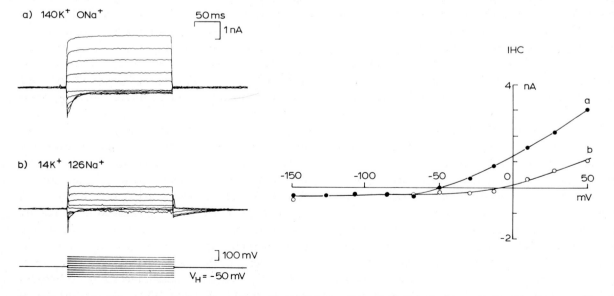

Fig. 1. Inner hair cell currents, whole-cell recording. Extracellular medium, L-15 (principal ions: Na$^+$ 145, K$^+$ 5.4, Ca^{2+} 1.3). Pipette contained major ions as shown (mM): (a) K$^+$ 140, closed circles; (b) K$^+$ 14, Na$^+$ 126, open circles. Ca(EGTA) 0.01 μM.

the membrane potential to be controlled by residual K(Ca) channels and an inward rectifying channel, which can be revealed by bath application of cadmium. The difficulties of buffering intracellular Ca near K(Ca) channels are well known (Marty and Neher, 1985) and the same difficulties arise with outer hair cells.

Fig. 2 shows an experiment in which the internal Ca buffering of the cell was increased by including BAPTA, theoretically estimated to reduce free Ca below 10 nM. However, the I – V curve of the cell shows an N-shaped form characteristic of a Ca and K(Ca) conductance system (Meech 1978). The distribution of the K(Ca) channels is likely to be non-uniform. Patch sampling may well be biassed towards certain channel types, but considerable

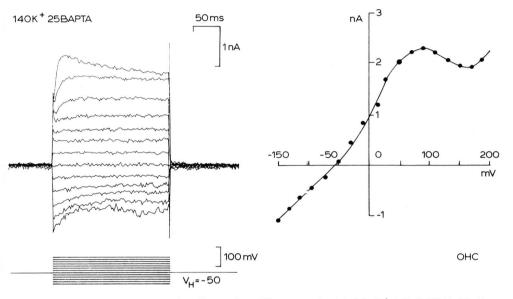

Fig. 2. Outer hair cell currents, whole-cell recording. Pipette contained (mM): K^+ 140, BAPTA 25. Currents measured at 200 ms. Cell RP, – 53 mV. Input slope conductance, 8 nS. The outward current is blocked by 1 mM Cd^+ (Ashmore and Meech, 1986), leaving a residual inward rectifier conductance, labelled g_i in Fig. 6.

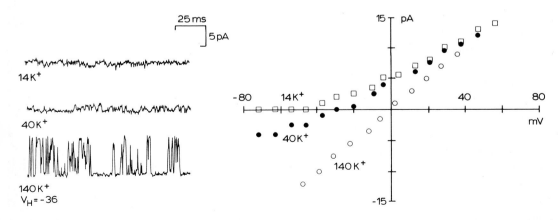

Fig. 3. Selectivity of a large Ca-activated K current from the outer hair cell base. Cell-detached patch. Pipette contained (mM): K^+ 140, Ca^{2+} 1.25, Mg^{2+} 2. Cytoplasmic K concentrations as shown; solutions contained 0.25 μM Ca. Channel membrane potential indicated, outward current upwards. Unit slope conductance (pS), K_i (mM): 250, 140; 161, 40; 149, 14.

single channel activity was found at the basal region of the cell where the efferent synaptic contacts are made. K(Ca) channels may be studied in cell detached patches, allowing the cytoplasmic concentration of Ca to be varied. Two types of Ca-activated K channel were found: one with a unit conductance of about 230 pS and the other smaller channel with a unit conductance of 45 pS in bilateral 140 mM K (Ashmore and Meech, 1986).

Fig. 3 shows an experiment in which the K was changed on the cytoplasmic surface of a patch in which there was a single 250 pS channel. The selectivity of the channel for K against Na was 8.6:1, comparable to the estimate for the inner hair cell membrane. Such experiments show that this channel type in outer hair cells has features in common with those found in other tissues. Although this selectivity ratio is high, it should be noted that a large, but still finite, K:Na selectivity ratio means that cells will tend to lose resting potential in the absence of K repletion. The observed selectivity implies that intracellular Na would rise in isolated cells at a rate of about 0.7 mM/s if permeating through these channels.

Mechano-electric transduction in mammalian hair cells

Until recently, inferences about the nature of the transducer in mammalian hair cells were based on results from intracellular recordings in vivo (Russell and Sellick, 1983; Dallos et al., 1982). Although the transducers of lower vertebrate hair cells have survived isolation procedures (Ohmori, 1985; Art et al., 1986), most studies have been based on isolated epithelia. Only recently have attempts been made to record from mammalian hair cells in vitro (Russell et al., 1986), in a preparation consisting of the developing mouse cochlea. These results show that the mechano-electric transducer is sensitive to movements measured in nanometers.

One difficulty is that organisation of stereocilia into a V-shaped geometry in outer hair cells makes an effective coupling between a displacing microprobe and the bundle hard to achieve. Fig. 4 shows

that a small mechanically induced current can be measured in isolated outer hair cells. The current was reversibly blocked by 300 μM streptomycin, a known ototoxic agent, when applied to the bath. This has been used as a detection criterion of the transducer channel in the frog saccular hair cells (Corey and Hudspeth, 1983). The novel feature of the outer hair cell current, however, is that it is a non-linear function of membrane potential. The currents generating the receptor potential in vivo are generated when about 160 mV is established across the apical transducer (Russell, 1983). Ex-

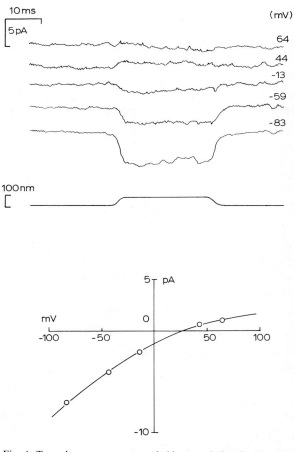

Fig. 4. Transducer currents recorded in outer hair cell. Currents activated by deflection of stereocilia in the conventional excitatory direction by a piezo-electric probe. Cell voltage-clamped at potentials indicated, all other currents subtracted. Cell in L-15, pipette as in Fig. 1a. Below, I–V curve for transducer current.

trapolating even the small currents in Fig. 4 yields estimates for the receptor potential of $1-2$ mV.

These measurements indicate that the outer hair cell transducer channels are likely to account for only about $5-10\%$ of the total membrane conductance. Thus current–voltage curves of outer hair cells will be dominated by the properties of the basolateral membrane. The comparable measurements for inner hair cells are not known. The quasi-linear $I-V$ curves for inner hair cells measured in vivo (Russell, 1983) are inconsistent with the measurements on inner hair cells in vitro (Fig. 1) and suggest that the transducer in inner hair cells accounts for a much larger fraction of the cell input resistance. This would certainly be required for the larger receptor potentials of inner hair cells.

Electro-mechanical coupling in outer hair cells

The most surprising feature of isolated outer hair cells is that they are motile (Brownell et al., 1985; Ashmore, 1987). Membrane depolarisation and hyperpolarisation shorten and lengthen the cells respectively (Fig. 5).

Patch recording methods provide good temporal control of the cell membrane potential and using a wide-band photosensor to detect movements, motile responses can be shown to follow command potentials at frequencies of up to at least 5 kHz (Ashmore, 1987). Although a variety of proposals for the mechanism have been made, the most likely explanation is the presence of a voltage-sensing mechanism in the outer hair cell plasmalemma, providing an electrostrictive mechanism whereby the cell can change shape against the surrounding viscous forces. The rate at which such movements can be induced, however, precludes a mechanism based solely on an interaction between actin and myosin but does indicate that the cells are capable of generating axial forces at acoustic frequencies. It is now appreciated that active mechanisms are involved in cochlear mechanics, mainly to counteract fluid damping of the basilar membrane (Neely and Kim, 1986). Properties of the outer hair cell

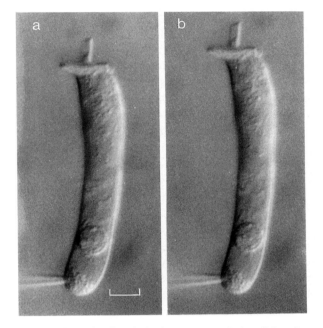

Fig. 5. Effect of cell polarisation on outer hair cell length. (a) Depolarised ($+50$ mV); (b) hyperpolarised (-150 mV). Scale, 10 μm.

thus fit the role of the cell as a force generating element within the cochlea. However, various attempts to reintegrate the cellular knowledge about hair cells into a full cochlear model are, because of the intrinsic non-linearity of the cochlear mechanics, likely to be faced with severe computational problems (e.g., Allen et al., 1985).

Discussion

The ionic properties of inner and outer hair cells reported here are seen to be quite different. Neither show any evidence of electrical tuning characteristic of lower vertebrate hair cells. Although it must be supposed that both cells detect a component of shear between the tectorial membrane and the reticular lamina, both cells have ionic channels designed to optimise K flow through the apical transduction channels. The role of the outer hair cell appears to be that of a device for boosting the motion of the basilar membrane near its best frequency.

Fig. 6 summarises the present results. The main feature is that both cell membranes are specialised to maximise the cell resting potential in the presence of a + 80 mV endocochlear potential. In such a scheme, one possibility is that Ca would enter via the transducer channel (Ohmori, 1985) to activate basal K channels outside the range of normal Ca channel thresholds.

Outer hair cells maintained in extracellular medium are found to have a relatively low initial resting potential, typically − 30 to − 15 mV. This is found even when recorded with microelectrodes (Brownell et al., 1985; Ashmore, unpublished). This suggests that the cells may exchange intracellular K for Na, when isolated. There are no definitive reports of an ATPase in either inner or outer hair cell, so that a likely explanation of the high resting potentials in vivo is that intracellular K levels may be maintained by loading through the transducer from the endolymph. The effective sodium pump for the cell would therefore be in the stria vascularis (Brownell et al., 1986).

The main function of such an arrangement is to reduce the metabolic load on such terminally differentiated cells. A high K flux passes through the cell: Brownell et al. (1986) have estimated the silent current as 500 pA (carried by K from the endolymph), on the assumption that none passes through the supporting cells. The present direct measurements of the transducer current reduce that estimate by a factor of about 5, but nevertheless a complete turnover of K in about 10 minutes in an apical outer hair cell would be anticipated. However, despite a high K endolymph which faces the transducer surface, there appears to be no evidence for a similar K loading from the endolymph in lower vertebrate cells.

Acknowledgements

This work was supported by the Medical Research Council, UK. I thank Rob Meech, who participated in the early experiments, Matthew Holley and Simon Pitchford for many helpful discussions.

References

Allen, J.B., Hall, J.L., Hubbard, A., Neely, S.T. and Tubis, A. (Eds.) (1985) Peripheral Auditory Mechanisms. Lecture Notes in Biomathematics, Vol 64. Springer-Verlag, Berlin.

Art, J.J., Crawford, A.C. and Fettiplace, R. (1986) Membrane currents in solitary turtle hair cells. In: B.C.J. Moore and R.D. Patterson (Eds.), Auditory Frequency Selectivity. Plenum Press, New York, pp. 81 − 88.

Ashmore, J.F. (1987) A fast motile event in outer hair cells isolated from the guinea pig cochlea. J. Physiol. (London), 388: 323 − 347.

Ashmore, J.F. and Meech, R.W. (1986) Ionic basis of membrane potential in outer hair cells of guinea pig cochlea. Nature (London), 322: 368 − 371.

Brownell, W.E., Bader, C.R., Bertrand, D. and de Ribaupierre, Y. (1985) Evoked mechanical responses of isolated cochlear outer hair cells. Science, 227: 194 − 196.

Brownell, W.E., Zidanic, M. and Spirou, G.A. (1986) Standing currents and their modulation in the cochlea. In: R.A. Altschuler, D.W. Hoffman and R.P. Bobbin (Eds.), Neurobiology of Hearing: The Cochlea. Raven Press, New York.

Cody, A.R. and Russell, I.J. (1987) The responses of hair cells in the basal turn of the guinea pig cochlea to tones. J. Physiol. (London), 383: 551 − 569.

Corey, D.P. and Hudspeth, A.J. (1983) Analysis of the microphonic potential of the bullfrog's sacculus. J. Neurosci., 3: 942 − 961.

Crawford, A.C. and Fettiplace, R. (1981) An electrical tuning mechanism in turtle cochlear hair cells. J. Physiol. (London), 312: 377 − 412.

Crawford, A.C. and Fettiplace, R. (1985) The mechanical pro-

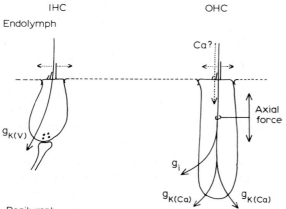

Fig. 6. Summary diagram of currents described in inner and outer hair cells.

perties of ciliary bundles of turtle cochlear hair cells. *J. Physiol. (London),* 364: 359 – 380.

Dallos, P., Santos-Sacchi, J. and Flock, A. (1982) Intracellular recordings from cochlear outer hair cells. *Science,* 218: 582 – 584.

Davis, H. (1983) An active process in cochlear mechanics. *Hearing Res.,* 9: 79 – 90.

Hamill, O., Marty, A., Neher, E., Sakmann, B. and Sigworth, F.J. (1981) Improved patch clamp techniques for high-resolution current recording from cells and cell-free membrane patches. *Pflügers Arch.,* 391: 85 – 100.

Holton, T. and Hudspeth, A.J. (1983) A micromechanical contribution to cochlear tuning and tonotopic organization. *Science,* 222: 508 – 510.

Lewis, R.S. and Hudspeth, A.J. (1983) Voltage- and ion-dependent conductances in solitary vertebrate hair cells. *Nature (London),* 304: 538 – 541.

Lim, D.J. (1986) Functional structure of the organ of Corti: a review. *Hearing Res.,* 22: 117 – 146.

Marty, A. and Neher, E. (1985) Potassium channels in cultured bovine adrenal chromaffin cells. *J. Physiol. (London),* 360: 117 – 142.

Meech, R.W. (1978) Calcium-activated potassium currents in nervous tissues. *Ann. Rev. Biophys. Bioengng.,* 7: 1 – 18.

Neely, S.T. and Kim, D.O. (1986) A model for active elements in cochlear biomechanics. *J. Acoust. Soc. Am.,* 79: 1472 – 1480.

Ohmori, H. (1985) Mechano-electrical transduction currents in isolated vestibular hair cells of the chick. *J. Physiol. (London),* 359: 189 – 218.

Russell, I.J. (1983) The origins of the receptor potential in hair cells of the mammalian cochlea, *Nature (London),* 301: 334 – 336.

Russell, I.J., Richardson, G.P. and Cody, A.R. (1986) Mechanosensitivity of mammalian auditory hair cells in vitro. *Nature (London),* 321: 517 – 519.

Weiss, T.F. (1982) Bidirectional transduction in vertebrate hair cells: a mechanism for coupling mechanical and electrical processes. *Hearing Res.,* 7: 431 – 438.

W. Hamann and A. Iggo (Eds.)
Progress in Brain Research, Vol. 74
© 1988 Elsevier Science Publishers B.V. (Biomedical Division)

CHAPTER 2

Mechano-electrical transduction of the chick hair cell

Harunori Ohmori

National Institute for Physiological Sciences, Myodaiji, Okazaki 444, Japan

Summary

A hair cell transduces mechanical energy applied to the apical hair bundle into an electrical signal, the transduction potential. The mechanical energy is most likely transduced into an electrical signal through mechanically gated ionic channels. Several features of the gate, ion selectivity and the discrete nature of the conductance are discussed.

Using the Ca-sensitive dye Fura-2 an inference was made on the site of mechano-electrical transduction.

Introduction

The sensory hair cell transduces mechanical energy applied to the apical hair bundle into an electrical signal (Hudspeth, 1983), through gatings of a mechanically gated ion channel. The coupling between the hair bundle displacement and the gating of the channel is still obscure. However, because of the high-speed switching properties of the mechano-electrical transduction (m-e.t.) channel (Corey and Hudspeth, 1983), a chance for a second messenger to be in direct operation in the gating mechanism seems small. Ionic selectivity, the discrete nature of conductance and some features of gatings have been demonstrated in detail in the mechano-electrical transduction channel of a chick vestibular hair cell (Ohmori, 1985, 1987). These three elements determine the nature of ion channels, in general (Hille, 1984).

Materials and methods

Hair cells were isolated from the vestibular organ of a chick, by partly enzymatic procedures, using papain, and partly mechanical procedures (Ohmori, 1984). The patch electrode voltage-clamp technique was applied to isolated hair cells. The experiment was performed at $28-30°C$.

A calibrated mechanical stimulation was applied exactly at a defined site on the hair bundle by a piezo-electrical mechanostimulator. Whole procedures could be observed and were recorded by using a contrast enhanced video-microscope system (AVEC/VIM system, Hamamatsu Photonics, Hamamatsu, Japan). Fig. 1A demonstrates one cycle of a mechanical stimulation applied to the hair bundle. The exact displacement of the hair bundle and the glass rod could be measured from a series of these pictures. They moved in complete synchrony. Fig. 1C shows a subtraction between the first frame (resting position) and the third frame (most bent position) of Fig. 1A. Moved parts during subtraction are indicated in white. The glass rod appears as a white band of constant width, and the hair bundle appears wedge-shaped, with the width at its tip exactly matching the width of the glass rod motion. It becomes narrower and disappears about the insertion to the cuticle. The hair bundle is, therefore, bent relative to the cuticle by exactly the amplitude of the glass rod motion.

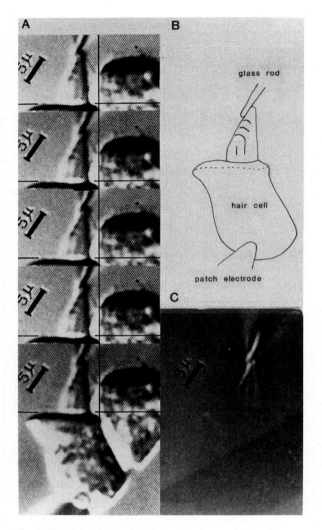

Fig. 1. Television images of a hair cell, the patch electrode and the stimulating probe. The distance between the glass rod contact and the hair bundle insertion to the cuticle is 7.5 μm. (A) Five frames demonstrate one cycle of the hair bundle displacement and return to the resting position. Cell debris is located at the right side of the hair cell. (C) Frame subtraction output. The images of two frames recorded near minimum and maximum displacement were subtracted. The moved parts in these two frames are illustrated white. The glass rod was focused only at its tip.

Results

Displacement vs. response relationship

In the following measurement of the displacement vs. transduction current amplitude relationship, the mechanical stimulation was applied to the hair bundle while tonically bending it by a very small amplitude – an extent which could be barely seen under a microscope. This procedure was used to ensure that every minute motion of the glass rod was transmitted to the hair bundle.

When a hair bundle was displaced towards the taller stereocilia, an inward going transduction current was generated at -50 mV (Fig. 2). When the displacement amplitude is small, the wave form of the m.-e.t. current resembles the driving signal (0.1 μm), but it becomes rounded with larger displacements. The displacement of the hair bundle towards the shorter stereocilia generated outward currents by closing the open channel. On average 12% of the transduction channels are open in the resting state. The amplitude of the outward current was saturated at small displacements. The overall displacement vs. transduction current relationship is S-shaped (Fig. 2B), and is similar to observations in other species (Hudspeth and Corey, 1977; Crawford and Fettiplace, 1985; Russell et al., 1986).

Mechanical stimulation was applied at exactly 5 μm above the insertion to the cuticle (Fig. 3). The amplitude of mechanical stimulation was changed from 0.1 μm to 0.01 μm in order to evaluate the lower limit of the m.-e.t. Since the glass rod is in maintained contact with the hair bundle, a 100 Å or even smaller displacement stimulus was likely to be transmitted to the hair bundle. Displacement vs. response relationship for the part towards taller stereocilia is demonstrated in Fig. 3B together with five other experiments after scaling. The mechano-electrical transducer generated currents that were linear to stimuli of up to about 0.6 μm, and saturated for much larger displacement. Since the minimum displacement which could generate transduction currents was 100 Å (Fig. 3A), and the

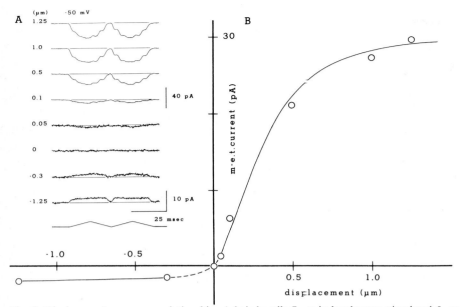

Fig. 2. Displacement – response relationship. A hair bundle 7 μm in lenght was stimulated 5 μm from the insertion to the cuticle. In this and succeeding figures displacements towards taller stereocilia have a positive sign. (A) Total averages of m-e.t. currents measured at −50 mV. Amplitudes of displacement are marked at each trace. The bottom trace indicates the time course of the mechanical stimulation. (B) Average amplitudes of two responses of the m-e.t. current are plotted against displacements. The curve is drawn through the points with a free hand.

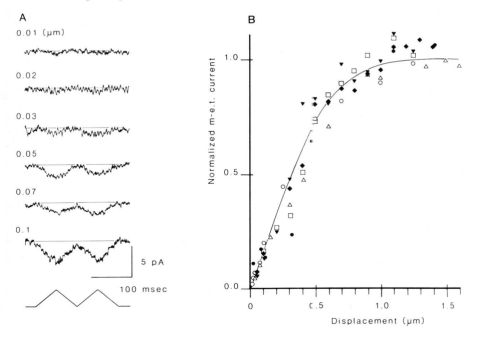

Fig. 3. Displacement – response relationship of the mechano-electrical transducer of hair cells of a short hair bundle group. (A) Total averages of the m-e.t. current generated by 0.01 – 0.1 μm deflection of the hair bundle, recorded at −52 mV. (B) M-e.t. currents recorded in six different cells by displacing the hair bundle at 5 μm above the insertion to the cuticle towards taller stereocilia are plotted after scaling. The solid line in B was drawn with a free hand.

14

stimulus was applied at 5 μm above the insertion to the cuticle, the mechano-electrical transducer of dissociated hair cells transduces the angular displacement of the hair bundle linearly from 0.1° to about 7°.

Angular displacement of the hair bundle determines gatings of the m-e.t. channel

In the vestibular organ, the length of a hair bundle varies systematically (Lewis and Li, 1975). The length is known to be related to the tuning properties in the basilar papilla of a lizard (Turner et al., 1981). Thus, the variation in the length of a hair bundle is likely to reflect sensitivity differences to mechanical stimulation applied to the tip of a hair bundle. Hair cells were, thus, roughly classified into two groups; one with a hair bundle shorter than 7.5 μm and the other with a hair bundle longer

than 12.5 μm. The displacement vs. response relationship presented in Fig. 3B is from the shorter hair bundle group. A comparison of sensitivities to mechanical displacement is made between these two groups of hair cells.

A cell with a 20 μm long hair bundle (Fig. 4) was mechanically stimulated at 10 μm from the hair bundle's insertion to the cuticle. The displacement vs. response relationship is illustrated in Fig. 4B, together with three other experiments. The overall response curve is similar to those in Figs. 2B and 3B. However, an almost linear increase of the transduction current is observed up to about 1.5 μm displacement. This is approximately twice as large as in the experiment made on the shorter hair bundle hair cells (Fig. 3B). The response curve measured from shorter hair bundle hair cells is illustrated here by a broken line.

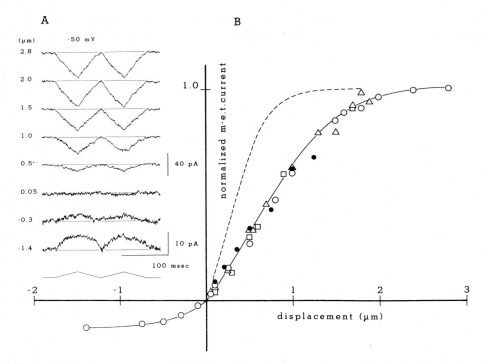

Fig. 4. Displacement – response relationship of the m-e.t. current recorded from hair cells of a long hair bundle group. (A) M-e.t. currents were generated at -50 mV by stimulation of a 20 μm long hair bundle at 10 μm from the insertion to the cuticle. Traces were total averages of 4 – 15 records. Average amplitudes of two responses of m-e.t. currents were plotted in B (open circles) against displacements with three other experiments after scaling. The broken line in B is the relationship determined in Fig. 3 for hair cells with a shorter hair bundle.

Since the distance of the site of mechanical displacement is twice as long in this case as in the previous 5 μm case, these two curves could determine a single displacement vs. response relationship, if the data were plotted against the angular displacement of the hair bundle at the insertion to the cuticle.

As a matter of fact, even a 20 μm long hair bundle could generate an exactly similar response curve to the 7 μm long hair bundle when both were stimulated at 5 μm above the insertion to the cuticle (Ohmori, 1987). These observations indicate that it is not the absolute displacement about the tip of the hair bundle but the angular displacement at the insertion to the cuticle that is the primary factor which governs the gatings of the transduction channel.

Unitary conductances

The unitary conductance is another element of a channel. The discrete nature of the mechano-electrical transduction current is demonstrated in Fig. 5. Transduction currents changed amplitude stepwise when a trapezoidal driving signal was applied to the hair bundle. Measurements were made in CsCl saline (160 mM CsCl, 2.5 mM CaCl$_2$, 10 mM HEPES buffered by TMA-OH to pH 7.4) at +50 mV while perfusing the cell with CsCl−EGTA medium (160 mM CsCl, 5 mM EGTA, 10 mM HEPES buffered by NaOH to pH 7.4), and the outward-going transduction currents were generated. By superimposing these traces, several conductance levels became clear. The amplitude histogram also demonstrates several peaks. This

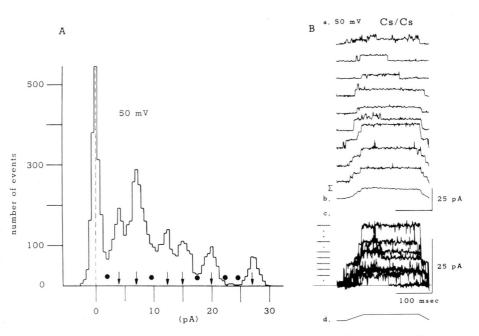

Fig. 5. M-e.t. responses to a trapezoidal driving signal in Cs−saline. The glass rod deflected the hair bundle by about 1 μm and was held at that position for 148 ms. (A) A probability density histogram for current amplitudes in B$_a$. The current levels corresponding to peaks are indicated by arrows on the abscissa. The current levels which are not obvious in the histogram as peaks but likely to exist are indicated by dots. B$_a$ shows individual traces, B$_b$ shows the total average of traces in a, B$_c$ shows superimposed traces and B$_d$ indicates the driving wave form.

histogram pattern and the superimposed current traces are most reasonably explained by assuming 11 channels of 50 pS unitary conductance.

Needless to say, these traces of only 11 conductance steps, thus of 11 channels, do not demonstrate a typical number of the m-e.t. channel of the chick hair cell (Holton and Hudspeth, 1986). Some cells generated much larger currents, but those cells with larger number of channels are inappropriate for demonstrations of stepwise events. The largest conductance of the whole cell transduction current was about 2 nS (Ohmori, 1985). Since the transduction channel is fairly vulnerable and is likely to be damaged during cell dissociation, even this 2 nS whole cell conductance must be taken as the lower limit of the whole cell transduction channel conductance.

Traces illustrated in Fig. $5B_a$ do not demonstrate fast open – close transitions, the so-called *flickering phenomenon* (Colquhoun and Sakmann, 1981). Thus, the open state of the m-e.t. channel might energetically be stable, and may not be allowed to flicker between the closed state. This may contradict the notion of the fast gating kinetics of the m-e.t. channel (Corey and Hudspeth, 1979, 1983; Hudspeth, 1985). The m-e.t. channel is gated by mechanical energy which influences the free-energy profile about the gate. The fast opening and non-flickering interstate transition might be explained by an assumption of a skewed potential energy profile about the gate, and its modification in a flip-flop manner by the externally applied mechanical force.

Smaller levels of conductance steps were observed in the isotonic Sr – saline (100 mM $SrCl_2$, 10 mM HEPES buffered by KOH to pH 7.4) while perfusing a cell with CsCl – EGTA medium. The conductance was about 30 pS and was 60% of that carried by Cs ions (Ohmori, 1985). The step conductance ratio is similar to the ratio of slope conductances between the outward current carried by Cs ions and the inward current carried by Sr ions (Fig. 6).

Ionic selectivity

The third property of the transduction channel is ionic selectivity, and this was studied from measurements of reversal potentials of the transduction currents. Since all the experiments were performed using CsCl as an internal solution, the

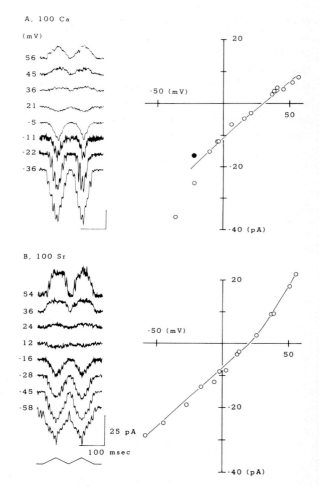

Fig. 6. M-e.t. currents in Ca and in Sr – saline. (A) The m-e.t. currents reversed polarity at + 30 mV in 100 mM Ca – saline. The rundown of the m-e.t. current was quick in this saline. (B) M-e.t. currents reversed polarity at + 20 mV in 100 mM Sr – saline. The I – V relationship showed clear outward-going rectification.

permeability coefficient was calculated as a reference to Cs ions.

Table 1 summarizes reversal potentials and the permeability coefficient relative to Cs ions. Among alkaline cations, the permeability coefficient does not show large differences, but certainly demonstrates a sequence of Li, Na, K, Rb to Cs. This is equal to the XIth sequence of the Eisenman series (Eisenman, 1962), suggesting the presence of a relatively high field strength, negatively charged binding site as a selectivity filter of the channel.

Ca ions and the other divalent cations demonstrated larger permeabilities than monovalent cations. Fig. 6 demonstrates m-e.t. currents carried by Ca ions and Sr ions. In Fig. 6A, transduction currents were generated in isotonic $CaCl_2$ – saline (100 mM $CaCl_2$, 10 mM HEPES buffered by KOH to pH 7.4). The inward-going transduction current was therefore carried by Ca

ions. The amplitude was plotted against membrane potentials, and the current reversed at +30 mV.

Sr ions also carried transduction currents. The reversal potential was +20 mV in isotonic $SrCl_2$ – saline (100 mM, $SrCl_2$, 10 mM HEPES buffered by KOH to pH 7.4). The slope conductance of the inward current carried by Sr ions is 54% of that of the outward current carried by Cs ions. This is due to the inefficiency of Sr ions as a current carrier through the transduction channel (Ohmori, 1985).

Mechano-electrical transduction and the Ca ion

The Ca ion is one of the cations that permeates most easily through the transduction channel (Table 1). Although the concentration of Ca^{2+} in the endolymph is small (Bosher and Warren, 1968), the presence of Ca ions is known to be essential for the mechano-electrical transduction to be in operation (Sand, 1975; Jorgensen, 1983; Ohmori, 1985). The recent development of the Ca-sensitive dye, Fura-2, enabled us to study the intracellular distribution of Ca ions within a very small cell (Grynkiewicz et al., 1985; Williams et al., 1985).

Hair cells were loaded with Fura-2, and excited at 340 nm to monitor fluorescence which is proportional to the intracellular Ca concentration, and at 380 nm to monitor fluorescence reciprocally proportional to the intracellular Ca concentration. By taking the ratio of fluorescence intensities at these two excitation wavelengths, the intracellular Ca concentrations could be estimated irrespective of the variation in the cellular thickness and the concentration of the dye. Fig. 7 demonstrates a Nomarski image (Fig. 7a), an epi-fluorescence image with bright field illumination (Fig. 7b) and an epi-fluorescence image after frame integration (Fig. 7c). Most of the cellular profile comes out in the fluorescence images (Fig. 7c). Fluorescence intensity was measured while displacing the hair bundle towards taller stereocilia and towards shorter stereocilia. The ratio intensity changed in the hair bundle and the cell body with stimulation. With displacements towards taller stereocilia, the ratio

TABLE 1

Reversal potentials and permeability ratios as a reference to Cs

Test cation	$E_{rev} \pm$ S.D. (number of cells) (mV)	P_x/P_{Cs}[a]
Li	+10.7 ± 1.3 (4)	1.39
Na	+7.0 ± 1.6 (12)	1.22
K	+6.8 ± 1.0 (2)	1.17
Rb	+5.9 ± 1.6 (4)	1.12
Cs + 2.5 Ca	+4.3 ± 0.5 (4)	0.96[b]
Cs + 20 μ Ca	+0.3 ± 0.6 (3)	0.99[b]
Choline	−17.0 ± 1.5 (5)	0.33
TMA	−23.5 ± 7.0 (3)	0.20
TEA	−25.3 ± 0.4 (2)	0.17
Ca	+28.2 ± 4.0 (3)	4.65
Sr	+20.6 ± 1.4 (5)	2.82
Ba	+20.2 ± 3.4 (7)	2.73
Mn	+19.0 ± 1.4 (2)	2.50
Mg	+18.0 ± 3.5 (2)	2.41

[a] Except for the calculation of P_{Ca}/P_{Cs} and P_{Sr}/P_{Cs}, the relative permeability coefficients for divalent cations were calculated by using the P_{Ca}/P_{Cs} value of 4.65. The relative permeability ratios of monovalent cations were then calculated by using the values of P_{Ca}/P_{Cs} and P_{Mg}/P_{Cs} in this table.
[b] Relative permeability ratio of external Cs to internal Cs.

intensity increased, while it decreased with displacement towards shorter stereocilia. With small amplitude sinusoidal stimulation at 1 kHz, the ratio intensity increased about the insertion of the hair bundle to the cuticle.

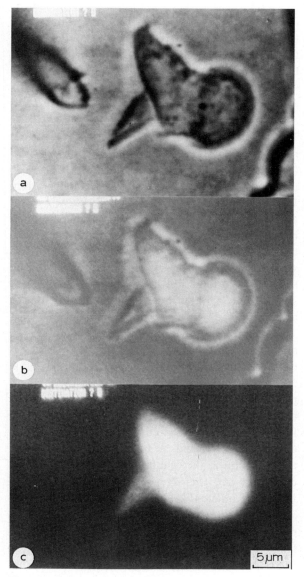

Fig. 7. A hair cell loaded with Fura-2, a Ca-sensitive dye. (a) Shows a hair cell and a stimulating puff pipette. The hair bundle is bent towards the taller stereocilium by puffing. (b) Shows the same hair cell as in (a) with ultraviolet illumination at 340 nm wavelength. (c) Shows epi-fluorescence image after frame integration.

Discussion

Site of m-e. transduction

Mechano-electrical transduction channels may not be located about the distal end of the individual stereocilium (Hudspeth, 1982). Electrophysiological experiments demonstrated that the angular displacement of the hair bundle was a primary factor regulating the steady-state gatings of the channel (Ohmori, 1987). Thus, if we assume a mechano-sensor in detecting angular displacement of the hair bundle and for the gating of the transduction channel, it would be located about the insertion of the stereocilium to the cuticle. Optical experiments detected Fura-2 fluorescence changes about the hair bundle's insertion to the cuticle when it was mechanically stimulated. Since the Ca ion is one of the cations that permeate most easily through the transduction channel, a change in the Fura-2 fluorescence could result from Ca influx through the transduction channel. These two lines of evidence are circumstancial, and we are not yet at a stage to pinpoint the exact site of the mechano-electrical transduction. However, we must take the hair bundle's insertion into the cuticle into consideration again as a candidate for the site of the m-e. transduction. Although the recent finding of the fine fibrous connections about the tip of each stereocilium may indicate a site of transduction there (Pickles et al., 1984), the tip of the stereocilium seems too far for a gate to be affected by the angular displacement of the hair bundle, and Ca ions to influence the fluorescence about the insertion to the cuticle.

Discrete nature of the m-e.t. conductance

I have already presented enough evidence to believe that unitary m-e.t. channels have a conductance of 50 pS in the chick hair cells in normal saline or in artificial Cs − saline (Ohmori, 1985). However, Holton and Hudspeth (1986) failed to record such stepwise current responses in a bullfrog hair cell. The main reasons for their failure could be (1) the low temperature of their experiments (10°C) and (2) relatively high level of background noise in their records. The noise is partly due to (3) the relatively large capacitance (15 pF) of their hair cell. (4) The relatively large transduction current in their preparation might have minimized a chance to disclose stepwise current events further because of the large number of transduction channels in activity.

We are not yet certain about the gating mechanism of the transduction channel. We feel that the channel may be in operation quite similarly to the voltage gated or to the ligand gated other ionic channels in the sense that the channel has a definite unitary conductance, ion selectivity and stochastically regulated kinetics. The most uncertain point about the transduction channel is how mechanical energy leads to gatings of the individual channel. There are at least two possibilities in the case of direct mechanical gatings of the channel (Hille, 1984). The first is that the displacement stimulus alters the potential energy field which uniformly influences the potential energy profile of each gate: namely, the displacement – response relationships measured in Figs. 2, 3 and 4 would represent an open probability of a single m.-e.t. channel in this first occasion. The second possibility is that the alteration of the potential energy field is systematically different from one channel to the other channel because only a fraction of the total displacement stimulus could actually be applied to the gate and that fraction changes systematically from channel to channel. This could happen when the channel locates in relation to the individual stereocilium and when the bundle of stereocilia has some sort of compliance in transmission of the mechanical energy from the tallest group to the shortest group. The displacement – response relationship would then represent a nature of the multiple of the transfer function of the mechanical energy within the ciliary bundle and the gating property of the individual m.-e.t. channel. The individual m.-e.t. channel will not be in a statistically equivalent condition in this second case. The situation that all the components are in statistical equivalence is the prerequisite for quantitative interpretation of stochastic events (Lee, 1960; DeFelice, 1981). In this sense, the mechano-electrical transduction channel may not be appropriate for the type of analysis of the current fluctuations.

References

Bosher, S.K. and Warren, R.L. (1968) Observations on the electrochemistry of the cochlear endolymph of the rat; a quantitative study of its electrical potential and ionic compositions as determined by means of flame spectrophotometry. *Proc. R. Soc. B,* 171: 227 – 244.

Colquhoun, D. and Sakmann, B. (1981) Fluctuations in the microsecond time range of the current through single acetylcholine receptor ion channels. *Nature (London),* 294: 464 – 466.

Corey, D.P. and Hudspeth, A.J. (1983) Kinetics of the receptor current in bullfrog saccular hair cells. *J. Neurosci.,* 5: 962 – 976.

Crawford, A.C. and Fettiplace, R. (1985) The mechanical properties of ciliary bundles of turtle cochlear hair cells. *J. Physiol. (London),* 364: 359 – 379.

DeFelice, L.J. (1981) *Introduction to Membrane Noise.* Plenum Press, New York, 500 pp.

Eisenman, G. (1962) Cation selective glass electrodes and their mode of operation. *Biophys. J.,* 2: 259 – 323.

Grynkiewicz, G., Poenie, M. and Tsien, R. (1985) A new generation of Ca^{2+} indicators with greatly improved fluorescence properties. *J. Biol. Chem.,* 260: 3440 – 3450.

Hille, B. (1984) *Ionic Channels of Excitable Membranes.* Sinauer, Sunderland, MA 426 pp.

Holton, T. and Hudspeth, A.J. (1986) The transduction channel of hair cells from bull-frog characterized by noise analysis. *J. Physiol. (London),* 375: 195 – 227.

Hudspeth, A.J. and Corey, D.P. (1977) Sensitivity, polarity and conductance change in the response of vertebrate hair cells to controlled mechanical stimuli. *Proc. Natl. Acad. Sci. U.S.A.,* 74: 2407 – 2411.

Hudspeth, A.J. (1982) Extracellular current flow and the site of transduction by vertebrate hair cells. *J. Neurosci.,* 2: 1 – 10.

Hudspeth, A.J. (1983) Mechanoelectrical transduction by hair cells in the acousticolateralis sensory system. *Ann. Rev. Neurosci.,* 6: 187 – 215.

Hudspeth, A.J. (1985) The cellular basis of hearing; the biophysics of hair cells. *Science,* 230: 745 – 752.

Jorgensen, F. (1983) Influence of Ca^{2+} on the mechanosensitivity of the hair cells in the lateral line organs of *Nectulus maculosus. Acta Physiol. Scand.,* 118: 423 – 431.

Lee, Y.W. (1960) *Statistical Theory of Communication.* John Wiley & Sons, New York, 509 pp.

Lewis, E.R. and Li, C.W. (1975) Hair cell types and distributions in the otolithic and auditory organs of the bull frog. *Brain Res.*, 83: 35 – 50.

Ohmori, H. (1984) Studies of ionic currents in the isolated vestibular hair cells of the chick. *J. Physiol. (London)*, 350: 561 – 581.

Ohmori, H. (1985) Mechano-electrical transduction currents in isolated vestibular hair cells of the chick. *J. Physiol. (London)*, 359: 189 – 217.

Ohmori, H. (1987) Gating properties of the mechano-electrical transducer channel in the dissociated vestibular hair cell of the chick. *J. Physiol. (London)*, 387: in press.

Pickles, J.O., Comis, S.D. and Osborne, M.P. (1984) Cross-links between stereocilia in the guinea-pig organ of Corti, and their possible relation to sensory transduction. *Hearing Res.*, 15: 103 – 112.

Russell, I.J., Richardson, G.P. and Cody, A.R. (1986) Mechanosensitivity of mammalian auditory hair cells in vitro. *Nature (London)*, 321: 517 – 519.

Sand, O. (1975) Effects of different ionic environments on the mechanosensitivity of lateral line organ in the mudpuppy. *J. Comp. Physiol.*, A102: 27 – 42.

Turner, R.G., Muraski, A.A. and Nielsen, D.W. (1981) Cilium length; influence on neural tonotopic organization. *Science*, 213: 1519 – 1521.

Williams, D.A., Fogarty, K.E., Tsien, R.Y. and Fay, F.S. (1985) Calcium gradients in single smooth muscle cells revealed by the digital imaging microscope using Fura-2. *Nature (London)*, 318: 558 – 561.

W. Hamann and A. Iggo (Eds.)
Progress in Brain Research, Vol. 74
© 1988 Elsevier Science Publishers B.V. (Biomedical Division)

CHAPTER 3

On the ionic mechanism of hair cells

A comparative study

Finn Jørgensen

Physiological Institute, Odense University, Campusvej 55, 5230 Odense M, Denmark

Summary

In this study the ionic mechanism of the transduction channels of the hair cells in the lateral line organs of *Xenopus laevis* and in the macula of the sacculus from *Rana esculenta* has been examined.

In the isolated voltage-clamped skin of Xenopus the magnitude of the receptor current was determined indirectly as the degree of synchronization (DOS) between the mechanical stimulation and the afferent spikes. The transepithelial voltage at which DOS attained a minimum value was considered equivalent to the reversal potential, where the receptor current was zero.

In the isolated voltage-clamped epithelium from the sacculus of the frog the summed receptor current from many hair cells activated by the mechanical displacement of the otolithic membrane was measured directly. The transepithelial voltage at which the receptor current was zero was considered equivalent to the reversal potential.

The influence of changes in the ionic content of the apical solution on the apparent reversal potential was presented and discussed in relation to results obtained by the direct determination of the reversal potential across the apical membrane.

Introduction

Hair cells are specialized epithelial cells with different properties of the apical and the basolateral membranes. The apical membrane is specialized for the transduction of mechanical energy into electrical signals. The basolateral membranes are responsible for cellular homeostasis, essential for the transduction as well as for the transmission link to the primary afferents by controlling the membrane potential and the ionic gradients.

By using the isolated voltage-clamped epithelium with the two sides of the hair cells perfused independently (Jørgensen, 1981, 1984) the properties of the two membranes of the hair cells may be examined. Furthermore, the dependence of the properties of the basolateral membranes on the function of the apical membrane may be examined as well.

This macroscopic analysis of hair cells integrated into the sensory epithelium may serve as a frame of reference for results obtained by using more direct methods on these extremely sensitive mechano-receptors.

Materials and methods

The determination of the ionic selectivity of membrane channels is based upon the determination of the reversal potential, E_{rev}, for the current through the channels and the influence of changes in the ionic gradient on this potential (Hille, 1984). In this study the transepithelial voltage at which the receptor current was zero or where the derived parameter, the degree of synchronization (DOS) between a certain phase of the mechanical stimulation and action potentials from the afferent axons (see Jørgensen, 1984) attained a minimum value, represented the reversal potential. The influence of changes in the ionic content of the apical solution on the change in this reversal potential provides an estimate of the ionic selectivity of the transduction channels.

The lateral line organs of Xenopus

The preparation and the mounting of the skin from *Xenopus laevis* containing the lateral line organs in an Ussing chamber have been described previously (Jørgensen, 1984).

The generation of action potentials in the afferent axons is controlled by the liberation of transmitter from the basolateral membranes of the hair cells. The voltage across these membranes controls the voltage dependent Ca channels (Ohmori, 1984) and thereby the liberation of transmitter. Changes in the membrane potentials of the hair cell may be achieved either by the displacement of the hair bundles, thus generating the receptor potentials, or by current injection across the hair cells.

The method of determining the DOS controlled by the injection of sinusoidal current across the hair cells was based on the generation of cycle histograms (Jørgensen, 1984).

The relationship between the electrically activated DOS and the magnitude of the sinusoidal current injection was determined for different values of the transepithelial voltage, V_t. In this way the influence of the transepithelial voltage on DOS at the same magnitude of current as well as on the magnitude of the current sufficient to obtain a constant DOS could be examined.

The macula of the sacculus of the frog

The preparation of the isolated macula from the sacculus of *Rana esculenta* followed the procedures described in the article of Corey and Hudspeth (1983). Instead of fixing the epithelium

mechanically the epithelium was glued across the hole connecting the two chambers of the Ussing chamber.

The two chambers were perfused separately, the lower chamber with perilymph and the upper chamber with endolymph. Care was taken to prevent movement of the epithelium during the perfusion. In a preliminary series of experiments where the influence of the concentration of K on the reversal potential was examined, sucrose was added to keep the osmolarity of the solution constant.

The receptor current, I_{rec}

The electrical potential difference across the apical membrane of the hair cells during the voltage-clamping is determined by the voltage divider ratio of the resistances of the apical and the basolateral membranes. This ratio was determined by Corey and Hudspeth (1983) to be 0.89. This value resembles the value usually found in the frog skin (Hellmann and Fisher, 1977).

The epithelium was voltage-clamped to different values and I_{rec} activated by the displacement of the otolithic membrane was averaged after suitable amplification. The frequency of this summed receptor current from many hair cells could be the same or the double frequency to that of the stimulus frequency, depending upon whether the group of hair cells being activated by the stimulus probe was of the same or of opposite morphological polarity (Corey and Hudspeth, 1983).

Experimental procedure

Before the relation between the I_{rec} and the V_t was examined the relation between the extracellularly recorded receptor potential and the displacement of the probe was determined. The displacement applied in each experiment was chosen as the displacement which caused near saturation of the receptor potentials. In this way most of the mechanically activated channels were in the active state.

Results

The lateral line organs of Xenopus laevis

In a previous study of the lateral line organs of *Xenopus laevis* (Jørgensen, 1984) the relation between the mechanically activated DOS and the transepithelial voltage, V_t, was examined. The V_t at which a minimum value of DOS was obtained was suggested to be equivalent to the E_{rev} for the I_{rec} across the apical membrane of the hair cells. This conclusion was mainly based upon the change in the mean phase of DOS of 180° around this potential suggesting that the receptor current had changed direction across the apical membranes. Fig. 1A shows an example of the relation between DOS and V_t.

The possible influence of the changes in the electrical potential difference across the basolateral

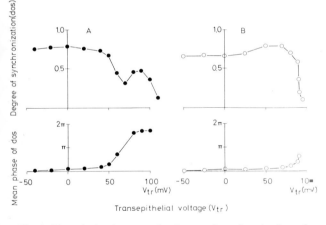

Fig. 1. The relation between the degree of synchronization of afferent spikes (DOS) from a lateral line organ of Xenopus and the transepithelial voltage (V_{tr}). (A) The magnitude of DOS controlled by the mechanical stimulation of the hair cells is plotted as a function of the transepithelial voltage. The corresponding change in the mean phase of DOS is also plotted as a function of the transepithelial voltage. Note that at the minimum value of DOS the afferent spikes are no longer time-locked to the mechanical stimulation. (B) The magnitude of DOS controlled by current injection across the epithelium is plotted as a function of the transepithelial voltage. The corresponding change in the mean phase of DOS is shown beneath. The magnitude of the injected current was 1.1 μA. Apical solution: 1 mM $CaCl_2$, 5 mM MOPS-KOH, pH = 7.1.

membranes on the mechanically activated DOS seen in Fig. 1A was examined by controlling the DOS by sinusoidal current injection and examining the influence of V_t on DOS. In this way the transduction channels of the apical membranes were not activated and the potential change across the basolateral membranes controlling the liberation of transmitter was instead produced by the current injection.

An example of these experiments is shown in Fig. 1B. The magnitude of DOS was not reduced in the range of V_t where the mechanically activated DOS was reduced. Instead a small increase was often seen. At values of V_t close to 100 mV the DOS was abruptly reduced as also seen in Fig. 1A. This reduction was probably caused by the hyperpolarization of the basolateral membranes since increased magnitude of the current could restore the coupling.

The corresponding changes in the mean phase of DOS was found to be a monotonous and non-linear function of the transepithelial voltage. Thus the continuous changes in the mean phase seen in Fig. 1A may have the same origin. An abrupt change in the mean phase of DOS of 180° as seen in Fig. 1A was never found.

Thus the changes in the mechanically activated DOS caused by the increase in the transepithelial voltage may be explained mainly by the reduction in the electrical potential difference across the apical membrane of the hair cells leading to a reduction in the receptor current.

The finding that changes in Ca_o shifted the reversal potential along the voltage axis (Jørgensen, 1984) may indicate that Ca^{2+} may carry a major fraction of the receptor current in the lateral line organs of Xenopus.

The sacculus of Rana esculenta

In the isolated voltage-clamped epithelium from the frog's sacculus it was possible to measure directly the receptor current from all the hair cells activated by the displacement of the otolithic membrane.

Fig. 2A shows an example of the influence of V_t on the summed I_{rec} from the voltage-clamped macula to mechanical displacement of the otolithic membrane (11 Hz). As the V_t was increased the magnitude of I_{rec} was reduced and became zero at 60 mV. The apical solution was K-endolymph. In Fig. 2B I_{rec} was plotted as a function of V_t showing that the relationship was non-linear. The non-linear relationship was usually found in preparations with large and moderate magnitudes of I_{rec}. In preparations with small I_{rec} a linear relationship was found.

In 14 experiments the mean reversal potential, V_{rev}, was found to be 48.6 mV + 7.4 mV (SD) when the apical solution was K-endolymph. When the K^+ was substituted by Na^+ the mean reversal potential was found to be 48.5 mV + 7.8 mV (SD), n = 11. Only the results of experiments where a double determination of I_{rec} at one or more values of V_t deviated less than 10% were included.

Influence of Ca_o on the E_{rev}

P_{Ca}/P_K of the transduction channels of the hair cells in the isolated epithelium from the sacculus of *Rana catesbeiana* was found by Corey and Hudspeth (1979) to be 0.3. This value was obtained by comparing the magnitude of the receptor current at $V_t = 0$ when the cation content of the apical solution was changed. In the isolated hair cells of the chick Ohmori (1985) found a value of $P_{Ca}/P_K = 4.1$ by direct determination of the reversal potential for the receptor current.

The extended Goldman, Hodgkin, Katz constant field equation including divalent cations (Lewis, 1979), assuming K^+ and Ca^{2+} as the sole charge carriers, may be written as

$$\exp(E_{rev}F/RT) = [K]_o/[K]_i + 4P_{Ca}[Ca]_o/P_K[K]_i$$
$$(1 + \exp(E_{rev}F/RT))$$

assuming that Ca_i is very small. As solution to this second order equation in $\exp(E_{rev}F/RT)$ the reversal potential may be written as

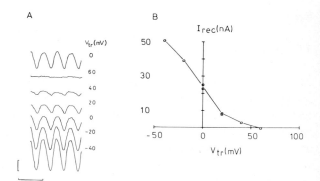

Fig. 2. The receptor current from hair cells of the isolated sacculus of *Rana esculenta* as a function of the transepithelial voltage. (A) the averaged receptor current from the hair cells activated by the displacement of the otolithic membrane is shown at different values of V_{tr}. The frequency of the receptor current is twice that of the mechanical stimulation. The calibration bars indicate 10 nA and 10 ms, respectively. (B) The results shown in Fig. 2A are plotted as a function of the transepithelial voltage. The transepithelial voltage at which the receptor current was zero, the reversal potential, V_{rev}, was determined directly in this experiment. Apical solution: 124 mM KCl, 2.5 mM NaCl, 0.26 mM $CaCl_2$, 5 mM MOPS, 5 mM glucose, pH = 7.1.

In Fig. 3 the calculated E_{rev} is plotted as a function of the external K concentration for two values of P_{Ca}/P_K. The relation was calculated for $Ca_o = 0.26$ mM, 2.6 mM and 26 mM.

Provided the receptor current through the transduction channels can be modelled by the extended constant field equation the figure shows that the expected change in the E_{rev} in normal K-endolymph (124 mM) with changes in Ca_o is small. Only when P_{Ca} is higher than P_K a 100-fold change in Ca_o may result in changes in the reversal potential which can be reliably recorded using this method.

Since isotonic concentrations of external Ca irreversibly influence the transduction mechanism (Ohmori, 1985) the influence of changes in K_o on V_{rev} was examined instead in a preliminary series of experiments. The changes in the reversal potential were measured with $K_o = 62$ mM and 5 mM

$$E_{rev} = \frac{RT}{F} \ln \frac{\dfrac{-([K]_i - [K]_o)}{[K]_i} + \sqrt{\left(\dfrac{[K]_i - [K]_o}{[K]_i}\right)^2 + 4\left(\dfrac{4P_{Ca}[Ca]_o}{P_K[K]_i} + \dfrac{[K]_o}{[K]_i}\right)}}{2}.$$

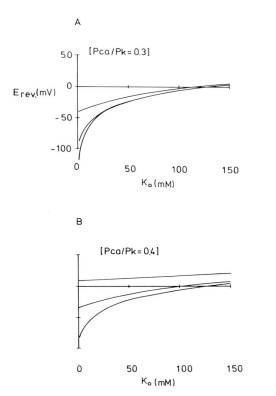

Fig. 3. The reversal potential, E_{rev}, calculated from the extended Goldman, Hodgkin, Katz constant field equation (see text) is plotted as a function of the external K^+ concentration. The relation was calculated for Ca_o = 0.26 mM, 2.6 mM and 26 mM. In A the ratio between P_{Ca} and P_K was 0.3 and in B the ratio was 4.

function of K_o. The calculated changes in the reversal potential for P_{Ca}/P_K = 0.3 and 4 are plotted as well. Although the changes in the reversal potential with $1/2$ K_o in the apical solution may be explained by transduction channels of both high and low P_{Ca} the changes in the reversal potential observed at K_o = 5 mM indicate that the transduction channels of the sacculus hair cells may have a higher P_{Ca} than determined by Corey and Hudspeth (1979).

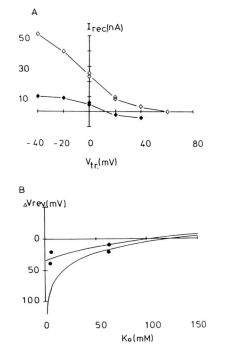

Fig. 4. The influence of the external K^+ concentration on the reversal potential, V_{rev}. (A) The receptor current is plotted as a function of the transepithelial voltage when the apical solution was normal K-endolymph (124 mM) (open symbols) and when the K concentration of the apical solution was reduced to 5 mM. The Ca^{2+} concentration was raised from 0.26 mM to 2.6 mM. The osmolarity of the solution was kept constant by addition of sucrose. (B) The changes in the reversal potential, V_{rev}, are plotted as a function of the K concentration in the apical solution. Also shown are the calculated changes in the reversal potential, E_{rev}, for two values of the ratio between P_{Ca} and P_K (0.3 and 4).

in the apical solution. The osmolarity of the apical solution was kept constant by adding sucrose.

At low concentrations of K in the apical solution the extracellular receptor potentials could be recorded for more than half an hour. After the relationship between the I_{rec} and V_t was determined, however, the magnitude of the receptor potentials was irreversibly reduced.

In Fig. 4A the effects of 5 mM K on the I_{rec} at different values of V_t is shown together with the results obtained at normal K concentration (124 mM). The relationship was shifted along the voltage axis and the receptor current was reduced as well.

In Fig. 4B the changes in V_{rev} are plotted as a

Discussion

The interpretation of the relation between the mechanically activated DOS and V_t has already been discussed at length in a previous article (Jørgensen, 1984). The change in DOS with the increase in V_t was considered to be the combined effect of the receptor current across the apical membrane and the non-linear relationship between the receptor potentials and I_{Ca} (Ohmori, 1984). The finding that the electrically activated DOS was not influenced by changes in V_t where the mechanically activated DOS attained a minimum value indicates that the change in the electrical potential across the basolateral membranes is small compared to the corresponding changes across the apical membrane. The reduction seen in the mechanically activated DOS may then be explained by the reduction in I_{rec}.

The non-linear reduction of DOS may then arise from the combined reduction in the magnitude of the receptor potential and the voltage dependent channels of the basolateral membranes.

The continuous change in the mean phase of DOS seen in both experiments arises from the hyperpolarization of the basolateral membranes and may be interpreted as a real time delay in contrast to the change in the mean phase of 180° of DOS around the minimum value which represents a change in the direction of the I_{rec}.

In the isolated voltage-clamped epithelium from the sacculus the I_{rec} was found to be non-linear in the preparations with the larger currents. This finding was not in agreement with results obtained from the same preparation using two glass microelectrodes or whole cell patch clamp (Corey and Hudspeth, 1979; Holton and Hudspeth, 1985) or from the isolated hair cells of the chick using whole cell patch clamp (Ohmori, 1985). It is unlikely that the observed non-linearity may arise from changes in the voltage divider ratio caused by opening of the voltage dependent channels of the basolateral membranes (Lewis and Hudspeth, 1984; Ohmori, 1984) since this would result in a non-linearity in the opposite direction from the one observed. But a more detailed examination of this finding is needed before a conclusion as to the origin of this non-linearity can be reached.

The demonstration in this study that the reversal potential was not changed by substituting K with Na ions is in agreement with previous demonstrations that the transduction channels of the hair cells are non-selective to monovalent cations (Corey and Hudspeth, 1979; Ohmori, 1985). Taking a value of -60 mV to -50 mV for the membrane potential (Hudspeth and Corey, 1977), a reversal potential across the apical membrane estimated from this study would be between -10 and 0 mV.

Although the role of Ca^{2+} in the transduction mechanism of hair cells is not fully elucidated it appears to carry receptor current in the lateral line organs of Necturus and Xenopus (Sand, 1975; Jørgensen, 1983, 1984) and in the isolated hair cells of the chick the P_{Ca} of the transduction channels is higher than the permeability to monovalent cations (Ohmori, 1985). The lower permeability of Ca in the transduction channels of the hair cells from the sacculus from *Rana catesbeiana* found by Corey and Hudspeth (1979) may be due to the method applied since the preliminary results presented here may indicate that also in this preparation the transduction channels appear to be more permeable to Ca than to monovalent cations. It should be emphasized that additional experiments are needed before a final conclusion can be drawn.

References

Corey, D.P. and Hudspeth, A.J. (1979) Ionic basis of the receptor potential in the vertebrate hair cell. *Nature (London),* 281: 675–677.

Corey, D.P. and Hudspeth, A.J. (1983) Analysis of the microphonic potential of the bullfrog's sacculus. *J. Neurosci.,* 3: 942–961.

Hellmann, S.T. and Fisher, R.S. (1977) Microelectrode studies of the active Na transport pathways of frog skin. *J. Gen. Physiol.,* 69: 571–604.

Hille, B. (1984) *Ionic Channels of Excitable Membranes.* Sinauer, Sunderland, MA.

Holton, T. and Hudspeth, A.J. (1986) The transduction channel of hair cells from bull-frog characterized by noise analysis. *J. Physiol. (London),* 375: 195 – 227.

Hudspeth A.J. and Corey, D.P. (1977) Sensitivity, polarity and conductance change in the response of vertebrate hair cells to controlled mechanical stimuli. *Proc. Natl. Acad. Sci. U.S.A.,* 74: 2407 – 2411.

Jørgensen, F. (1981) Effect of Ca on the voltage dependent mechanosensitivity of lateral line organs of *Xenopus laevis. VII Int. Biophysics Congress,* Mexico City (abstract).

Jørgensen, F. (1983) Influence of Ca on the mechanosensitivity of the hair cells in the lateral line organs of *Necturus mac. Acta Physiol. Scand.,* 118: 423 – 431.

Jørgensen, F. (1984) Influence of Ca^{2+} on the voltage dependent mechanosensitivity of lateral line organs of Xenopus laevis. *Acta Physiol. Scand.,* 120: 481 – 488.

Lewis, C.A. (1979) Ion concentration dependence of the reversal potential and the single channel conductance of ion channels of the frog neuromuscular junction. *J. Physiol. (London),* 286: 417 – 445.

Lewis, R.S. and Hudspeth, A.J. (1983) Voltage- and ion-dependent conductances in solitary vertebrate hair cells. *Nature (London),* 304: 538 – 541.

Ohmori, H. (1984) Studies of ionic currents in the isolated vestibular hair cell of the chick. *J. Physiol. (London),* 350: 561 – 581.

Ohmori, H. (1985) Mechano-electrical transduction currents in isolated vestibular hair cells of the chick. *J. Physiol. (London),* 359: 189 – 217.

Sand, O. (1975) Effects of ionic environments on the mechanosensitivity of lateral line organs in the mudpuppy. *J. Comp. Physiol.,* 102: 27 – 42.

W. Hamann and A. Iggo (Eds.)
Progress in Brain Research, Vol. 74
© 1988 Elsevier Science Publishers B.V. (Biomedical Division)

CHAPTER 4

Classification of a calcium conductance in cold receptors

Klaus Schäfer[1], Hans A. Braun[2] and Ludgera Rempe[1]

[1]*Institut für Zoophysiologie, Universität Hohenheim, D-7000 Stuttgart 70, and* [2]*Institut für Physiologie, Universität Marburg, D-3550 Marburg, FRG*

Summary

The small size of mammalian cold sensors, which have been shown to be free nerve endings, has so far prevented any attempt to study their transducer processes directly. However, recently developed techniques such as discharge pattern analysis and reliable isolated organ preparations have allowed to gain some insight into the conditions under which afferent activity in cold receptors is initiated.

Afferent activity of mammalian cold sensors is generated by periodic receptor membrane processes. Frequency and amplitude of the impulse triggering cyclic membrane events are temperature dependent; the processes are supposed to be controlled by calcium currents and calcium-sensitive outward conductances. External menthol ($10-50$ μmol/l) induces changes of mean activity and discharge pattern qualitatively similar to those effected by reduced extracellular calcium concentrations.

In molluscan neurons calcium currents are reversibly reduced by external menthol ($100-500$ μmol/l). The mode of action appears to be a specific interaction of menthol with calcium channels, since the effect is stereochemically selective and cannot be evoked by intracellular application. Of the three classes of calcium conductances identified in dorsal root ganglion cells so far, menthol acts on the low-voltage-activated (LVA) type and high-voltage-activated (HVA) type only. These two calcium conductances differ in their potential range of activation, their kinetics, and their sensitivity to calcium channel modulators. For instance, the LVA-type conductance has been shown to be rather inert against verapamil and 1,4-dihydropyridine-type channel modulators.

External verapamil ($10-100$ μmol/l) either does not affect cold sensor discharges or inhibits afferent activity. These observations are at variance with the expected stimulating action of compounds interfering with calcium conductances (such as menthol).

Analysis of the temporal pattern of cold sensor activity indicates that the cyclic sensory processes are independent of the release of action potentials. Interspike intervals of 'irregular' discharges are even-numbered multiples (up to 8) of the oscillation period. Likewise, the oscillation period of grouped discharges is constant in spite of a varying number of impulses per group.

These various observations indicate that a verapamil-sensitive, action-potential-activated calcium conductance (such as the HVA type) is absent in cold sensors. The data suggest instead the existence of a calcium channel with properties of the LVA type.

Introduction

Mammalian cold sensors are free nerve endings (Hensel et al., 1974), and their small size has so far prevented any direct study of their transducer processes. However, various indirect experimental approaches have recently allowed to gain some insight into the conditions under which afferent activity of cold receptors is initiated (Braun et al., 1980, 1984; Schäfer et al., 1982, 1984, 1986; Schäfer, 1987). In particular the application of discharge pattern analysis and the development of a reliable isolated organ preparation have been proved to be effective techniques.

Afferent activity of mammalian cold sensors is generated by periodic receptor membrane processes (Braun et al., 1980). Frequency and amplitude of the impulse triggering cyclic events are temperature dependent. The periodic processes are supposed to be controlled by calcium currents and calcium-stimulated outward conductances (Schäfer et al., 1986). Changes of cold receptor activity induced by various levels of external calcium are in agreement with the hypothesis of calcium-sensitive conductances being present in cold receptors (Schäfer et al., 1982). In quantitative experiments by use of an isolated organ preparation these changes accord fairly well with the known properties of the corresponding neuronal channels, namely with the non-linear dependence of these conductances on the extracellular calcium concentration (Schäfer, 1987).

These various observations suggest that mammalian cold sensors might possess ionic conductances similar to those known to exist in other neurons. In avian and mammalian dorsal root ganglion cells three different classes of calcium currents have been recently identified (Carbone and Lux, 1984; Nowycky et al., 1985; Swandulla et al., 1987). They can be differentiated by their potential range of activation, by their kinetics of inactivation, and by their sensitivity to calcium channel modulators.

The aim of the present study was to identify the type of calcium channel present in cold sensors by application of so-called calcium entry blockers along with an analysis of the induced changes of afferent activity. A successful classification of the type of calcium conductance involved in sensory transduction is considered to signify a substantial progress in our understanding of sensory processes.

Calcium control of afferent activity

In various cold receptor populations beating activity and burst (grouped) discharges have been observed at maintained temperatures and during rapid cooling (Hensel, 1981). In all populations studied so far, analysis of the impulse activity revealed a cyclic pattern of impulse generation suggesting the existence of an underlying receptor potential oscillation, which initiates impulses in the afferent nerve when it exceeds a threshold value (Braun et al., 1984; Schäfer et al., 1984, 1986). An example of afferent impulse activity together with the corresponding interval distribution of a single cold receptor at various constant temperatures is represented in Fig. 1. From the data shown in this figure the burst frequency (i.e., oscillation frequency) and number of impulses induced during each cycle can be calculated (Braun and Hensel, 1977; examples of such a calculation are given in Schäfer et al., 1986). Consequently, the mean discharge rate is a function of the burst frequency, which increases with warming, and the number of impulses per burst, which increases with cooling. As a result, when the number of impulses per burst is multiplied by the burst frequency, the well-known parabolic relation between mean activity and temperature is obtained (Braun et al., 1980).

A calcium-stimulated outward current, acting as a negative feedback system, is generally viewed as an essential link in the cycle of events controlling periodic neuronal activity (Eckert and Lux, 1976; Gorman et al., 1982). Therefore, all experimental measures interfering with the availability of calcium to enter the receptive structure markedly affect the burst frequency, the number of impulses per burst, and, hence, the mean discharge rate (Schäfer et al., 1982, 1984, 1986; Schäfer, 1987). In our experiments, calcium supply was impaired by application of calcium chelators in whole animals, by perfusion of isolated organ preparations with solutions containing reduced calcium levels, and by application of menthol, which has been shown to selectively interfere with neuronal calcium channels (Swandulla et al., 1986). Nevertheless, the induced changes of afferent activity are rather uniform, independently of the kind of treatment applied. As can be seen in Fig. 2, the effects of either reduced external calcium concentrations or of impairment of calcium entry into the receptor are qualitatively similar in experiments on whole animals and isolated organ preparations, which indicates the involvement of a common mechanism in all cases.

Calcium conductances of sensory neurons

Three different classes of calcium channels have been recently characterized in vertebrate sensory neurons (Carbone and Lux, 1984; Nowycky et al., 1985). One of them, activated at high voltages (HVA type), resembles the classical calcium channel of other excitable cells. A second channel, activated at low voltages (LVA type), differs both kinetically and pharmacologically from the classical one. Its time-dependent inactivation is fast and complete, and it is rather inert against large doses

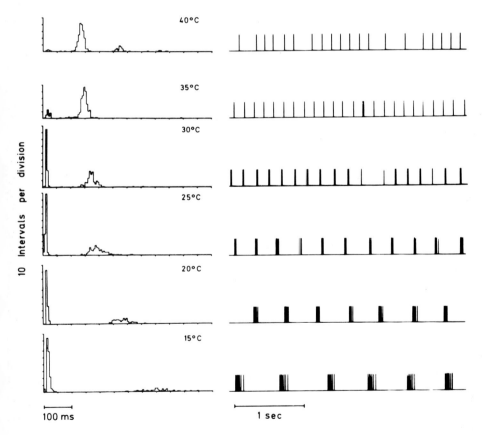

Fig 1. Discharge pattern of a feline lingual cold receptor at various constant temperatures. Left diagrams: interval distribution; right diagrams: impulse activity. The mean discharge rates (in s⁻¹) are: 5.4 (40°C); 7.2 (35°C); 9.2 (30°C); 10.4 (25°C); 12.0 (20°C); 11.0 (15°C). Intervals shorter than 100 ms are intraburst intervals. Dimensions of graphs and stimulus temperatures as indicated. (Methods are given in Braun et al., 1980; Schäfer et al., 1986).

of organic calcium channel modulators such as verapamil and 1,4-dihydropyridine derivatives (Boll and Lux, 1985). In mammalian sensory neurons, LVA channels occasionally contribute more than HVA channels to the total calcium current of the cell membrane (Swandulla et al., 1987).

Observations in molluscan neurons and in avian and mammalian dorsal root ganglion cells suggest a specific impeding action of menthol (2-isopropyl-5-methyl-cyclohexanol) on calcium currents (Swandulla et al., 1986, 1987). The effects of menthol develop in seconds, they are fully reversible and stereochemically selective, and they cannot be evoked by intracellular application. Related compounds, such as cyclohexanol, fail to produce any comparable effect, even in considerably higher concentrations, which suggests a specific interaction of menthol with calcium channels. Menthol reduces currents through two types of calcium channels present in sensory neurons by different mechanisms. The high-voltage-activated, long lasting conductance (HVA type) is impaired by an accelerated inactivation, whereas the low-voltage-activated, transient current (LVA type) is reduced without its inactivation time course being affected. Menthol has practically no effect on a third type of calcium current recently identified by Nowycky et al. (1985) in the same preparation. This fast inactivating channel activates at high voltages and deactivates at low voltages (N type).

Calcium conductance of cold sensors

Reduced extracellular calcium levels induce depolarizing shifts of membrane potential in invertebrate and vertebrate bursting neurons, whereas elevated calcium levels result in hyperpolarization; the induced changes of potential are

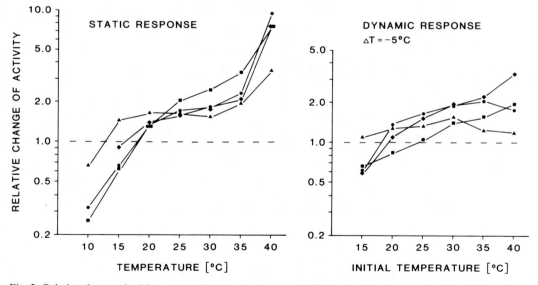

Fig. 2. Relative change of cold receptor activity induced by menthol and by reduced external calcium. Control values are represented by '1.00'. Left diagram: static firing rate; right diagram: dynamic peak frequency following 5°C cooling from adapting temperature. Circles, lingual cold receptors, isolated organ preparation, 0.5 mmol/l calcium (n = 11), data from Schäfer (1987); diamonds, lingual cold receptors, isolated organ preparation, 50 μmol/l menthol (n = 3), data from Schäfer et al. (1986); squares, nasal cold receptors, whole animal, 0.57 ± 0.11 mg/kg/min menthol i.v. (n = 8), data from Schäfer et al. (1986); triangles, nasal cold receptors, whole animal, 0.77 ± 0.29 mg/kg/min EDTA i.v. (n = 9), data from Schäfer et al. (1982). EDTA chelates calcium ions. Methods are given in the cited references.

associated with concomitant modifications of discharge rate (Gola and Selveston, 1981; Legendre et al., 1985). Activity of these neurons is controlled by calcium currents and by calcium-sensitive conductances. Cold receptor activity is comparably suppressed by excess external calcium and enhanced by reduced calcium (Schäfer et al., 1982; Schäfer, 1987). The considerable conformity of the calcium-induced changes of either the neuronal membrane potential or the sensory afferent discharge supports the view that the activity of both cell types is controlled by identical mechanisms, namely by calcium-stimulated outward conductances. Calcium seems not to be in-

volved in affecting the membrane potential as a current carrier, since elevation of external calcium neither induces depolarization nor increases afferent activity. The data indicate that a calcium-activated outward current is involved, which masks the direct effect of the calcium current by its considerably higher conductance (Akaike et al., 1978; Lux and Hofmeier, 1982).

Figs. 2 and 3 show that the menthol-induced changes of cold receptor discharge are fairly identical to those induced by reduced external calcium. Both menthol and reduced calcium exert their effects on the mean firing rate by comparable modifications of cyclic receptor activity (Schäfer et al.,

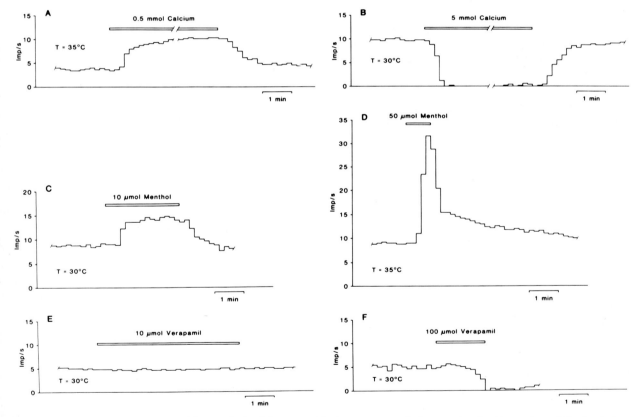

Fig. 3. Effect of reduced external calcium and of calcium entry blockers on mean discharge rate of cold receptors. Data from six lingual cold receptors out of a total of 43 which were studied. Isolated organ preparation. T, thermode temperature; discharge rate was averaged over periods of 10 s. The isolated organ preparation was perfused for the periods indicated by bars with solutions containing either reduced or elevated calcium levels (A, B), various menthol concentrations (C, D), or various verapamil concentrations (E, F). Under control conditions, the isolated organ preparation was perfused with a modified Krebs solution (for details, see Schäfer, 1987).

1986; Schäfer and Braun, unpublished). Since menthol has been proved to selectively impair the calcium entry, we compared menthol with the classical calcium entry blocker, verapamil. When tested in six specific cold receptors, either external verapamil in doses of $10-500$ μmol/l was ineffective or cold receptor discharge was inhibited. In every case the observed effects were at variance with the expected stimulating action of compounds interfering with the calcium entry such as menthol (Fig. 3). Since verapamil is mainly effective in reducing current through the ubiquitous calcium channel (HVA type) (Boll and Lux, 1985), these data do not support the view of an action-potential-activated calcium conductance being present at the cold receptor membrane. Cyclic receptor activity, however, is strongly controlled by calcium. If calcium entry through the HVA-type conductance is negligible, the periodic receptor activity should be independent of the release of afferent impulses by the sensor. In fact, various analyses of the temporal pattern of cold receptor discharges have indicated the existence of an endogenously

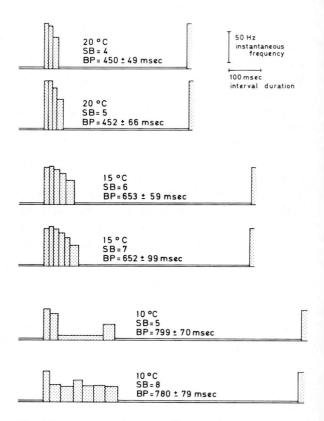

Fig. 5. Instantaneous frequency diagram of the temporal pattern of grouped (burst) discharges. Ordinate, instantaneous frequency in s^{-1} (reciprocal value of the duration of successive intervals); abscissa, time in ms. Data of a 2 min period at every constant temperature. BP, burst period (i.e., period of the underlying cyclic receptor events); SB, impulses per burst. Method of calculation is given in Braun et al. (1980).

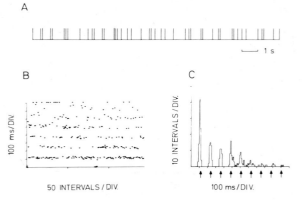

Fig. 4. Temporal pattern of cold receptor discharge. Lingual cold receptor, isolated organ preparation. Perfusion with a solution containing 0.5 mmol/l calcium (for details, see Schäfer, 1987). Thermode temperature, 40°C. (A) Impulse activity. (B) Duration of successive intervals. (C) Interval distribution. Arrows indicate the basic period of the cyclic receptor events and the even-numbered multiples. Values were calculated from the data presented in C (the method of calculation and examples are given in Braun et al., 1980; and in Schäfer et al., 1986; respectively).

oscillating receptor process (Braun et al., 1980, 1984; Schäfer et al., 1986). At higher adapting temperatures, these cyclic processes occasionally fail to initiate the appropriate impulse, which results in 'irregular' discharges. In that case, all interspike intervals are even-numbered multiples of the oscillation period, and sporadically intervals of a duration up to 8 times the oscillation period are seen (Fig. 4). At lower adapting temperatures, the periodic receptor processes mainly initiate groups of impulses during each cycle (Braun et al., 1980; Schäfer et al., 1986). At a given temperature, burst period (i.e., oscillation period) and burst duration are fairly constant in spite of a varying number of impulses induced per group (Fig. 5). This additionally accords with the assumption that action potentials do not contribute to the initiation and maintenance of cyclic sensory processes. Moreover, it indicates that cyclic activity might be differently controlled in cold receptors and in molluscan bursting pacemaker neurons. In these neurons, which have been repeatedly proposed as models for cold receptor function (Braun et al., 1980, 1984; Schäfer et al., 1982, 1986), the maintenance of cyclic activity evidently depends on the initiation of action potentials (Kramer and Zucker, 1985).

Taken together, these various observations indicate that calcium channels of cold receptors are menthol-sensitive, but verapamil-insensitive, and that action potentials contribute only insignificantly, if at all, to the calcium entry into the sensor. The data strongly suggest that the cold receptor membrane possesses calcium channels with properties of the recently characterized LVA channel. Since the action of menthol is rather specific, it can be concluded that the N-type calcium conductance is absent in cold receptor membranes. In this connection it might be of interest that the LVA type of calcium channel is assumed to be involved in the maintenance of rhythmic neuronal activity (Llinas and Yarom, 1981). Therefore, for the first time, by application of indirect methods of investigation, it was possible to identify a type of ionic conductance involved in sensory transduction of thermoreceptors.

Acknowledgement

This work was supported by the Deutsche Forschungsgemeinschaft.

References

Akaike, N., Lee, K.S. and Brown, A.M. (1978) The calcium current of Helix neuron. *J. Gen. Physiol.*, 71: 509 – 531.

Boll, W. and Lux, H.D. (1985) Action of organic antagonists on neuronal calcium currents. *Neurosci. Lett.*, 56: 335 – 339.

Braun, H.A. and Hensel, H. (1977) A computer program for identification and analysis of neuronal burst discharges. *Pflügers Arch.*, 368: R48.

Braun, H.A., Bade, H. and Hensel, H. (1980) Static and dynamic discharge patterns of bursting cold fibres related to hypothetical receptor mechanisms. *Pflügers Arch.*, 386: 1 – 9.

Braun, H.A., Schäfer, K., Wissig, H. and Hensel, H. (1984) Periodic transduction processes in thermosensitive receptors. In: W. Hamann and A. Iggo (Eds.), *Sensory Receptor Mechanisms.* World Sci. Publ. Corp., Singapore, pp. 147 – 156.

Carbone, E. and Lux, H.D. (1984) A low voltage-activated calcium conductance in embryonic chick sensory neurons. *Biophys. J.*, 46: 413 – 418.

Eckert, R. and Lux, H.D. (1976) A voltage-sensitive persistent calcium conductance in neuronal somata of Helix. *J. Physiol. (London)*, 254: 129 – 152.

Gola, M. and Selverston, A. (1981) Ionic requirements for bursting activity in lobster stomatogastric neurons. *J. Comp. Physiol.*, 145: 191 – 207.

Gorman, A.L.F., Hermann, A. and Thomas, M.V. (1982) Ionic requirements for membrane oscillations and their dependence on the calcium concentration in a molluscan pacemaker neurone. *J. Physiol. (London)*, 327: 185 – 218.

Hensel, H. (1981) *Thermoreception and Temperature Regulation.* Academic Press, London.

Hensel, H., Andres, K.H. and v. Düring, M. (1974) Structure and function of cold receptors. *Pflügers Arch.*, 352: 1 – 10.

Kramer, R.H. and Zucker, R.S. (1985) Calcium-induced inactivation of calcium current causes the interburst hyperpolarization of Aplysia bursting neurones. *J. Physiol. (London)*, 362: 131 – 160.

Legendre, P., McKenzie, J.S., Dupouy, B. and Vincent, J.D. (1985) Evidence for bursting pacemaker neurones in cultured spinal cord cells. *Neuroscience*, 16: 753 – 767.

Llinas, R. and Yarom, Y. (1981) Properties and distribution of ionic conductances generating electroresponsiveness of mammalian inferior olivary neurones in vitro. *J. Physiol. (London)*, 315: 569 – 584.

Lux, H.D. and Hofmeier, G. (1982) Properties of a calcium- and voltage-activated potassium current in *Helix pomatia* neurons. *Pflügers Arch.*, 394: 61 – 69.

Nowycky, M.C., Fox, A.P. and Tsien, R.W. (1985) Three types of neuronal calcium channel with different calcium agonist sensitivity. *Nature (London)*, 316: 440 – 443.

Schäfer, K. (1987) A quantitative study of the dependence of feline cold receptor activity on the calcium concentration. *Pflügers Arch.*, 409: 208 – 213.

Schäfer, K., Braun, H.A. and Hensel, H. (1982) Static and dynamic activity of cold receptors at various calcium levels. *J. Neurophysiol.*, 47: 1017 – 1028.

Schäfer, K., Braun, H.A. and Hensel, H. (1984) Temperature transduction in the skin. In: J.R.S. Hales (Ed.), *Thermal Physiology,* Raven Press, New York, pp. 1 – 11.

Schäfer, K., Braun, H.A. and Isenberg, C. (1986) Effect of menthol on cold receptor activity. Analysis of receptor processes. *J. Gen. Physiol.*, 88: 757 – 776.

Schäfer, K., Braun, H.A. and Kürten, L. (1987) Analysis of discharge pattern of cold- and warm-receptor activity of vampire bats and mice. *Verh. Dtsch. Zool. Ges.,* 80: 279.

Swandulla, D., Schäfer, K. and Lux, H.D. (1986) Calcium channel current inactivation is selectively modulated by men-thol. *Neurosci. Lett.,* 68: 23 – 28.

Swandulla, D., Carbone, E., Schäfer, K. and Lux, H.D. (1987) Effect of menthol on two types of calcium currents in cultured sensory neurons of vertebrates. *Pflügers Arch.,* 409: 52 – 59.

W. Hamann and A. Iggo (Eds.)
Progress in Brain Research, Vol. 74
© 1988 Elsevier Science Publishers B.V. (Biomedical Division)

CHAPTER 5

Calcium channel blockers and Merkel cells

E.G. Pacitti and G.S. Findlater

Department of Preclinical Veterinary Sciences, University of Edinburgh and Department of Anatomy, University of Edinburgh Medical School, Teviot Place, Edinburgh, UK

Introduction

It has been suggested for some time that slowly adapting type 1 (SA1) mechanoreceptors respond to mechanical stimulation by the release of a transmitter substance, possibly stored within Merkel cell dense cored vesicles. This concept was first suggested after the observation that there was a large number of dense cored vesicles between the nucleus and the subjacent nerve terminal (Iggo and Muir, 1969). The Merkel cell – neurite complex contains other ultrastructural characteristics which imply a neurosecretory function. Dense cored vesicles have been seen concentrated around areas of the Merkel cell membrane which are closely apposed to the subjacent terminal, where they have also been seen to fuse (Chen et al., 1973). Met-enkephalin-like immunoreactivity is associated with the dense cored vesicles of rodent Merkel cells (Hartschuh et al., 1979) and vasoactive intestinal polypeptide-like immunoreactivity is associated with dense cored vesicles of other mammalian Merkel cells (Hartschuh et al., 1983). Since these peptides are putative transmitters in other areas of the nervous system they may have a similar function in SA1 mechanoreceptors. More recent evidence indicates that the met-enkephalin-like substance is not the transmitter substance in rats but appears to have a modulatory function (Pacitti and Iggo, unpublished).

Analysis of the discharge pattern of SA1 mechanoreceptors shows that it is best described by an irregular oscillator model and the most likely cause of this is the release of transmitter substance from the Merkel cell (Horch et al., 1974).

Under hypoxic conditions feline SA1 mechanoreceptors failed progressively to respond to mechanical stimulation and this was correlated with a reduction in the number of dense cored vesicles in the Merkel cell, an effect reversed by return to normoxic conditions (Findlater et al., 1987). This is further evidence that the presence of dense cored vesicles is a requirement for the normal function of touch domes.

Calcium has been implicated in the transduction process in SA1 mechanoreceptors (Iggo and Findlater, 1984) since its presence is necessary for the release of a wide variety of molecules including neurotransmitters (Rubin, 1970). We have tested this idea using three calcium channel blockers in three experimental models.

Methods

Three experimental procedures were used to test electrophysiologically the effect of cobalt chloride ($CoCl_2$), cadmium chloride ($CdCl_2$) and verapamil hydrochloride on the response of SA1 mechanoreceptors to mechanical stimulation: (1) isolated hind limb perfusion in the cat; (2) intradermal injection under individual feline SA1 mechanoreceptors; (3) isolated superfused rat skin nerve preparation.

In models 1 and 2 cats were initially anaesthetised with a 4% mixture of halothane in O_2 and anaesthesia was maintained using chloralose in saline (70 mg/kg i.v. of a 10 mg/ml solution). Single unit recordings of the responses to standardised mechanical stimuli were made from afferent fibres in the saphenous nerve and stored on an FM tape recorder (Ampex). Afferent fibres innervating the touch domes were electrically stimulated at 1.2 times threshold by inserting fine electrodes into the skin on either side of the receptor.

Model 1

A detailed description of this model has been published (Iggo and Findlater, 1984). Constant displacement mechanical stimulation (250 μm, probe tip diameter 0.5 mm) of suitable identified touch domes consisted of either (a) 1.5 s stimulus duration, 1 s interstimulus interval or (b) 5 s stimulus duration, 25 s interstimulus interval for a total time of 10 min. $CoCl_2$ (2.0, 3.0 and 5.0 mM) and verapamil (30 μM) were tested under conditions a above and $CdCl_2$ (0.5, 1.0 and 2.5 mM) under conditions b. The concentrations of drugs used are the estimated final concentrations circulating in the hind limb. These responses were compared with saline controls.

Model 2

Touch domes were stimulated as described under a above. $CoCl_2$ (125, 250 and 500 pM) and verapamil (0.01 pM) were injected under individual touch domes and the responses obtained compared to saline controls. Afferent fibres innervating the touch domes were stimulated as described above.

Model 3

Albino-Wistar rats were anaesthetised with urethane (25% w/v, 0.7 ml/kg i.p.) and supplementary doses given as required. A midline incision was made in the dorsal lumbar region exposing the 4th and 5th dorsal cutaneous nerves. One nerve was transected at its point of entry into the

paraspinal muscles then it and the area of skin it innervated (10 × 20 mm) were dissected from the rat. The preparation was fixed epidermis uppermost onto a flat stainless steel mesh disc (26 mm diameter) located over a well in the superfusion chamber, with the nerve on a black perspex plate attached to the platform. The preparation was superfused (12 ml/min) with a physiological salt solution containing (mM): NaCl, 116; KCl, 5.4; $MgCl_2$, 1.2; $CaCl_2$, 2.5; dextrose, 5.6; HEPES, 10. The pH was adjusted to 7.4 prior to use and the solution heated to 31°C by passing it through a coil of polythene tubing sitting in a thermostatically controlled water bath surrounding the chamber. The epineurium was slipped back from the nerve. The tip of a glass micropipette was broken back so its internal diameter was slightly larger than the nerve's. The nerve was sucked into the pipette by creating a negative pressure with a 1 ml syringe attached to a polythene suction tube. A small amount of silicone grease was sucked into the space between the nerve and the pipette, thus creating a good seal which facilitated signal recording by improving the signal to noise ratio.

Touch domes were stimulated as described under b above. Appropriate quantities of drugs were added to the superfusing solution to give final concentrations of 0.05, 0.1, 0.5 or 1.0 mM $CdCl_2$ or 20, 50 or 100 μM verapamil. These responses were compared to control values.

Histology

In models 1 and 2 the hind limb was perfused with a 4% paraformaldehyde/2.5% glutaraldehyde/0.1 M cacodylate buffer fixative (pH = 7.4). Tissue was removed for normal processing for electron microscopical examination.

Data and statistical analysis

All data were analysed on a Cromemco System 3 microcomputer. Results were normalised to eliminate inherent variation between individual mechanoreceptors. All results are expressed as mean ± SEM. Student's *t*-test was used for statistical analysis of the data.

Results

In all experimental models the overall effect of the calcium channel blockers was to decrease the response to mechanical stimulation.

Model 1, isolated hind limb perfusion

When 0.15 M NaCl was injected the response of the touch domes to mechanical stimulation never failed, even after 40 min of stimulation. With $CoCl_2$ the changes in the response of the SA1 mechanoreceptors were consistent between experiments but the time course of events varied. In all experiments there was a transient increase in afferent fibre activity within 30 s of the start of the injection which was unrelated to mechanical stimulation. Eventually the touch domes failed to respond to mechanical stimulation and the time to failure was concentration dependent: 2.0 mM caused failure in approximately 9 min (n = 3) and 3.0 and 5.0 mM caused failure in 3.5 – 4 min (n = 2). Measurement of serum Co^{2+} concentration showed that the peak value occurred around the time of receptor failure (0.97, 1.4 and 2.05 mM respectively). The effects of the two smallest doses were reversed by restoring the general circulation

to the limb. In these experiments, though the response to mechanical stimulation had failed, there was still background activity associated with the afferent fibre under investigation.

When verapamil (30 μM) was injected the response declined gradually to 25% of control value after 10 min and fluctuated around this value for the rest of the experiment (n = 1).

$CdCl_2$ was given in a 1 ml bolus dose after the fifth mechanical stimulation. A summary of results is given in Table 1. One minute after injection, 0.5 mM $CdCl_2$ significantly increased the response of the touch domes to mechanical stimulation. With this exception $CdCl_2$ caused a dose dependent decline in the response of the SA1 mechanoreceptors. When the response to mechanical stimulation failed the afferent fibre still responded to electrical stimulation.

Model 2, intradermal injection

When 100 μl of 0.15 M NaCl was injected intradermally under the touch domes the response to mechanical stimulation continued for as long as the touch domes were stimulated. Injection of 125 and 250 pM of $CoCl_2$ caused a transient increase in the response of touch domes to mechanical stimulation. The time to receptor failure depended on the concentration: 125 pM reduced the response to 25% of controls after 6.5 min and 250 and 500

TABLE 1

Percent response at 1, 2, 5 and 8 min after $CdCl_2$ (0.5, 1.0 and 2.5 mM)

Time after $CdCl_2$ (min)	% response			
	Control	0.5 mM	1.0 mM	2.5 mM
1	99.6 ± 7.7	130.0 ± 8.7*	97.6 ± 15.9	65.4 ± 2.1**
2	93.4 ± 8.9	115.2 ± 3.0	88.4 ± 8.3	13.4 ± 7.0***
5	103.1 ± 7.6	100.9 ± 15.7	82.4 ± 0.9*	0.0 ± 0.0***
8	97.9 ± 8.8	95.4 ± 0.6	78.8 ± 3.8	0.0 ± 0.0***

Values are given as mean ± SE of mean; n = 5 for control response and n = 2 for others.
* $P < 0.05$, ** $P < 0.01$, *** $P < 0.001$ (*t*-test).

pM caused receptor failure at 3 min and 25 s respectively. When the response to mechanical stimulation failed, electrical stimulation of the afferent fibre innervating the touch dome still produced an action potential.

Histology

There was a significant decrease in the number of granules present in the cytoplasm adjacent to the nerve terminal in Merkel cells exposed to $CoCl_2$ and verapamil (Table 2). The remaining vesicles were generally found close to the cell membrane. There was also a significant increase in the number of 'synapse-like' structures observed in Merkel cells exposed to $CoCl_2$.

Model 3, isolated skin nerve preparation

Five stimulations were given before the preparation was exposed to drugs to ensure that the touch domes were responding in the usual way. $CdCl_2$ caused a dose dependent attenuation in the response of the SA1 mechanoreceptors to mechanical stimulation (Fig. 1). The higher concentrations caused the decline in response most quickly. Fifteen minutes after application the responses were reduced to 59.7 ± 7.9, 50.1 ± 2.7, 31.7 ± 10.4 and $23.0 \pm 5.6\%$ by 0.05, 0.1, 0.5 and 1.0 mM

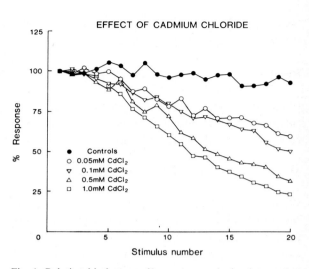

Fig. 1. Relationship between % response and stimulus number with increasing concentrations of cadmium chloride. Superfusing solution containing drug is given after stimulus 5. Stimuli are applied twice per minute for 5 s each. Response reduced after stimulus 8 ($P < 0.05$ at 0.05 mM, $P < 0.001$ at 0.1, 0.5 and 1.0 mM).

$CdCl_2$, respectively ($P < 0.01$ at 0.05 mM and $P < 0.001$ at 0.1, 0.5 and 1.0 mM). Verapamil also reduced the response to mechanical stimulation dose dependently: 69.6 ± 1.7, 45.0 ± 4.5 and $31.6 \pm 10.7\%$ by 20, 50 and 100 μM ($P < 0.001$) 15 min after application (Fig. 2).

Discussion

It is now well established that several divalent cations including Co^{2+} and Cd^{2+} compete with Ca^{2+} for its channel binding site (Hurwitz, 1986). The dose dependent and reversible effect of Co^{2+}, with the exception of the highest concentration, on the evoked response of SA1 mechanoreceptors to mechanical stimulation is similar to that in the frog sciatic nerve – sartorius muscle preparation (Weakly, 1973; Kita and Van den Kloot, 1973). Increasing concentrations of Co^{2+} produced a progressive decrease in the end-plate potential (epp) which almost disappeared at bath concentrations of 1 mM Co^{2+}. This value is similar to the con-

TABLE 2

The vesicle density and the number of 'synaptic-like' structures in Merkel cells after saline, cobalt chloride or verapamil hydrochloride

Drug (mM)	Granule density (number/μm)		Synapses (number/section)	
Saline control	12.1 ± 1.5	(13)	0.6 ± 0.25	(13)
$CoCl_2$ (2.0)	4.3 ± 0.8**	(17)	2.1 ± 0.40*	(17)
Verapamil (0.03)	6.8 ± 0.8*	(18)	–	

Values are given as mean $\pm$ SE of mean, with number of observations in parentheses.
* $P < 0.01$, ** $P < 0.001$ (t-test).

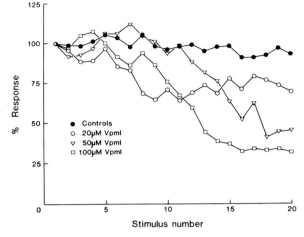

Fig. 2. Relationship between % response and stimulus number with increasing concentrations of verapamil (Vpml). Superfusing solution containing drug is given after stimulus 5. Stimuli are applied twice per minute for 5 s each. Response reduced after stimulus 8 ($P< 0.01$ at 20 and 100 μM) and stimulus 14 ($P< 0.01$ at 50 μM).

centrations measured in the blood serum when the touch domes failed to respond to mechanical stimulation. The effect of Co^{2+} was reversed by washing the preparation in a Co^{2+}-free solution and antagonised by elevating the external Ca^{2+} concentration (Weakly, 1973). Weakly (1973) suggested Co^{2+} inhibited neuromuscular transmission by competitive antagonism of Ca^{2+} leading to failure of transmitter release.

Cobalt (3 mM) also blocked the K^+ evoked release of substance P from cultured rat dorsal root ganglion neurones, [^{3}H]noradrenaline from cultured rat sympathetic neurones (Preney et al., 1986) and dopamine from isolated hypothalamic tuberoinfundibular neurones (Annunziato et al., 1986). The similarities between the effect of Co^{2+} in the Merkel cell − neurite complex and the neuromuscular junction (NMJ) and the demonstration that it can block evoked neurotransmitter release in vitro suggest that Co^{2+} may be blocking Ca^{2+} channels on the Merkel cell membrane, preventing release of a transmitter substance.

Cobalt produced an increase in activity in afferent fibres innervating the touch domes. Co^{2+} has been found to cause an increase in miniature end-plate potentials (mepps) produced by an increase in spontaneous transmitter release at the NMJ (Kita and Van den Kloot, 1973; Weakly, 1973). If Co^{2+} increased spontaneous transmitter release from each Merkel cell in a touch dome, then sufficient may be released to initiate action potentials in the afferent fibre.

In later experiments in model 1 and in all model 3 experiments, Co^{2+} was replaced by Cd^{2+} because it is a more selective Ca^{2+} blocker and to avoid the complications associated with Co^{2+}. The general effect of Cd^{2+} was very similar to Co^{2+}, i.e., a dose dependent decline in response, possibly due to prevention of transmitter release.

Acetylcholine or K^+ evoked release of catecholamines from perfused adrenal glands was inhibited by verapamil and methoxyverapamil (D600) at ID_{50}s of at least 10 μM (Arqueros and Daniels, 1978; Pinto and Trifaro, 1976). D600 (50 and 100 μM) inhibited the K^+ evoked release of dopamine from tuberoinfundibular neurones in vitro (Annunziato et al., 1986). Similar concentrations of verapamil reduced the response of touch domes to mechanical stimulation in our experiments, providing further evidence that transmitter release is involved.

At receptor failure there was a significant decrease in the number of dense cored vesicles present in Merkel cells after exposure to $CoCl_2$ or verapamil. If their only action was to block Ca^{2+} entry then an increase in the number of dense cored vesicles would be expected. In bullfrog dorsal root ganglion neurones it has been shown that fast axonal transport, but not protein synthesis, was inhibited by bathing the neurones in Co^{2+}-containing or Ca^{2+}-free solutions (Lavoie and Bennet, 1983). They suggested that Ca^{2+} was required for proteins to leave the Golgi region in transit for the fast axonal transport system. A similar process may operate in Merkel cells, thus preventing transit of proteins from the Golgi region.

Conclusions

These results suggest that Ca^{2+} is a necessary requirement for the normal function of SA1 mechanoreceptors, possibly via the Merkel cell. This is further evidence supporting the concept of transmitter release from Merkel cells.

References

Annunziato, L., Amoroso, S., Tagliatela, M., De Natale, G. and Di Renzo, G.F. (1986) Effect of different organic and inorganic blockers of calcium entry on the release of endogenous dopamine from tuberoinfundibular neurons. *Neuropharmacology,* 25: 527 – 532.

Arqueros, L. and Daniels, A.J. (1978) Analysis of the inhibitory effect of verapamil on adrenal medullary secretion. *Life Sci.,* 23: 2415 – 2422.

Chen, S.Y., Gerson, S. and Meyer, J. (1973) The fusion of Merkel cell granules with synapse-like structures. *J. Invest. Dermatol.,* 61: 290 – 292.

Findlater, G.S., Cooksey, D., Anand, A., Paintal, A.S. and Iggo, A. (1987) The effects of hypoxia on slowly adapting type I (SAI) cutaneous mechanoreceptors in the cat and rat. *Somatosensory Res.,* 5: 1 – 17.

Hartschuh, W., Weihe, E., Buchler, M., Helmstaeder, V., Feurle, G.E. and Forssmann, W.G. (1979) Met-enkephalin-like immunoreactivity in Merkel cells. *Cell Tissue Res.,* 201: 343 – 348.

Hartschuh, W., Weihe, E., Yanaihara, N. and Reinecke, M. (1983) Immunohistochemical localization of VIP in Merkel cells of various mammals: evidence for a neuromodulator function of the Merkel cell. *J. Invest. Dermatol.,* 81: 361 – 364.

Horch, K.W., Whitehorn, D. and Burgess, P.R. (1974) Impulse generation in type 1 cutaneous mechanoreceptors. *J. Neurophysiol.,* 37: 267 – 281.

Hurwitz, L. (1986) Pharmacology of calcium channels and smooth muscle. *Ann. Rev. Pharmacol. Toxicol.,* 26: 225 – 258.

Iggo, A. and Muir, A.R. (1969) Structure and function of a slowly adapting touch corpuscle in hairy skin. *J. Physiol. (London),* 200: 763 – 796.

Iggo, A. and Findlater, G.S. (1984) A review of Merkel cell mechanisms. In: W. Hamann and A. Iggo (Eds.), *Sensory Receptor Mechanisms,* World Scientific Publ. Co., Singapore.

Kita, H. and Van den Kloot, W. (1973) Action of Co^{2+} and Ni^{2+} at the frog neuromuscular junction. *Nature, New Biol.,* 245: 52 – 53.

Lavoie, P.A. and Bennet, G. (1983) Accumulation of [^{3}H]fucose labelled glycoproteins in the Golgi apparatus of dorsal root ganglion neurons during inhibition of fast axonal transport caused by exposure of the ganglion to Co^{2+} containing or Ca^{2+} free medium. *Neuroscience,* 8: 351 – 362.

Perney, T.M., Hirning, L.D., Leeman, S.E. and Miller, R.J. (1986) Multiple calcium channels mediate neurotransmitter release from peripheral neurons. *Proc. Natl. Acad. Sci. U.S.A.,* 83: 6656 – 6659.

Pinto, J.E.B. and Trifaro, J.M. (1976) The different effects of D600 (methoxyverapamil) on the release of adrenal catecholamines induced by acetylcholine, high potassium or sodium deprivation. *Br. J. Pharmacol.,* 57: 127 – 132.

Rubin, R.P. (1970) The role of calcium in the release of neurotransmitter substances and hormones. *Pharmacol. Rev.,* 22: 389 – 428.

Weakly, J.N. (1973) The action of cobalt ions on neuromuscular transmission in the frog. *J. Physiol. (London),* 234: 597 – 612.

W. Hamann and A. Iggo (Eds.)
Progress in Brain Research, Vol. 74
© 1988 Elsevier Science Publishers B.V. (Biomedical Division)

CHAPTER 6

Responsiveness of slowly adapting cutaneous mechanoreceptors after close arterial infusion of neomycin in cats

K.I. Baumann, W. Hamann and M.S. Leung

Department of Physiology, Faculty of Medicine, The Chinese University of Hong Kong, Shatin, N.T., Hong Kong

Summary

Slowly adapting type 1 and type 2 cutaneous mechanoreceptors were studied in anaesthetised cats. Standard mechanical stimuli comprising a 200 ms ramp and a 2.0 s plateau phase of 20 mN constant force were applied every 30 s. Nervous activity in single unit afferent fibres dissected from the saphenous nerve supplying the receptor under investigation was recorded. During test periods neomycin was infused at a rate of 2.5 mg/min through a side branch into the blood stream of the femoral artery. During control periods the same volume (0.025 ml/min) of saline was infused.

Within minutes after switching from saline to neomycin infusion nervous responses dropped in both types of receptor reaching a minimum at the end of the usually 20 min period of neomycin infusion. Responsiveness of type 1 (Merkel cell) receptors was suppressed to about 25% of the control level. In contrast, type 2 receptors (Ruffini endings) maintained close to 70% of their initial responsiveness. Interspike interval histograms of the type 2 receptors showed only a shift of the main classes of intervals by 10 ms to higher values whereas the typical Poisson shape of the interspike interval distribution of type 1 receptors was totally distorted.

The present results support the notion that neomycin acts on two sites in type 1 receptors: the mechano-electric transduction process in the Merkel cell and the putative synaptic transmission to the afferent nerve terminal. In contrast, in type 2 receptors the receptor endings are likely to be the main target sites of action.

Introduction

Close arterial infusion of the aminoglycoside neomycin strongly suppresses the excitability of slowly adapting type 1 (SA1) cutaneous mechanoreceptors in the cat (Baumann et al., 1986). Assuming that mechano-electric transduction takes place in the Merkel cells, there are two possible target sites for the action of neomycin, the transducer itself as well as the synaptic link between Merkel cell and nerve terminal. There appears to be no acute effect of neomycin on transmission through myelinated nerve fibres (Chan et al., 1985). However, voltage dependent plugging for small ions by neomycin has been described by Ohmori (1985) at the chick hair cell, and synaptic transmission at the neuromuscular junction is reduced in the presence of neomycin (Prado et al., 1978; Singh et al., 1978). The present investigation is a comparison between the acute effects of neomycin on cutaneous mechanoreceptors of primary (Ruffini endings) and secondary type

(Merkel cell receptors), with the aim of determining whether or not Merkel cells are the site of mechano-electric transduction in SA1 receptors and of furthering the understanding of the mode of action of aminoglycosides on secondary receptors.

Methods

Cats of both sexes weighing 1.5 – 2.5 kg were anaesthetised initially with thiopental sodium (60 mg/kg, i.p.) and anaesthesia was subsequently maintained with 1.5% pentobarbital i.v. as necessary. The body temperature was kept constant at about 37°C with a thermostatically controlled blanket. The left carotid artery was cannulated for monitoring of arterial blood pressure and the left jugular vein was cannulated for venous access. A catheter was inserted into the medial circumflex femoris artery in a retrograde fashion for close arterial infusion of neomycin into the femoral artery of the right leg, without substantial change in femoral blood flow. A paraffin pool was made at the medial part of the right thigh for the dissection of fine nerve strands from the saphenous nerve. Single unit recordings were made from afferent nerve fibres in the saphenous nerve supplying either SA1 or SA2 receptors in the skin of the anterior part of the right leg.

Standard mechanical stimuli were applied every 30 s, through a perspex stylus with a spherical tip (diameter 1 mm) attached to a Statham (UC2) force transducer, which was driven by an electromechanic transducer (Bruehl and Kjaer No. 4810). Each stimulus rose from a contact force of 0.5 mN within 200 ms to a peak force of 20 mN and was kept constant for a duration of 2.0 s (plateau phase). The displacements needed for the stimulation were recorded with a Sangamo displacement transducer (Schlumberger). Original recordings of nervous responses, forces and displacements of stimulation were made with an FM tape recorder (Hewlett Packard 3964A). Cumulative spike counts during individual stimuli, displacements, and forces were recorded with a Graphtec chart recorder. Spike trains were analysed for interspike intervals using the last second of the plateau phase (1200 – 2200 ms after the beginning of the mechanical stimuli). Normal saline was infused at a flow rate of 0.025 ml/min into the femoral artery throughout the experiments except during the period of neomycin infusion.

After the identification of an SA1 or SA2 unit by their typical response and discharge pattern (Chambers et al., 1972; Horch et al., 1974), repetitive mechanical stimuli were applied for at least half an hour with saline infusion to ensure steady state responses. Neomycin sulphate (Mycifradin, Upjohn) was then infused usually for 20 min at the same rate of 0.025 ml/min delivering 2.5 mg neomycin/min (total amount: 50 mg). After switching back to saline infusion responses to repetitive mechanical stimulation were recorded for at least another 1.5 h. At the end of an experiment, methylene blue was infused to see whether the receptor was positioned within areas of skin well supplied by the close arterial infusion.

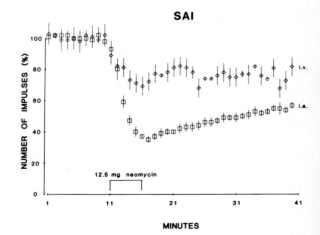

Fig. 1. Responsiveness of SA1 receptors to standard mechanical stimuli (200 ms ramp followed by a 2 s plateau of 20 mN constant force) every 30 s. Neomycin was infused between min 15 and 20, either into the femoral artery (i.a.) or into the jugular vein (i.v.), at a rate of 2.5 mg/min (total amount: 12.5 mg). Before and after neomycin infusion normal saline was infused at the same rate of 0.025 ml/min. Responses during the last 10 min before neomycin infusion were taken as 100%. Mean ± SEM of two units employing close arterial infusion and one unit with intravenous infusion.

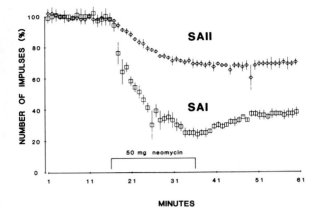

Fig. 2. Responsiveness of SA1 and SA2 receptors to standard mechanical stimuli every 30 s. Neomycin was infused at a rate of 2.5 mg/min into the femoral artery between min 15 and 35 (total amount: 50 mg). Mean responses during the last 10 min before neomycin infusion were taken as 100%. Mean ± SEM of three SA2 and two SA1 units.

Results

The effects of 5 min infusion of 2.5 mg/min neomycin (total amount: 12.5 mg) on type 1 receptors when given either into the jugular vein or into the femoral artery are compared in Fig. 1. The mean values of the steady state nervous responses during the last 10 min before the neomycin infusion were taken as the 100% control value. Within minutes after neomycin reached the circulation, the responsiveness of the SA1 receptors began to decrease. This drop in mean number of nervous impulses was much more pronounced when neomycin was infused into the femoral artery than when the same amount was administered intravenously. After switching back to saline infusion a slight recovery of nervous responses following close arterial infusion could be observed. However, responses did not reach the same level as after intravenous infusion in spite of about the same final plasma concentration of neomycin in either case.

Fig. 2 shows the effects of 20 min of close arterial infusion of 2.5 mg/min neomycin (total amount: 50 mg neomycin) on the responsiveness of SA1 and SA2 receptors. The time mark at 15 min

indicated the time when the neomycin first reached the circulation. The number of nerve impulses of both types of receptor began to drop as soon as neomycin got into the femoral artery and continued to decrease throughout the neomycin infusion. Recovery after switching back to saline infusion was only minimal in either type of receptor. The mean number of nerve impulses obtained from SA2 receptors was reduced to about 70% of the control level before neomycin infusion. In contrast, the responsiveness of SA1 receptors was reduced to approximately 25% of their control value, indicating a more drastic effect of neomycin of SA1 than on SA2 receptors.

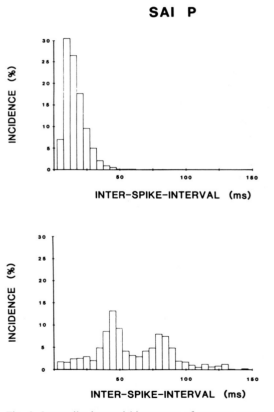

Fig. 3. Interspike interval histograms of nervous responses of two SA1 receptors obtained during the late plateau phase (1200 – 2200 ms) of 10 constant force stimuli each before and after close arterial infusion of neomycin, respectively. Upper part: control period with normal saline infusion, lower part: after 20 min of 2.5 mg/min neomycin infusion.

The distribution of the interspike intervals during the plateau phase of the constant force mechanical stimulation is shown in Figs. 3 and 5 for the SA1 and SA2 receptors, respectively. The upper part of Fig. 3 shows the distribution of the interspike intervals from the SA1 units during the control period before neomycin infusion. It resembles a Poisson distribution with a relatively high incidence of short intervals. The results in the lower part of Fig. 3 were obtained from the 10 stimuli with the lowest number of impulses after neomycin infusion. The pattern of distribution was severely distorted and spread over a large range of intervals, i.e., between 1 and 150 ms. Principally the same tendency of distortion of the interspike interval distribution was already obtained after a much smaller degree of suppression in responsiveness as observed after 5 min of intraveneous infusion (Fig. 4).

The distribution of the interspike intervals for the SA2 receptors during the plateau phase of mechanical stimuli (Fig. 5) showed, as expected, a different pattern of distribution compared with the SA1 receptors. As shown in the upper graph, the discharge pattern of the type 2 receptors is much more regular with the highest incidence at intervals of 30 and 35 ms. After the infusion of neomycin

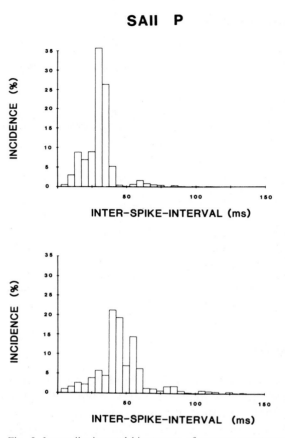

SAII P

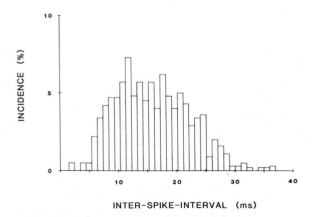

Fig. 4. Interspike interval histogram for 10 responses during the late plateau phase (1200 – 2200 ms) obtained from the SA1 unit shown in Fig. 1 at the time of maximal suppression in responsiveness shortly after 5 min of intravenous neomycin infusion at a rate of 2.5 mg/min.

Fig. 5. Interspike interval histograms of nervous responses of three SA2 receptors during the late plateau phase (1200 – 2200 ms) of 10 constant force stimuli each before and after close arterial infusion of neomycin. Upper part: control period with normal saline infusion, lower part: after 20 min of 2.5 mg/min neomycin infusion.

the distribution of the interspike intervals is broadened and the highest incidence shifted to between 40 and 45 ms reflecting the 30% decrease in responsiveness of the SA2 receptors.

Discussion

The present study is a comparison between acute effects of neomycin on SA1 and SA2 receptors in cats with the aim of determining whether or not Merkel cells are the site of mechano-electric transduction in SA1 receptors. Responsiveness of both types of receptor to the same mechanical stimuli applied at the skin surface was found to be reduced within minutes after the start of close arterial infusion of 2.5 mg/min neomycin into the femoral artery. At the end of the 20 min infusion period nervous responses of type 1 receptors were reduced to about 25% of their original level while type 2 receptors maintained approximately 70% of their control responsiveness. No changes in the displacements of the probe required to maintain the 20 mN force of stimulation were observed during that time in either type of receptor. Thus, neomycin-induced alterations in force transmission from the skin to the receptor can be excluded as a possible cause of the suppressed responsiveness.

Within the infusion period of 20 min effective concentrations of neomycin at the receptor site can be assumed to reach similar levels in both types of receptor in spite of the different anatomical structure and position of the receptors within the skin. Femoral blood flow was not measured in the present experiments. In analogy to data obtained in dogs (Mason and Ledsome, 1974) the femoral blood flow in the cats of this study is assumed to be 5 – 10 ml/min. Thus, the transient plasma concentrations reaching the leg are estimated to fall into the range of 250 – 500 mg/l and are likely to equilibrate quickly with the interstitial fluid. In both types of receptor responsiveness starts decreasing within minutes of switching the infusion to neomycin. As shown in Fig. 1 the short period (5 min) of high concentration of neomycin in the femoral blood flow is more effective in suppressing nervous activity in SA1 receptors than a gradual build-up to reach the same final plasma concentration in the general circulation after infusing neomycin at the same rate and for the same duration into the jugular vein instead of the femoral artery. It has also been shown previously that responses of type 1 receptors are less severely affected if the close arterial neomycin infusion of 2.5 mg/min is given only for 5 or 10 min rather than for 20 min (Baumann et al., 1987a).

In the present results a marked difference was observed in the degree of suppression of nervous responses. Neomycin is known to affect mechano-electric transduction in vestibular hair cells by voltage dependent plugging of transduction channels (Ohmori, 1985). This acute electrostatic interaction of aminoglycosides with the hair cell membrane has also been described by Schacht (1986). It appears that neomycin impairs mechano-electric transduction also in cutaneous mechano-receptors. A similar degree in suppression of responses would be expected for both types of receptors investigated, if only the transducer membrane was affected by neomycin. The finding that nervous responses of SA1 receptors are much more severely suppressed than those of SA2 receptors cannot be explained by the assumption of a direct effect on the transducer membrane alone. The interspike interval histograms of type 2 receptors show only a slight broadening and a shift of the range of intervals with the highest incidence from 30 to 40 ms corresponding to the increase in mean firing interval with the reduced number of nerve impulses. The coefficient of variance of the three SA2 receptors shown in Fig. 5 was 0.40 during the control period and 0.44 after the infusion of neomycin. These values are well above those obtained in our experiments during ongoing activity at contact force (0.095) and also usually reported for fully adapted type 2 receptors (Chambers et al., 1972), indicating that in the present experiments with analysis of the spike trains after 1.2 – 2.2 s the adaptation process is still going on. In contrast, the typical Poisson-like distribution of the interspike interval histogram of type 1 receptors (Iggo and Muir, 1969; Horch et al., 1974) is totally distorted after 20 min of neomycin infusion at 2.5 mg/min. Already after 5 min of intraveneous infusion at the same rate that resulted in a less drastic reduction of nervous impulses, the normal Poisson-like distribution is deformed (Fig. 4).

Schacht (1986) has proposed a dual mode of action of aminoglycosides on inner ear hair cells. Neomycin could affect the hair cells acutely by electrostatic interaction of the drug with the cellular membrane. Neomycin might also get into the cells and exert long lasting changes inside the

48

cells. These could include an interaction with the metabolism of phosphoinositides (Schacht, 1974). These substances are believed to play an important role as a second messenger system in hair cells and other sensory receptors (Berridge, 1984; Yanagisava et al., 1984). The latter mode of action appears to be involved in the reduction of responsiveness of SA1 receptors observed in rats chronically treated with neomycin (Baumann et al., 1987b).

Slowly adapting type 1 receptors are believed to be secondary receptors with the mechano-electric transduction process taking place in the Merkel cell and synaptical transmission to the adjoining nerve terminal (Andres, 1966; Anand et al., 1979; Cooksey et al., 1984a,b; Iggo and Findlater, 1984; Yamashita et al., 1986). Neomycin is known to affect transmission at the neuromuscular junction (Wright and Collier, 1977; Singh et al., 1978), whereas the conduction velocity of myelinated nerve fibres appears to be unaffected by acute exposure to neomycin in concentrations up to 350 mg/l (Chan et al., 1985). In contrast, in type 2 receptors mechano-electric transduction is known to take place in the terminal branches of the afferent nerve fibre within the Ruffini corpuscle.

The larger reduction in responsiveness of SA1 receptors after close arterial neomycin infusion supports the hypothesis of synaptic transmission between the Merkel cell and the adjoining nerve terminal (Iggo and Findlater, 1984) critically depending on the metabolic condition of the Merkel cells. Acute hypoxia resulted in a sharp decrease in responsiveness of SA1 receptors with good recovery after the cessation of hypoxia (Anand et al., 1979; Cooksey et al., 1984a). Application of calcium antagonists reduced responsiveness of SA1 receptors in both mammals and amphibians (Cooksey et al., 1984b; Yamashita et al., 1986).

Our results are in good support of the hypothesis of a synaptic transmission between the Merkel cell and afferent nerve terminal. Assuming that both SA1 and SA2 receptors employ similar ionic transduction mechanisms, one would expect similar degrees of suppression if only the transducer was affected by neomycin. The greater reduction in responsiveness in SA1 than in SA2 receptors is in support of the idea that in the SA1 receptors neomycin acts on two target sites: the mechano-electric transducer in the Merkel cell and the putative synapse between the Merkel cell and the adjoining nerve terminal.

References

Anand, A., Iggo, A. and Paintal, A.S. (1979) Lability of granular vesicles in Merkel cells of the type I slowly adapting cutaneous receptors of the cat. *J. Physiol. (London),* 296: 19P – 20P.

Andres, K.H. (1966) Uber die Feinstruktur der Rezeptoren an Sinushaaren. *Z. Zellforsch.,* 75: 339 – 365.

Baumann, K.I., Hamann, W. and Leung, M.S. (1986) Reduced responsiveness of touch (SAI) receptors in the cat following close arterial infusion of neomycin. *Brain Res.,* 377: 160 – 162.

Baumann, K.I., Hamann, W. and Leung, M.S. (1987a) Dynamic and static responses of cat s.a. I mechanoreceptors after close arterial infusion of different doses of neomycin. *J. Physiol. (London),* 382: 76P.

Baumann, K.I., Cheng-Chew, S.B., Hamann, W. and Leung, M.S. (1987b) Responsiveness of s.a.I receptors in degenerative skin conditions and ageing in the rat and the cat. In: L.M. Pubols and B.J. Sessle (Eds.), *Effects of Injury on Trigeminal and Spinal Somatosensory Systems. Neurology and Neurobiology,* Vol 30. Alan Liss, New York, pp. 29 – 36.

Berridge, M.J. (1984) Inositol triphosphate and diacylglycerol as second messengers. *Biochem. J.,* 220: 345 – 360.

Chambers, M.R., Andres, K.H., Von Düring, M. and Iggo, A. (1972) The structure and function of the slowly adapting type II mechanoreceptors in hairy skin. *Quart. J. Exp. Physiol.,* 57: 417 – 445.

Chan, W.S., Cheng-Chew, S.B., Hamann, W. and Ng, K.C. (1985) Acute exposure of myelinated nerve fibres to neomycin. *Neurosci. Lett.,* Suppl. 20: S41.

Cooksey, E.J., Findlater, G.S. and Iggo, A. (1984a) A limb-perfusion preparation allowing manipulation of the internal and external environment of cutaneous receptors in cats. *J. Physiol. (London),* 346: 14P.

Cooksey, E.J., Findlater, G.S. and Iggo, A. (1984b) The responses to mechanical stimulation of SAI receptors of cats and rats in the presence of calcium antagonists. *J. Physiol. (London),* 357: 30P.

Horch, K.W., Whitehorn, D. and Burgess, P.R. (1974) Impulse generation in type I cutaneous mechanoreceptors. *J. Neurophysiol.,* 37: 267 – 281.

Iggo, A. and Muir, A.R. (1969) The structure and function of a slowly adapting touch corpuscle in hairy skin. *J. Physiol. (London)*, 200: 763 – 796.

Iggo, A. and Findlater, G.S. (1984) A review of Merkel cell mechanisms. In: W. Hamann and A. Iggo (Eds.), *Sensory Receptor Mechanisms*. World Scientific, Singapore, pp. 117 – 131.

Mason, J.M. and Ledsome, J.R. (1974) Effects of obstruction of the mitral orifice or distention of the pulmonary vein-atrial junctions on renal and hind-limb vascular resistance in the dog. *Circ. Res.*, 35: 24 – 32.

Ohmori, H. (1985) Mechanoelectric transduction currents in isolated vestibular hair cells of the chick. *J. Physiol. (London)*, 359: 189 – 217.

Prado, W.A., Corrado, A.P. and Marseillan, R.F. (1978) Competitive antagonism between calcium and antibiotics at the neuromuscular junction. *Arch. Int. Pharmacodyn.*, 231: 297 – 307.

Schacht, J. (1974) Interaction of neomycin with phosphoinositide metabolism in guinea pig inner ear and brain tissues. *Am. Otol.*, 83: 613 – 618.

Schacht, J. (1986) Molecular mechanism of drug-induced hearing loss. *Hearing Res.*, 22, 297 – 304.

Singh, Y.N., Harvey, A.L. and Marshall, I.G. (1978) Antibiotic-induced paralysis of the mouse phrenic nerve-hemidiaphragm preparation, and reversibility by calcium and by neostigmine. *Anesthesiology*, 48: 418 – 424.

Wright, J.M. and Collier, B. (1977) The effects of neomycin upon transmitter release and action. *J. Pharmacol. Exp. Ther.*, 200: 576 – 587.

Yamashita, Y., Ogawa, H. and Taniguchi, K. (1986) Differential effects of manganese and magnesium on two types of slowly adapting cutaneous mechanoreceptors afferent units in frogs. *Pflügers Arch.*, 406: 218 – 224.

Yanagisawa, K., Yoshioka, T. and Katsuki, Y. (1984) Sound transducer mechanism and phospholipids in the hair cell of the ear. In: W. Hamann and A. Iggo (Eds.), *Sensory Receptor Mechanisms*. World Scientific, Singapore, pp. 109 – 116.

W. Hamann and A. Iggo (Eds.)
Progress in Brain Research, Vol. 74
© 1988 Elsevier Science Publishers B.V. (Biomedical Division)

CHAPTER 7

Evidence that the Merkel cell is not the transducer in the mechanosensory Merkel cell—neurite complex

J. Diamond, L.R. Mills and K.M. Mearow

Department of Neurosciences, McMaster University, 1240 Main Street West, Hamilton, Ontario, L8N 3Z5, Canada

The problem of the Merkel cell as a transducer

Merkel, discussing the cutaneous cell he discovered that now bears his name, regarded it as a 'touch cell' that was analogous to the specialized cells he assumed to be associated with other sensory modalities such as taste, hearing, and vision (Merkel, 1880). The touch cells were taken to be the actual transducers, i.e., they detected the primary energy change in the environment, and converted it to a form appropriate to excite impulses in the sensory nerves. An alternative possibility, that the Merkel cell might simply convey (and perhaps modify en route) the stimulus to the ending, itself the actual transducer, seems not to have been discussed by Merkel.

The application of electron microscopy (EM) (Munger, 1965), used with correlative electrophysiology (Iggo and Muir, 1969), confirmed some of Merkel's original observations and suggestions. His assumption that the 'Merkel cell' was the transducer was reinforced by the finding of simple morphological synapses (Fig. 2) between Merkel cells and their associated nerve endings, and the presence of some dense cored granules (dcgs) concentrated in the Merkel cell cytoplasm opposite the nerve ending. In the mammal the synapses are structurally polarized in the direction Merkel cell—neurite (Fig. 2), but in lower vertebrates the synapses can be reciprocal (Fox and Whitear, 1978; Mearow and Diamond, 1983; Diamond et

al., 1987). Gradually the concept has emerged of a mechanosensory complex in which the Merkel cell reacts to a mechanical deformation of the epidermis, probably by generating a receptor potential, and excites the nerve ending presumably via the synaptic release of a transmitter present in the dcgs. During a maintained stimulus the continued release of transmitter would produce the slowly adapting discharge characteristic of the mammalian sensory structures known to contain Merkel cells (e.g., Iggo and Muir, 1969).

There are, however, a number of difficulties with this view of Merkel cell function. First, aside from older observations suggesting that the mechanosensory nerve endings are likely to be excitable by acetylcholine (Gray and Diamond, 1957), there is no plausible candidate for the role of the putative transmitter. The chemical nature of the Merkel cell granules is still unknown, although recently immunocytochemical evidence has suggested the presence of peptides (Hartschuh et al., 1979, 1983), and no convincing correlation has been established between the occurrence or density of the granules and mechanosensory function. Second, chemical synaptic transmission was thought to be too slow to explain the ability of mechanosensory units in the vibrissae of the cat to 'follow', one-to-one, a high frequency (up to 1500 Hz) vibratory stimulus (Gottschaldt and Vahle-Hinz, 1981). Third, if the Merkel cell is the transducer then it should itself be mechanosensitive; Cooper and Nurse (1986) studied Merkel cells dissociated from neonatal rat vibrissae, and failed to detect membrane current or voltage changes in response to a mechanical stimulus. Finally, although Merkel cell morphology is essentially similar in all vertebrates, the mechanosensory responses of Merkel cell – neurite complexes in the salamander (Cooper and Diamond, 1977; Parducz et al., 1977) and in Xenopus (Mearow and Diamond, 1983) are *rapidly* adapting. It is worth noting here that in the rat the normal slowly adapting discharge from a touch dome is not achieved by successive recruitment of possibly rapidly adapting single Merkel cell – neurite complexes; when only a fraction of the available Merkel cell – neurite complexes within a dome are activated the discharge is still slowly adapting (Yasargil et al., 1988).

Is there a chemical transmission step in the initiation of the mechanosensory response?

To study this possibility an isolated nerve skin preparation was devised that allowed the function of single Merkel cell complexes in salamander skin to be studied under relatively controlled conditions in vitro (Diamond et al., 1986). Two tests were of special interest: the effects of altering temperature, and of altering the concentrations of certain divalent ions in the extracellular environment. The latency of the afferent impulse, whether it was evoked mechanically or by an electrical stimulus applied via the mechanical prodder, had a small Q_{10} (1.3 – 2), i.e., similar to the value for axonal conduction in frogs, and was in marked contrast to the relatively large temperature coefficient ($Q_{10} = 3$) of chemical transmission (Katz and Miledi, 1965). The latency of the mechanically evoked impulse was always some 0.5 – 2.5 ms longer than that evoked electrically; thus, this extra component, *which included the transduction step*, was relatively temperature insensitive. In the second test, Ca^{2+} was removed from the fluid bathing the isolated nerve skin preparation, while Mg^{2+} was simultaneously increased (to 10 – 40 mM), a pro-

cedure which effectively depresses or completely blocks transmitter release at conventional chemical synapses (Katz, 1969); the mechanosensitivity of the salamander Merkel cell – neurite complexes was totally unaffected.

These results not only indicated that a conventional chemical synapse was not involved in the initiation of the impulse, but also coincidentally excluded a possible 'unifying' hypothesis (Diamond et al., 1986) which supposed that in the lower vertebrate the reciprocal synapses provided an inhibitory feedback mechanism that transformed the slowly adapting discharge characteristic of mammals, to the rapidly adapting one characteristic of lower vertebrates (cf. McDonald and Mitchell, 1975).

Mechanosensitivity after selective elimination of Merkel cells

Despite the findings described above, in principle the Merkel cell might still act as a mechanosensory transducer, responding to the stimulus and exciting

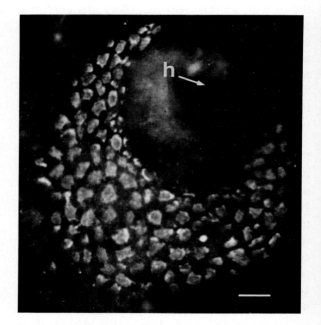

Fig. 1. Touch dome in a whole mount of skin from a rat that had received quinacrine (15 mg/kg, i.p.) 24 h earlier. h = tylotrich hair. (Reproduced from Nurse et al., 1983.) Scale bar = 20 μm.

the nerve by unconventional mechanisms. To answer these (and other) possibilities we have attempted to selectively eliminate the Merkel cell from the complex, then test for residual mechanosensitivity. The technique we used took advantage of our finding that Merkel cells can be selectively labeled by the fluorochrome quinacrine (e.g., Fig. 1; Nurse et al., 1983). Thus it seemed possible, by appropriately irradiating the skin of an animal loaded with quinacrine, to damage the Merkel cells selectively.

Such experiments have now been done on the Merkel cell – neurite complexes in touch domes of rats, and on those located at the gland openings in Xenopus skin (Mills et al., 1985). In both preparations (studied in vivo), the initial investigations were directed at finding an irradiation regime that 'bleached' the quinacrine fluorescent Merkel cells but did not simultaneously damage the nerve endings or the neighboring keratinocytes. When examined *immediately* following such an irradiation, both the mechanosensitivity and the fine structural appearances of the Merkel cells and associated nerve endings seemed always to be unchanged. A particularly intriguing finding, however, came from preliminary studies of touch domes examined at 2 – 5 days post irradiation, and in areas of Xenopus skin examined at 3 – 13 days post irradiation. In these instances mechanosensory function seemed to be normal, yet in the EM no Merkel cells could be found except for a very few obviously dying or dead ones. Some of the touch domes in these experiments had been examined prior to their fixation by a systematic mapping of the mechanosensitivity across them; the technique utilized a vertical 'prodder' of 16 μm tip diameter, which had a spatial resolution of about 50 μm in the plane of the epidermis (Yasargil et al., 1988). Thus, if a mechanosensitive area of about 50 μm or more radius, for example, was subsequently found to be devoid of Merkel cells, then Merkel cells could not have been implicated in the evoked response.

We have now completed the EM reconstruction of one such mapped dome, that physiologically was almost indistinguishable from nearby unirradiated, normally responsive, domes; in this irradiated dome examination of serial sections revealed only seven, grossly pathological, Merkel cells, out of the normal complement of 90 or so (Nurse and Diamond, 1984). When the correlation was made, it was clear that near-normal responses were evoked at many locations where the nearest of the seven abnormal Merkel cells was 150 – 200 μm away. Significantly, numerous 'isolated' nerve endings were observed in the dome epidermis, including these Merkel cell-free areas (Fig. 3), with about the same frequency of occurrence as that of Merkel cell – neurite complexes in normal domes; this finding was common in the irradiated domes we examined. The presence, just above the basal lamina, of these large, mitochondria-rich terminals was striking, since individual nerve endings unassociated with Merkel cells are rare anywhere in the normal epidermis (e.g., Kruger et al., 1981), and in particular are never seen within normal touch domes (our unpublished observations).

Analogous results have come from irradiated Xenopus skin, i.e., normal rapidly adapting responses were evoked from irradiated skin regions (thresholds were sometimes slightly higher than normal), that subsequent EM examination showed to be devoid of Merkel cells.

We conclude that the initiation of mechanosensory responses from Merkel cell – neurite complexes, both in the rat touch dome and in Xenopus skin, does not require the presence of the Merkel cell, and, therefore, that *the Merkel cell is not the mechanosensory transducer*. Rather this function must be ascribed to the nerve ending itself. The adaptation character too appears to be an intrinsic property of the nerve ending, since its expression did not require the presence of the Merkel cell.

The suggested function(s) of the Merkel cell

The enigma of the Merkel cell's function is, if anything, heightened by the evidence that the cell is not the primary mechanosensory transducer. However, there is no shortage of putative roles for this intriguing cell, none of them exclusive of the others.

(1) The Merkel cell as a target

This is now well established. In both salamanders (Scott et al., 1981) and Xenopus (new findings) Merkel cells differentiate de novo in skin that has newly regenerated in a nerve-free limb; when nerves are allowed to regenerate into this skin (which has no pre-existing neural pathways), the Merkel cells become innervated, and normal mechanosensory function is established. Similarly, in the glabrous skin of rat footpads denervated at or shortly after birth, the Merkel cells can develop independently of nerves, and subsequently become innervated if regenerating nerves arrive (Mills et al., 1984); however, if the hairy skin of rats is denervated at birth, Merkel cells fail to develop in the touch domes. Nevertheless, even in touch domes it seems that the Merkel cells may well be the final targets for the arriving terminals of the very nerves that appear to induce their differentiation.

This target role for Merkel cells implies that their distribution determines the distribution of the mechanosensory endings associated with them.

Thus the Merkel cells are responsible for the selective location of these endings within the epidermis, their organization into characteristic groups, and their concentration at strategic locations where active exploration of the environment occurs such as the fingertips, lips, toes, vibrissae etc. Exactly what determines the distribution of the Merkel cells themselves is unknown; certainly in mammalian glabrous skin they appear well in advance of other 'organizing' structures, e.g., the rete ridges (Dell and Munger, 1986). To date this target role is the only proven role for the Merkel cell, and although the mechanisms involved are unknown it seems plausible that the presumed synaptic release sites could be the means by which such target influences are exerted.

(2) Other trophic functions

Although our results indicate that the presence of the Merkel cell is not necessary for the generation of normal mechanosensory responses, the Merkel cell may nevertheless have an essential role in ensuring that these responses can occur. As has been

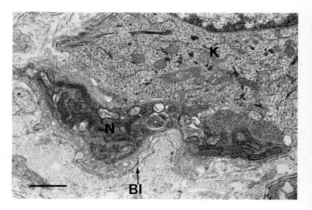

Fig. 3. Electron micrograph from a touch dome that had been irradiated 3 days earlier, in a rat that had received quinacrine. The isolated nerve ending (N), lying above the basal lamina (Bl) and adjacent to a normal keratinocyte (K), was typical of those seen in Merkel cell-free regions of such domes; the local mechanosensitivity was essentially normal in the region that included this ending, and the nearest Merkel cell, that appeared to be dying or dead, was about 175 μm distant. Scale bar = 1 μm.

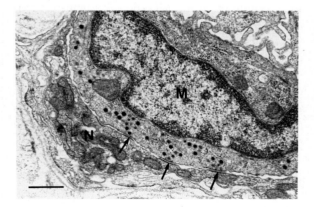

Fig. 2. Electron micrograph of a normal Merkel cell – neurite complex from an adult rat dome. There are three 'synaptic' zones present (arrows). M = Merkel cell. N = nerve ending. (Reproduced from Yasargil et al., 1987.) Scale bar = 0.5 μm.

mentioned, the general scarcity of nerve endings in the epidermis is noteworthy, and to some extent may reflect an inadequate or even inimical environment; the Merkel cell may have a function in providing necessary metabolic support to the mechanosensitive, and judging by their relatively high density of mitochondria (Figs. 2 and 3) highly biochemically active, nerve endings. Our irradiation experiments did not test the *long-term* ability of Merkel cell-free nerve endings to function as mechanoreceptors.

(3) The Merkel cell as a 'fine tuner' of the terminal's mechanosensitivity

When quinacrine-loaded Merkel cells in Xenopus and rat skin were selectively eliminated by irradiation, the mechanosensory thresholds of the surviving nerve endings were often high (though many were within the normal range). Of course this could well have simply reflected damage of the nerve endings, and we know from EM observations that in many instances this definitely occurred. However, the possibility exists that in some way the Merkel cell is responsible for ensuring the characteristic low threshold of the Merkel cell — neurite complex, and that in its absence the nerve ending expresses only an intrinsically higher threshold mechanosensitivity. We attempted to answer this by crushing the nerves to the skin in Xenopus, and following the recovery of cutaneous mechanosensitivity with correlative EM (Mearow and Diamond, 1983). Although high threshold rapidly adapting responses were observed prior to the nerve endings contacting the Merkel cells, it seemed that full recovery was approximately coincident with the reestablishment of a morphological synaptic relationship between the cells and neurites. Two quite different mechanisms that could be considered here are (1) that Merkel cells continuously secrete a substance that lowers the mechanosensory threshold of the nerve endings, and (2) that the cells *induce* the characteristic low threshold mechanosensitivity to develop in the nerve ending.

A potential role that none of our findings have

excluded is that the Merkel cell is specifically involved in *modulating* other aspects of the mechanosensory response, e.g., the ability of the mechanoreceptor to resist fatigue, or to recover rapidly after a stimulus.

(4) The Merkel cell as a possible mediator of positional information

A great deal of evidence now exists which indicates that the development of the somatosensory nervous system, and especially the organization of the somatosensory cortex, is critically influenced by information arriving along afferent nerves (Kaas et al., 1983), in accord with the original idea that sensory nerves convey 'positional information' (Wolpert, 1971) to the developing central nervous system, that relates to the region they supply, and which eventually is utilized in the construction of the appropriate central circuitry (Sperry and Miner, 1949). Intriguingly, all of the peripheral nerves that have been implicated in influencing the development of the somatosensory nervous system in vertebrates contain mechanosensory axons that supply Merkel cells. Could these cells be involved in the 'positional labeling' of these nerves? Such a role would be a logical extension of their function as the specific targets of these axons, i.e., the Merkel cells would both regulate the exact location of the nerve endings, and instruct them as to where in the body this is.

Conclusion

In view of the clearly successful evolution of specialized nerve terminals that are intrinsically mechanosensitive, it is not surprising that the Merkel cell is turning out to have specialized functions, in particular that of acting as a specific target cell, other than that of mechanosensory transduction. Given the importance of locating and appropriately distributing the highly sensitive touch modality associated with the Merkel cells, in what may be the most important sensory interface the animal has with its environment (Diamond, 1987), it is not surprising that a target cell with the particular characteristics of the Merkel cell has evolved. It can be expected that the elucidation of its still undetermined cell lineage will throw further light on the role(s) of this remarkable cell.

Acknowledgements

This work was supported by grants from MRC (Canada) and from the Public Health Service (Grant NS 15592).

References

Cooper, E. and Diamond, J. (1977) A quantitative study of the mechanosensory innervation of the salamander skin. *J. Physiol. (London),* 264: 695 – 723.

Cooper, E. and Nurse, C.A. (1986) Studies on isolated Merkel cells using patch and whole cell recording. *Soc. Neurosci. Abstr.,* 16: 18.2.

Dell, D.D. and Munger, B.L. (1986) The early embryogenesis of papillary (sweat duct) ridges in primate glabrous skin: the dermatotopic map of cutaneous mechanoreceptors and dermatoglyphics. *J. Comp. Neurol.,* 244: 511 – 532.

Diamond, J. (1987) Plasticity and stability in the sensory innervation of skin. In: L.M. Pubols and B.J. Sessle (Eds.), *Effects of Injury on Trigeminal and Spinal Somatosensory Systems.* Alan R. Liss, New York, pp. 43 – 48.

Diamond, J., Holmes, M. and Nurse, C.A. (1986) Are Merkel cell-neurite reciprocal synapses involved in the initiation of tactile responses in salamander skin?. *J. Physiol. (London),* 376: 101 – 120.

Fox, H. and Whitear, M. (1978) Observations on Merkel cells in amphibians. *Biol. Cell.,* 32: 223 – 232.

Gottschaldt, K.M. and Vahle-Hinz, C. (1981) Merkel cell receptors; structure and transducer function. *Science,* 214: 183 – 186.

Gray, J.A.B. and Diamond, J. (1957) Pharmacological properties of sensory receptors and their relation to those of the autonomic nervous system. *Br. Med. Bull.,* 13: 185 – 188.

Hartschuh, W., Weihe, E., Buchler, M., Helmstaedter, V., Feurle, G.E. and Forssmann, W.G. (1979) Met-enkephalin-like immuno-reactivity in Merkel cells. *Cell. Tiss. Res.,* 201:343 – 348.

Hartschuh, W., Weihe, E., Yanaihara, N. and Reinecke, M. (1983) Immunohistochemical localization of vasoactive intestinal peptide (VIP) in Merkel cells of various animals. *J. Invest. Dermatol.,* 81: 361 – 364.

Iggo, A. and Muir, A.R. (1969) The structure and function of a slowly-adapting touch corpuscle in hairy skin. *J. Physiol. (London),* 200: 763 – 796.

Kaas, J.H., Merzenich, M.M. and Killackey, H.P. (1983) The reorganization of somatosensory cortex following peripheral nerve damage in adult and developing mammals. *Ann. Rev. Neurosci.,* 6: 325 – 356.

Katz, B. (1969) *The Release of Neural Transmitter Substances.* Charles C. Thomas, Springfield, IL.

Katz, B. and Miledi, R. (1965) The effect of temperature on the synaptic delay at the neuromuscular junction. *J. Physiol. (London),* 181: 659 – 670.

Kruger, L., Perl, E.R. and Sedivec, M.J. (1981) Fine structure of myelinated mechanical nociceptor endings in cat hairy skin. *J. Comp. Neurol.,* 198: 137 – 154.

McDonald, D.M. and Mitchell, R.A. (1975) The innervation of glomus cells, ganglion cells and blood vessels in the rat carotid body: a quantitative ultrastructural analysis, *J. Neurocytol.,* 4: 177 – 230.

Mearow, K.M. and Diamond, J. (1983) The development of mechanosensory function and synaptic morphology when regenerating axons arrive at nerve-free Merkel cells in Xenopus skin. *Soc. Neurosci. Abstr.,* 9: 228.12.

Merkel, F. (1880) *Über die Endungen der sensiblen Nerven in der Haut der Wirbelthiere.* H. Schmidt, Rostock.

Mills, L.R., Nurse, C.N. and Diamond, J. (1984) Regional differences in the sensory nerve dependence of Merkel cell development in rat skin. *Soc. Neurosci. Abstr.,* 14: 307.15.

Mills, L.R., Mearow, K.M., Diamond, J. and Visheau, B. (1985) Are Merkel cells the mechanosensory transducers in rat touch domes and Xenopus touch spots?. *Soc. Neurosci. Abstr.,* 15: 36.3.

Munger, B.L. (1965) The intraepidermal innervation of the snout skin of oppossum. A light microscopic study with observations on the nature of Merkel's tastzellen. *J. Cell Biol.,* 26: 79 – 97.

Nurse, C.A. and Diamond, J. (1984) A fluorescent microscopic study of the development of rat touch domes and their Merkel cells. *Neuroscience,* 11: 509 – 520.

Nurse, C.N., Mearow, K.M., Holmes, M., Visheau, B. and Diamond, J. (1983) Merkel cell distribution in the epidermis as determined by quinacrine fluorescence. *Cell Tiss. Res.,* 228: 511 – 524.

Parducz, A., Leslie, R., Cooper, E., Turner, C. and Diamond, J. (1977) The Merkel cells and the rapidly adapting mechanoreceptors of the salamander skin. *Neuroscience,* 2: 511 – 521.

Scott, S.A., Cooper, E. and Diamond, J. (1981) Merkel cells as targets of the mechanosensory nerves in salamander skin. *Proc. R. Soc. Lond. B.,* 211: 455 – 470.

Sperry, R.W. and Miner, N. (1949) Formation within sensory nucleus V of synaptic associations mediating cutaneous localization. *J. Comp. Neurol.,* 90: 403 – 424.

Wolpert, L. (1971) Positional information and pattern formation. *Curr. Top. Dev. Biol.,* 6: 183 – 229.

Yasargil, G.M., Macintyre, L., Doucette, R., Visheau, B., Holmes, M. and Diamond, J. (1988) Axonal domains within shared touch domes in the rat: a comparison of their fate during conditions favoring collateral sprouting and following axonal regeneration. *J. Comp. Neurol.,* in press.

W. Hamann and A. Iggo (Eds.)
Progress in Brain Research, Vol. 74
© 1988 Elsevier Science Publishers B.V. (Biomedical Division)

Mechanisms of Transduction I: Summary and discussions

A. Iggo

The meeting, after the opening welcoming address by Professor Choa, Founding Dean of the Faculty of Medicine and pro-Vice-Chancellor, moved to a consideration of the mechanisms of transduction. The first three papers dealt with the mechanisms of hair cells in the cochlea of mammals (Ashmore), birds (Ohmori) and amphibia (Jørgensen), a topic also taken up again by Å. Flock in a later session. This structure is a very well researched example of a mechanoreceptor and the ability to isolate it as a viable single cell has greatly aided analysis of ionic mechanisms by patch clamp methods, that permit not only the examination of the characteristics of single ionic channels, but also, using whole cell patches, to change the internal composition of the cell. The latter technique allowed Ohmori to perfuse the cell with Fura-2 and thereby explore the role of Ca^{2+} in transduction. This powerful tool established that the ionic movement through transduction channels in the apical region of the cell was strongly selective for divalent cations, particularly Ca. Displacement/response relationships, measured using hair bundles of different length, were independent of hair length, but were correlated with angular displacement of the bundle about its insertion. This fact, taken together with localised fluorescence changes to limited mechanical stimulation at the point of hair bundle insertion, is good evidence that the mechano-electric transducer channels are localised to the region of insertion. The question of the subsequent steps in transduction, especially the transfer of excitation from the hair cell to the subjacent afferent nerve terminal, was not addressed by Dr Ohmori, even though he was asked whether his normal point of patch clamp cell attachment at the base of the hair

cell might influence his interpretation. The hair cells, in response to a question from B.H. Pubols, were not acting as frequency encoders but rather as mechanical analysers detecting movement of the basilar membrane, although inner and outer hair cells differ in their ability to follow high frequencies of sound.

Although Ashmore's paper preceded that of Ohmori, his topic dealt with aspects of the hair cell mechanisms that might be seen as consequences of the primary mechano-electric transduction conductance changes reported by Ohmori. In particular, differences in membrane properties between inner and outer hair cells in the guinea pig cochlea exist. Once again isolated hair cells conferred great benefits on examination of the ionic conductances, presumably of the non-transducer channels. Of particular significance were voltage-dependent K currents, which would be active in the normal physiological range of inner hair cells. The latter are connected to the great majority of the cochlea afferent fibres and activation of these channels is presumably involved in the release of the, as yet, unidentified transmitters responsible for onward transfer of sensory activity to the cochlea afferent fibres.

The outer hair cells have K currents that probably require the entry of Ca ions for them to be activated. This Ca could enter through the apical transducer site reported by Ohmori. Of particular interest was the possible mechanical function of the outer hair cells. They receive most, if not all, of the afferent cochlea fibres and it was quite sensational to witness Ashmore's demonstration, using isolated hair cells, of their ability to change shape when they were depolarised at frequencies in the range of both pop and classical music. These electro-mechanical properties of the outer hair cells could, as described by Ashmore, and given their location, strongly influence the tuning properties of the basilar membrane in relation to the inner hair cells in a way that could account for the highly frequency-selective properties of the cochlea afferent fibres.

Hair cell mechanisms were further elaborated using the whole sensory epithelium of the sacculus of the frog by Jørgensen, by examining transepithelial voltages in bathing solutions of different ionic composition. This experimental approach failed to demonstrate any dependence of transepithelial voltage on Ca ion concentration and the independence of the reversal potential for transepithelial current flow in K- and Na-endolymph led Jørgensen to suggest that the transduction channels were non-selective for monovalent cations. There was some difficulty in establishing the concordance of these results with the previous studies using isolated hair cells.

The role of calcium in transduction was further developed in the next papers. The afferent discharge from mammalian cold receptors may occur in temperature-dependent bursts. Schäfer's presentation dealt with the possible kinds of Ca conductances that could underly the Ca currents and conductances that might be responsible for the discharge patterns. Drawing on an analogy with the Ca conductances identified in dorsal root ganglion cells and considering the temporal pattern of cold receptor activity he drew the conclusion that the cold receptors have only the low-voltage activated type of calcium channels. The difficulty of gaining access to the sensory terminals of the cold receptors was clearly a serious impediment to the prospect of testing the hypothesis by direct measurements of the kind used with isolated hair cells. Matthews raised the question whether the analysis depended on the assumption that two processes were involved, to which Schäfer agreed in the sense that there was more than one process — a basic ionic electrogenic pump plus an oscillatory process. By a consideration of the electron micro-scopical studies of cold receptors, it could be suggested that the oscillator exists at one place on the receptor terminal and the generator at a more distal location.

Calcium channel blockers were used by Pacitti and Findlater to explore the role of Ca ions in the SA1 mechanoreceptor. They reported a significant reduction in the responses of such mammalian receptors in the presence of Ca channel blockers, cadmium chloride, cobalt chloride and verapamil. These changes were unrelated to any detectable excitatory change in the afferent axon. The reduction in number of dense-cored vesicles in SA1 Merkel cells in receptors fixed for histological examination at the time of receptor failure indicated a possible link between the release of such granules and transducer function in these sensory receptors. This topic was further explored by Ogawa and Yamashita in frog Ft1 and Ft2 mechanoreceptors. Manganese in low concentrations strongly suppressed the tonic responses of Ft1 units to mechanical stimulation while higher concentrations affected both Ft1 and Ft2 units. Furthermore, ω-conotoxin, a presynaptic Ca channel blocker, irreversibly decreased tonic responses to mechanical stimulation, results leading to the conclusion that Ft1 units have a Ca requiring process at both transducer and transmitter sites.

The studies on mammalian receptors did not include a comparison of the effects of Ca channel blockers on SA2 receptors. Munger questioned the specificity of cobalt and cadmium actions since both agents are toxic. However, at the concentrations used the afferent axons were still conducting normally so that toxic effects could be discounted.

The SA1/SA2 slowly adapting mechanoreceptors were also examined by Baumann, Hamann and Leung to explore their sensitivity to neomycin, a drug known to block transduction in hair cells of the acoustico-lateralis system. Neomycin was more effective against SA1 than SA2 and the greater responsiveness of the SA1 led to the conclusion that there were two target sites in the SA1 compared with the SA2, a result consistent with the view that the Merkel cells have a direct role in mechano-electric transduction. A conclusion not, however, supported by Diamond in a later presentation.

The neomycin concentrations at SA1 and SA2 receptors, because of the locations of the receptors, might have been different, but since it is not protein-bound and various doses and durations of exposure were used this was not considered by Hamann to be a factor. The use of very high doses of neomycin was not tried since they would have been fatal.

In general discussion Paintal commented on the failure so far to identify any chemical transmitter for either hair cells or Merkel cells, to which Flock responded by citing studies on the cochlea indicating that small amino acids such as aspartate, glutamates and purines were current candidates. He also stressed the point that the synapses were extremely fast. For the frog ampulla, Ashmore stated that NMDA-like receptor binding sites existed and that in the retina there may be a nonvesicular release of transmitter.

A second item of general interest from the point of view of the transduction process was the question of how stretch of a membrane (a mechanical event) affects the transduction channel in the membrane. Flock reported that a small angular displacement of the stereocilia by 0.1° leading to a 2 Å stretch of the membrane could affect the permeability of the membrane and that this small movement might be sufficient to affect gating currents and thus alter conductivity of ionic channels. This brought the discussion around to the property of channel proteins which seemed to be setting up questions or themes for the next symposium on sensory transduction.

Mechanisms of Transduction II

W. Hamann and A. Iggo (Eds.)
Progress in Brain Research, Vol. 74
© 1988 Elsevier Science Publishers B.V. (Biomedical Division)

CHAPTER 8

Mechano-electric transduction in the slowly adapting cutaneous afferent units of frogs

H. Ogawa and Y. Yamashita

Department of Physiology, Kumamoto University Medical School, Honjo 2-2-1, Kumamoto 860, Japan

Summary

To elucidate the mechano-electric transduction mechanism of the frog type 1 slowly adapting (SA) units, we examined effects of Ca antagonists on responses of the frog type 1 (Ft1) units to both mechanical and electrical stimulation in the receptive field.

On the basis of receptive properties of the SA units to DC stimulation, we considered that anodal stimulation activated the receptor cells of the Ft1 units and cathodal stimulation the nerve terminals of the Ft2 units.

There was a tendency that manganese at 3 and 10 mM decreases responses of the Ft1 units to mechanical stimulation more heavily than those to electrical stimulation. It was suggested that there is a highly Ca requiring process at the mechano-electric transduction of the Ft1 units.

Concentrated verapamil decreased responses of Ft1 units to both electrical and mechanical stimulation. Because of the high concentration, it was considered that the action of this drug is not due to its specific blockade of the Ca channel.

Synthetic ω-conotoxin GVIa, a Ca channel blocker at the presynaptic region, decreased responses of the Ft1 units to mechanical stimulation. It is suggested that another Ca requiring process may also be involved in synaptic transmission from the receptor cells to nerve terminals in Ft1 units, although this problem remains to be studied in the future.

Introduction

It has been suggested that Ca ions play an important role in mechano-electric transduction of some mechanoreceptors, e.g., frog muscle spindles (Ito et al., 1981), slowly adapting (SA) type 1 mechanoreceptive afferent units of mammals (Cooksey et al., 1984) and vestibular hair cells of chicken (Ohmori, 1984).

In frogs there are two kinds of cutaneous mechanoreceptive SA units: irregularly discharging frog type 1 (Ft1) and regularly discharging frog type 2 (Ft2) units (Ogawa et al., 1984). Since Merkel cells are present in the frog skin (Fox and Whitear, 1978), we assumed that Merkel cells are the receptor cells of the Ft1 units, as in the SA1 units of mammals (Iggo and Muir, 1969). Previously we reported that Ft1 units have highly Ca requiring processes in comparison with Ft2 units (Yamashita et al., 1986). However, we could not locate these Ca requiring processes either for mechano-electric transduction, for synaptic transmission or for both. Recently we found that DC electrical stimulation, applied to the skin in the receptive field (RF), may activate the receptive regions of the cutaneous SA units of frogs (Yamashita and Ogawa, 1986), skipping the mechano-electric transduction process.

The aim of the present study was to clarify the property of mechano-electric transduction process of the Ft1 units by examining the effects of Ca antagonists on their responses to mechanical and electrical stimulation. In this paper, we first describe the response properties of frog SA units to DC stimulation, and then effects of Ca antagonists on the responses of the SA units, especially the Ft1 units.

Methods

American bullfrogs, *Rana catesbeiana,* weighing 200–400 g, were used. Experimental procedures, except the method for electrical stimulation of the receptive field with a long pulse (1 s), were the same as used in the previous studies (Yamashita et al., 1986). After anesthesia with urethane (3 g/kg, i.p.), the animals were placed in a prone position on the table, and the left foot was attached to the wooden plate with surgical plaster. Cutaneous SA units innervating the plantar surface of the left foot were isolated from a small strand of the sciatic nerve at the thigh. Calibrated von Frey hairs and a moving coil transducer (Ling MSE 101 vibrator) were used to apply mechanical stimulation to the receptive field. Glass pipettes (0.45 and 0.25 mm in outer and inner diameter, respectively), filled with physiological saline – agar, were used for stimulating electrodes, and an indifferent Ag – AgCl wire electrode was inserted under the skin near the fifth finger of the left foot. The stimulating electrode was placed on the skin in the receptive field of the SA unit under study, and a small amount of anodal or cathodal current was applied to the unit through this electrode. After the Ft1 and Ft2 units were identified on the basis of patterns of impulse discharges in response to mechanical skin indentation, the left common iliac artery and vein were cannulated in the abdominal cavity to perfuse the left leg. Perfusates were pumped into the arteries by using a peristaltic pump at 40 peristalses/min. Mean flow rates were 3.3 ml/min. The normal Ringer solution used had the following composition: 66 mM NaCl, 2.5 mM KCl, 1.8 mM CaCl$_2$, 10 mM glucose, 5% dextran (MW 70 000; Pharmacia, Uppsala, Sweden), 40 mM sucrose, 15 mM Na lactate, 125 U/ml heparin and 18 mM NaHCO$_3$ (255 mOsm, pH 7.4 when bubbled with

a mixture of 5% CO$_2$ and 95% O$_2$). Manganese was added in the form of chloride salts and the osmolarity was kept constant by decreasing the sucrose content. Other drugs, e.g., verapamil and synthetic ω-conotoxin GVIa (ω-CTX; Peptide Institute, Minoo, Japan), were added without decreasing the sucrose content, because of their small concentration.

Results

Most of the Ft1 units studied innervated the warty skin, and unless otherwise stated, the Ft1 units had RFs on the warty skin. All of the Ft2 units innervated the non-warty skin.

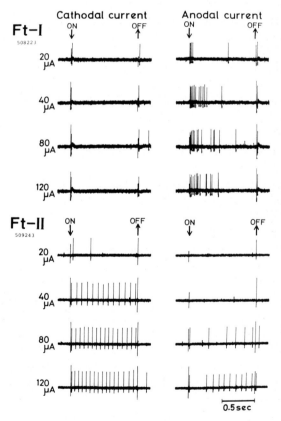

Fig. 1. Responses of two types of SA units (Ft1 and Ft2 units) in frogs to DC stimulation (1 s in duration).

Responses of SA units to DC stimulation of a long duration

When a small current was applied, both the Ft1 and Ft2 units produced single spikes in response to cathodal pulses with a short latency but not to anodal pulses (Fig. 1). The threshold current was $12.4 \pm 8.9 \, \mu A$ (n = 30) in the Ft1 units and $17.6 \pm 11.7 \, \mu A$ (n = 6) in the Ft2 units. However, when a greater intensity ($> 40 \, \mu A$) of current pulses (duration 1 s) was used, Ft1 units gave rise to long-lasting discharges in response to anodal DC stimulation only. On the other hand, Ft2 units produced tonic responses to both anodal and cathodal DC stimulation, but cathodal DC stimulation was more effective. The number of spikes discharged increased and the latency of the first spikes decreased with an increased intensity of DC stimulation. Ft1 units produced irregular discharges after the distinct phasic discharges in response to DC stimulation, and Ft2 units gave rise to regular discharges without a clear burst at the onset (Fig. 1). The response features of these units are quite similar to those seen in response to mechanical stimulation.

RFs for DC stimulation to produce long-lasting discharges were located on those for mechanical stimulation in both types of SA units. After perfusion of the leg for a long period with normal perfusate, rarely cathodal stimulation was found to be effective at the margin of the RF for mechanical stimulation in the Ft1 units, although anodal current was effective at the most sensitive area of the RF.

The present findings indicate that DC stimulation activates the receptive site of these units directly, but not the spike generation site, to produce maintained discharges.

Effects of Ca antagonists on responses of Ft1 units to both mechanical and electrical stimulation

Manganese

A perfusion of the foot with a perfusate contain-

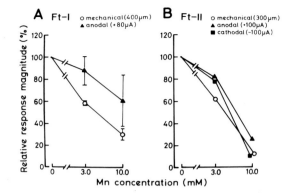

Fig. 2. Effects of manganese ions on responses of two types of SA units in frogs to both mechanical and DC stimulation. (A) Ft1 units (n = 4) in warty skin. Vertical bars represent SEM. (B) Ft2 units (n = 3) in non-warty skin. Open circles, responses to mechanical stimulation (400 μm for Ft1 units and 300 μm for Ft2 units); solid triangles, responses to anodal stimulation (80 μA, 1 s in Ft1 units; 100 μA in Ft2 units); solid squares, responses to cathodal stimulation (100 μA, 1 s). Responses are expressed by the total number of spike discharges during stimulation.

ing Mn decreased responses of Ft1 units to mechanical stimulation more heavily than those to electrical stimulation (Fig. 2A). Manganese decreased responses of Ft1 units to both mechanical and electrical stimulation dose-dependently. Although Mn had a tendency to decrease responses to mechanical stimulation more heavily than those to electrical stimulation, no significant difference was noticed between the two responses in any concentration of Mn ($P > 0.05$, Student's t-test) because of the small number of units tested.

On the other hand, Mn decreased responses of the Ft2 units to mechanical stimulation and both anodal and cathodal stimulation dose-dependently and by almost the same ratios (Fig. 2B).

Latencies of the responses to both types of stimulation were delayed in the presence of Mn, e.g., by about 10 – 15 ms in 10 mM Mn.

Verapamil

Verapamil, 100 μM, depressed both phasic and tonic responses of Ft1 units to mechanical stimulation in three Ft1 units. The average ratio of

66

decrease in responses was about $80-90\%$. In one unit, effects of $10-100$ μM verapamil on responses to both mechanical and electrical stimulation were tested, and 30 μM was the threshold concentration to decrease responses of the Ft1 units (Fig. 3). No differential effects of verapamil on responses to mechanical and electrical stimulation were noticed. No changes in the latency of responses to either type of stimulation were observed in the presence of verapamil.

ω-Conotoxin

To ascertain the possibility that concentrated Mn (10 mM) affected the mechanical responses of Ft1 units through synapses between receptor cells (probably Merkel cells) and nerve terminals as well, we examined the effects of ω-CTX, a Ca channel blocker at the presynaptic region (Kerr and Yoshikami, 1984), on these responses (Fig. 4). ω-CTX (0.2 μM) slowly but irreversibly decreased the tonic response of Ft1 units. This slow and irreversible action was not due to deterioration of the preparation, because Mn reversibly decreased the response of the same preparation, but this is characteristic of the drug used (Enomoto et al., 1986). Latencies of the responses were not affected by this drug.

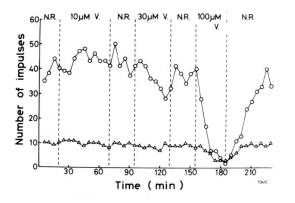

Fig. 3. Effects of various concentrations of verapamil on responses of Ft1 units to mechanical stimulation (300 μm, 3 s). Open circles, tonic responses (150 ms to 3 s after the onset of stimulation); open triangles, phasic responses (0 – 150 ms after the onset of stimulation). N.R. represents a normal Ringer solution, V indicates verapamil.

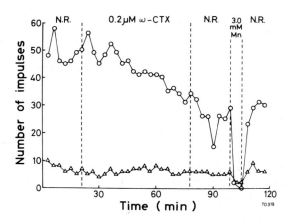

Fig. 4. Effects of ω-conotoxin on responses to Ft1 units to mechanical stimulation (200 μm, 3 s). For symbols, see legend to Fig. 3.

Discussion

Anodal stimulation has been found to produce maintained discharges in mechanoreceptors of toads and frogs (Maruhashi et al., 1952; Loewenstein, 1956), but they did not specify the types of SA units activated. In the present study, we showed that anodal stimulation was effective in Ft1 units and both anodal and cathodal stimulation were effective in Ft2 units in producing maintained discharges. Since many investigators have studied mechanoreceptors in the warty skin of amphibians where only Ft1 units are present, the present finding is partly consistent with those previous results.

On the basis of the receptive properties of both Ft1 and Ft2 units to DC stimulation, we considered that the receptor cells of the Ft1 units and the nerve terminals of the Ft2 units were activated by electrical stimulation to produce maintained discharges. Our conclusion is consistent with previous findings: cathodal DC stimulation is effective to the sensory nerve terminals such as the muscle spindle (Edwards, 1955; Ito, 1970), but anodal DC stimulation is effective to sensory units with receptor cells such as lateral line organs and taste units (Katsuki et al., 1950, Bujas et al., 1979).

Manganese, a Ca antagonist, tended to affect responses of the Ft1 units to mechanical and electrical stimulation differentially. It is suggested that Ca ions are highly required at the mechano-electric transduction process in Ft1 units. In the present study, Mn affected responses of both Ft1 and Ft2 units to mechanical stimulation by the same degree. Since Ft1 units in the present study had RFs on the warty skin, the present finding was rather consistent with the previous finding (Yamashita and Ogawa, 1986).

Another Ca antagonist, verapamil, decreased the responses of the Ft1 units to both types of stimulation dose-dependently. It is reported that, although verapamil acts on the Na channel at almost the same concentration as the drug affects the Ca channel, 10 μM verapamil decreases Ca entry at the skeletal muscle of frogs without affecting NaCl (Hagiwara and Byerly, 1981). Since the threshold concentration of this drug to decrease the responses to mechanical stimulation was rather high (30 μM), the effect of verapamil was probably attributed to a blockade of both Na and Ca channels in the receptor cells as well as spike generation sites of the Ft1 units.

Recently three types of Ca channel were identified: the T-, L- and N-type. The N-type Ca channel is found only in neuronal cells (Nowycky et al., 1985). A presynaptic Ca channel blocker, ω-CTX (Kerr and Yoshikami, 1984), has been found to irreversibly block the N-type channel, but also reversibly blocks other types of Ca channel (Kasai et al., 1987). In the present study, ω-CTX decreased the responses of Ft1 units to mechanical stimulation irreversibly, which suggests the presence of active chemical synapses between the receptor cells and nerve terminals in the Ft1 units. However, because of the limited number of our experiments with this drug, we are not sure that decreased responses of Ft1 units in the presence of ω-CTX were caused by merely a blockade of N-type Ca channels in the presynaptic region of the receptor cells. The problem remains to be studied in the future.

References

Bujas, Z., Frank, M. and Pfaffmann, C. (1979) Neural effects of electrical taste stimuli. *Sens. Proc.*, 3: 353–365.

Cooksey, E.J., Findlater, G.S. and Iggo, A. (1984) The responses to mechanical stimulation of SA I receptors of cats and rats in the presence of calcium antagonists. *J. Physiol. (London)*, 357: 30P.

Edwards, C. (1955) Changes in the discharge from a muscle spindle produced by electrotonus in the sensory nerve. *J. Physiol. (London)*, 127: 636–640.

Enomoto, K., Sano, K., Shibuya, Y. and Maeno, T. (1986) Blockade of transmitter release by a synthetic venom peptide, ω-conotoxin. *Proc. Japan Acad.*, 62: 267–270.

Fox, H. and Whitear, M. (1978) Observations of Merkel cells in amphibians. *Biol. Cell.*, 32: 223–232.

Hagiwara, S. and Byerly, L. (1981) Calcium channel. *Annu. Rev. Neurosci.*, 4: 69–125.

Iggo, A. and Muir, A.R. (1969) The structure and function of a slowly adapting touch corpuscle in hairy skin. *J. Physiol. (London)*, 200: 763–796.

Ito, F. (1970) Effects of polarizing currents on long lasting discharges in the frog muscle spindle. *Jpn. J. Physiol.*, 20: 697–710.

Ito, F., Komatsu, Y. and Katsuta, N. (1981) Effects of calcium blockers on the discharge pattern of muscle spindle. *Brain Res.*, 218: 388–392.

Kasai, H., Aosaki, T. and Fukuda, J. (1987) Presynaptic Ca-antagonist ω-conotoxin irreversibly blocks N-type Ca-channels in chick sensory neurons. *Neurosci. Res.*, 4: 228–235.

Katsuki, Y., Yoshino, S. and Chen, J. (1950) Action currents of the single lateral-line nerve fiber of fish. 2. On the discharge due to stimulation. *Jpn. J. Physiol.*, 1: 179–194.

Kerr, L.M. and Yoshikami, D. (1984) A venom peptide with a novel presynaptic blocking action. *Nature (London)*, 308: 282–284.

Loewenstein, W.R. (1956) Modulation of cutaneous mechanoreceptors by sympathetic stimulation. *J. Physiol. (London)*, 132: 40–60.

Maruhashi, J., Mizuguchi, K. and Tasaki, I. (1952) Action currents in single afferent nerve fibres elicited by stimulation of the skin of the toad and the cat. *J. Physiol. (London)*, 117: 129–151.

Nowycky, M.C., Fox, A.P. and Tsien, R.W. (1985) Three types of neuronal calcium channel with different calcium agonist sensitivity. *Nature (London)*, 316: 440–443.

Ogawa, H., Yamashita, Y., Nomura, T. and Taniguchi, K. (1984) Functional properties of mechanoreceptors in frogs. In: W. Hamann and A. Iggo (Eds.), *Sensory Receptor Mechanisms*, World Scientific Publ., Singapore, pp. 169–178.

Ohmori, H. (1984) Studies of ionic currents in isolated vestibular hair cells of the chick. *J. Physiol. (London),* 350: 561 – 581.

Yamashita, Y. and Ogawa, H. (1986) Responses to electrical stimulation of mechanoreceptor afferent units in the frog skin. *J. Physiol. Soc. Japan,* 48: 313.

Yamashita, Y., Ogawa, H. and Taniguchi, K. (1986) Differential effects of manganese and magnesium on two types of slowly adapting cutaneous mechanoreceptor afferent units in frogs. *Pfluger's Arch.,* 406: 218 – 224.

W. Hamann and A. Iggo (Eds.)
Progress in Brain Research, Vol. 74
© 1988 Elsevier Science Publishers B.V. (Biomedical Division)

CHAPTER 9

The ultrastructure and receptor transduction mechanisms of dentine

B. Matthews and S.H.S. Hughes

Department of Physiology, The Medical School, University of Bristol, Bristol BS8 1TD, UK

Introduction

A discharge of impulses can be recorded from intradental nerves of experimental animals when a variety of different stimuli are applied either to the crown of an intact tooth, to dentine after removing the overlying enamel, or to exposed dental pulp (review: Matthews, 1985). The stimuli which excite these nerves cause pain if applied in a similar manner in man. Of particular interest is the fact that responses can be evoked in nerves in a cat canine tooth by gently touching the outer dentine at the tip of the tooth using a fire-polished glass probe (diameter 0.5 mm) or a von Frey hair (diameter 10 – 100 μm, bending force 10 – 100 mg), provided that the dentinal tubules are not obstructed. The exposed dentine surface may be 1.5 mm or more above the pulp cornu. Nerves appear to penetrate approximately 100 μm into the dentinal tubules in this region (Holland et al., 1987), therefore the contents of the outer parts of the tubules must be involved in the transduction mechanism of the receptors. The present experiments were carried out to investigate the contents of the tubules which lead from the pulp cornu to the tip of this tooth. Holland (1976b) and Holland et al. (1987) examined the tubules alongside the pulp cornu but not those directly above it.

We have also investigated the effects of different methods of fixation since there are always uncertainties about whether the lack of cellular material

in outer dentine might be due to inadequate preservation. Recent experience has emphasised that the tubule contents are not fixed rapidly after vascular perfusion, and that sufficient time must be allowed for diffusion of fixative into the tubules. In experiments designed to detect horse-radish peroxidase (HRP) transported to the teeth in nerves, we perfused the animals in the normal way then washed out the fixative after half an hour to preserve the HRP. The pulps were well fixed, including the cornua, but not the contents of the dentinal tubules.

Methods

Specimens were taken from the tips of the cusps of the upper and lower permanent canine teeth of young adult cats (age: 8 – 12 months). The cats were anaesthetised with sodium pentobarbital (induction: 42 mg/kg i.p., maintenance: 2 mg/kg i.v. as required). The samples were removed after either vascular perfusion of the head of the animal with fixative, or without prior fixation.

Animals were perfused through the common carotid arteries with 5% glutaraldehyde in 0.1 mol/l phosphate buffer for 20 – 30 min using the method described by Holland et al. (1987), except that no dextran was added to the perfusates. The slices and core samples taken from the teeth of these animals were immersed overnight in the same fixative. All the slices and core samples that were removed without prior fixation were immersed overnight in a solution of 5% glutaraldehyde and 4% paraformaldehyde in 0.1 M phosphate buffer (Karnovsky, 1965).

The samples were removed in one of two ways. With the first technique, two transverse slices approximately 0.8 mm thick were cut from the tip of each tooth using a fine diamond disc (Komet, type 943) in a conventional dental handpiece. The disc was cooled and lubricated with a stream of Ringer solution. The movement of the handpiece was controlled accurately by attaching it to a sturdy micromanipulator with Vernier scales, which was fixed to a heavy metal base. The skull of the cat was also fixed to the same base and the mandible fixed to the maxilla (Horiuchi and Matthews, 1974). The diamond disc was lined up initially at right angles to the long axis of the crown and with one face just in contact with the tip of the tooth. Three transverse cuts were then made after advancing the disc along the long axis of the crown to 0.5, 1.5 and 2.5 mm from this initial position. The thickness of the disc is 0.1 mm and each cut removed approximately 0.2 mm of tissue, giving three slices of 0.8 mm thickness. The slice which included the tip of the tooth was discarded. The enamel was approximately 0.2 mm thick over the tip of the tooth and the dentine about 2.0 mm (slightly more in the upper canine than the lower). Thus the slice which extended from 1.5 to 2.3 mm from the tooth tip contained the pulp cornu.

With the second technique, a core sample was taken from the tooth using a diamond-coated tube drill. The drill (ID approx. 1.0 mm; A.D. Burs Ltd., Gloucester, England) was mounted in a surgical handpiece (Kavo, no. 6) which enabled a stream of Ringer to be passed through the bore of the drill. A special chuck was made to fit the tube drill to the handpiece. Without the internal cooling, relying only on an external flow of Ringer, the tube drill caused overheating of the sample. The handpiece was attached to a micromanipulator, as above. The drill was centred on the long axis of the crown of the tooth and advanced slowly to 2.5 mm below the tooth tip. The disc described above was then used to make transverse cuts at 0.5 and 2.5 mm from the tip, to give a cylindrical sample 1 mm diameter and 1.8 mm long which included the pulp cornu.

Immediately after being removed, all slices and core samples were immersed in 5% citric acid for 30 s, to ensure that the ends of the dentinal tubules were patent. They were then washed in Ringer and immersed in fixative overnight.

The samples were decalcified in 0.1 mol/l EDTA and 4% glutaraldehyde (Baird et al., 1967) at room temperature on a rotor. Each slice or core sample was placed in approximately 5 ml of decalcifying solution which was changed every 1 − 3 days. The progress of decalcification was monitored by determining the calcium content of these solutions by atomic absorption spectroscopy. Decalcification was stopped when the calcium content reached a stable, minimal value of around 5 ppm. This took 10 − 14 days.

After decalcification, the samples were washed, osmicated, and dehydrated in ethanol, then embedded in Araldite or Epon. Blocks were orientated and trimmed so that ultra-thin and 1 μm, semi-thin sections could be cut at right angles to the long axis of the tooth crown. For each tooth, sectioning began at the pulpal surface of either the second slice or the core sample, and progressed outwards towards the tip of the crown. The distance of each section from the pulp cornu (i.e., where pre-dentine first appeared in the centre of the block) was determined from measurements of the block which were made with a micrometer gauge. Ultra-thin sections were stained with lead acetate and uranyl acetate, and examined in a Philips 300 electron microscope. Semi-thin sections were stained with methylene blue for light microscopy.

Results

Electron microscopy

In sections taken from the slice samples, the ultrastructure of the contents of the dentinal tubules was essentially the same irrespective of whether the animals had been perfused or not. Damage caused by slicing the teeth was confined to the surface of each block. The odontoblast cell bodies were not separated from the pre-dentine and there was no evidence of odontoblast nuclei being displaced into the tubules. Similar results have been obtained with the core samples although so far the dentine in these blocks has only been examined up to 0.5 mm from the pulp cornu.

All the samples were fully decalcified and we have found that measuring the calcium content of decalcifying solutions by atomic absorption spectroscopy is a much more precise and reliable method of determining the end-point of decalcification than radiography, particularly with small samples.

Evidence on the changes which occur in the contents of the dentinal tubules with distance from the pulp was obtained from slice specimens in two ways: by examining tubule profiles along a radius of a single transverse section through a region close to the pulp cornu, and also the profiles in the centre of each of a sequence of sections from over the cornu. With the first method, the tubules would have been sectioned at different (although unknown) distances from the pulp, but at similar diffusional distances from the surface of the block. They therefore would have had a similar exposure to fixative. With the second method, the distance from the section to the pulp surface was known, and since the tubules in this region run an almost straight course from the pulp towards the tip of the crown, the approximate distance along the tubule was also known. The same group of tubules would also have been examined at each level, but the diffusional distances from the surface of the block to the points of section of each tubule would not have been the same. Nevertheless, we found the same sequence of changes in structure of the tubule contents with increasing distance from the pulp in both sets of data, indicating that all the material was equally well fixed and that poor fixation was not responsible for the structures seen.

The thickness of the pre-dentine over the pulp cornu was approximately 10 μm. Examples of the tubules at five points along the radius of a section at the level of the predentine over the cornu are shown in Fig. 1.

The small processes in the dentinal tubules (Fig. 1, top), which were identified as nerves by Holland et al. (1987), were present up to 100 μm above the pulp cornu. Close to 100% of tubules contained nerves in this region.

Odontoblast processes extended 200 – 300 μm into the tubules above the pulp cornu. Beyond the ends of the odontoblast processes, from 300 to 500 μm, the tubules appeared empty (Fig. 1). Throughout the remainder of their length (a distance of approx. 1.5 mm), they were filled with an almost structureless, electron-dense material which was not surrounded by a cell membrane (Fig. 1, bottom). This material was much more electron-dense than plasma in pulpal vessels of samples that had not been perfused. In some tubules it appeared to contain fibres cut in cross-section.

As has been shown previously, the tubules decreased in diameter as they passed out from the pulp towards the enamel (Fig. 1). In the predentine, their mean diameter was approximately 2 μm and in the outer dentine, where they were filled with the electron-dense material, they ranged from having a diameter of 1 μm to being almost totally occluded. The reduction in diameter could only partly be accounted for by the formation of peritubular dentine. An electron-dense layer, called the limiting membrane by Thomas (1979), was present throughout the calcified dentine. Apart from immediately adjacent to the predentine, it formed the inner border of the peritubular dentine and therefore appeared to line the lumen of each tubule. It was more electron-dense than the material in the outer ends of the tubules.

The peritubular dentine, being highly calcified and containing little organic matrix, is almost totally lost in decalcified material. It was represented by an almost structureless space containing variable amounts of a radially arranged matrix. It lined the tubules within the matrix of the inter-

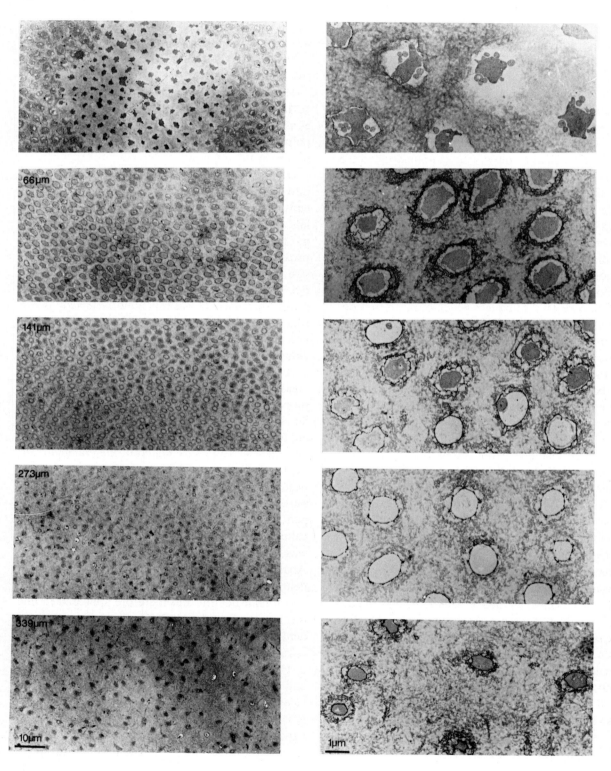

tubular dentine and was present throughout the calcified dentine, surrounding the odontoblast processes and also the empty spaces and electron-dense material beyond the ends of the processes (Fig. 1). The thickness of the peritubular dentine tended to be less where the lumen was empty than where it was filled with electron-dense material. In the calcified dentine adjacent to the pre-dentine, the space between the limiting membrane and the cell membrane of the odontoblast process also contained radially arranged filaments which appeared to be the organic matrix produced as a first stage in the formation of the peritubular dentine. Where the limiting membrane lined the peritubular dentine it had a scalloped outline, as if tethered out by the radial filaments. In many regions, there was an annulus of intertubular dentine around the peritubular dentine in which the randomly arranged matrix stained more densely than in the rest of the intertubular dentine (Fig. 1). The outer diameters of both this annulus and the peritubular dentine became smaller as the diameter of the lumen of the tubule decreased in the outer dentine. Also, in the outer dentine, both diameters tended to be smaller than those of the tubules in the calcified dentine adjacent to the pre-dentine. Thus, if either of these interfaces represents the outline of the tubule when it was first formed, it follows that the tubule increased in diameter as more primary dentine was laid down.

Light microscopy

Some of the nerves in the pre-dentine and inner calcified dentine could be seen in semi-thin sections in the light microscope, although they were at the limit of its resolution. They were stained more deeply by methylene blue than the odontoblast processes. The odontoblast processes were easily resolved. The tubules beyond the end of the odontoblast processes, where they appeared empty in the electron microscope, were unstained and the electron-dense material in the remainder of each tubule was stained by methylene blue.

Discussion

Since the same sequence of changes in structure of the tubule contents with increasing distance from the pulp was found irrespective of the method of fixation and the distance over which the fixative had to diffuse, it seems safe to conclude that the results are not due to delayed or inadequate fixation. Holland (1976a) used several other methods and also concluded that the lack of cellular material in the outer dentine was not due to poor fixation.

We have confirmed that only the innermost 100 μm of cat dentine above the pulp cornu is innervated, and that in this region almost all the tubules contain nerve endings (Holland et al., 1987). The odontoblast processes extended only 200 – 300 μm into these tubules. This is substantially less than Holland (1976b) found. He examined dentine from cat canine teeth, although not directly above the pulp cornu. He estimated that the processes were about one-third of the length of the dentinal tubules in the mid-crown region, but because of the curvature of the tubules in this region he would have been unable to measure their lengths directly. In dentine from the crowns of human teeth, Thomas (1979), Thomas and Payne (1984) and Thomas and Carella (1984) showed that the odontoblast processes extended no further than the inner one-third of the dentine, and in a scanning electron microscope study of fractured specimens, Brann-

Fig. 1. Electron micrographs from five areas at different distances from the centre of a transverse section of dentine from the canine tooth of a cat. The section was taken through the pre-dentine over the cornu of the pulp. The micrographs on the left are all at the same magnification and, from above down, were centred at the following distances from the mid-axis of the tooth: 0, 66, 141, 273, and 339 μm. The total radius of the dentine in this plane is approximately 750 μm. The micrographs on the right are at 8 times higher magnification and show details of regions from the corresponding micrographs on the left, the upper one being at the pre-dentine/dentine junction.

strom and Garberoglio (1972) estimated that the processes were no longer than $400-700$ μm. It is claimed that some studies on freeze-fractured specimens have demonstrated odontoblast processes in outer as well as inner dentine, although they were inexplicably absent in the central part of the tubules (Kelley et al., 1981; Grossman and Austin, 1983). It seems likely that the material in outer dentine was the same as the electron-dense core which we found. Thomas and Carella (1984) have suggested that it was the limiting membrane, but this extends throughout the calcified dentine.

The outer three-fourths of the length of the tubules was filled with an electron-dense material which also stained with methylene blue. Little attention has been paid to this material in the past, although it has been noted that the outer ends of the tubules contained a finely granular or hyaline material (Tsatas and Frank, 1972; Holland, 1975, 1985; Thomas, 1979). Our data confirm that this electron-dense material is not simply the remains of poorly fixed odontoblast processes. The nature of the material is unknown but it seems unlikely that it has the same composition as extracellular fluid elsewhere in the body. Its staining properties suggest that it may contain large amounts of protein or polysaccharide. In some tubules it appeared to have a fibrous structure, similar to the collagen described by Frank and Voegel (1980) in tubules under caries. Collagen has also been described in the outer ends of tubules in normal dentine (Thomas, 1979). The region of the tubule which appeared empty, between the end of the odontoblast process and the electron-dense material, presumably contains extracellular material of different composition. Holland (1985) has noted the presence of this intermediate region in which the tubules appeared empty.

The radially arranged matrix of the peritubular dentine is similar to that described by Takuma (1967) and Thomas and Carella (1984) in human dentine.

A very different account of the contents of the tubules of outer dentine has been given by LaFleche et al. (1985). They examined by transmission electron microscopy sections from teeth that had been frozen in liquid nitrogen immediately after extraction. They claim to have identified odontoblast processes and nerves in this region. They suggest that these structures retract towards the pulp when the dentine is exposed or fixed without prior freezing. Tubulin has been demonstrated immunocytochemically in the outer dentine of rat and human molars (Sigal et al., 1984a, b) and this also suggests that the odontoblast processes extend to the ends of the tubules. Resolution of these apparent conflicts must await further experimentation.

We suggest that the tubules in outer dentine contain extracellular material in the form of a viscous fluid or gel (rather than a non-viscous fluid or solid). This is consistent with other observations on the physical and chemical properties of the tubule contents. Human dentine, including outer dentine, is permeable to dyes such as Evans blue (Anderson and Ronning, 1962). Also, fluid can be sucked out of the tubules of human dentine by subjecting them to reduced pressure, particularly close to the enamel (Stevenson, 1965). Samples of fluid extracted by centrifugation from porcine dentine were shown to contain protein (1.1 g/100 ml), glycoprotein and polysaccharides (Paunio and Nanto, 1965), and those from human dentine contained Na, K and Cl ions in concentrations similar to extracellular fluid and co-coagulated readily on exposure to air (Coffey et al., 1970). It has also been shown that stimuli which cause pain in man can cause movement of fluid through dentine (Brannstrom, 1968; Horiuchi and Matthews, 1973). Warshawsky and Josephsen (1981) showed that labelled fucose, a constituent of glycoprotein, was present in even the outer ends of the dentinal tubules of rat incisors $1-4$ days after injection, indicating that there is a constant turn-over of the tubule contents. It is not known, however, how far the odontoblast processes extend into these tubules.

When a mechanical stimulus is applied to exposed outer dentine and evokes a discharge of nerve impulses, the material within the tubules must provide the link between the stimulus and the receptors. The receptors are assumed to be either the nerve endings at the pulpal ends of the tubules or others in the pulp. From histological evidence and studies on pain in human subjects, Brannstrom (1963) concluded that the receptors were excited by displacement of the contents of the dentinal tubules. Although it is clear that the tubule contents can be displaced under certain conditions, it seems unlikely that some of the less intense stimuli which will evoke pain in man or nerve impulses in experimental animals have this effect (Matthews, 1985), particularly if the tubules contain a viscous fluid or gel throughout most of their length. It seems more likely that the effective stimulus transmitted through the tubules is a pressure change, rather than bulk flow of their contents. Such as mechanism could generate nerve impulses by acting on pressure-sensitive ion channels in the receptor membrane. The nerve endings in the tubules would be in the best position for this. Both the odontoblast processes and the surrounding extracellular fluid would transmit pressure changes through the inner dentine without necessarily moving within the tubules. Other forms of stimulus, including thermal, could also produce pressure changes within the tubules and activate the receptors similarly. The material which we found in the tubules in the outer dentine could also act as a form of semi-permeable membrane across which osmotic stimuli have their effect. Some interesting parallels exist in these respects between the properties of the ampullae of Lorenzini of elasmobranchs and certain other fish (Murray, 1960, 1974) and the dentinal tubules of mammals.

References

Anderson, D.J. and Ronning, G.A. (1962) Dye diffusion in human dentine. *Arch. Oral Biol.,* 7: 505–512.

Baird, I.L., Winborn, W.B. and Bockman, D.E. (1967) A technique of decalcification suited to electron microscopy of tissues closely associated with bone. *Anat. Rec.,* 159: 281–290.

Brannstrom, M. (1963) A hydrodynamic mechanism in the transmission of pain-producing stimuli through the dentine. In: D.J. Anderson (Ed.), *Sensory Mechanisms in Dentine,* Pergamon, Oxford, pp. 73–79.

Brannstrom, M. (1968) Physio-pathological aspects of dentinal and pulpal response to irritants. In: N.B.B. Symons (Ed.), *Dentine and Pulp: Their Structure and Reactions,* Livingstone, Edinburgh, pp. 231–246.

Brannstrom, M. and Garberoglio, R. (1972) The dentinal tubules and the odontoblast process: a scanning electron microscope study. *Acta Odont. Scand.,* 30: 291–311.

Coffey, C.T., Ingram, M.J. and Bjorndal, A.M. (1970) Analysis of human dentinal fluid. *Oral Surg. Oral Med. Oral Path.,* 30: 835–837.

Frank, R.M. and Voegel, J.C. (1980) Ultrastructure of the human odontoblast process and its mineralisation during dental caries. *Caries Res.,* 14: 367–380.

Grossman, E.S. and Austin, J.C. (1983) Scanning electron microscope observations on the tubule content of freeze-fractured, peripheral, vervet monkey dentine (*Cercopithecus pygerythrus*). *Arch. Oral Biol.,* 28: 279–282.

Holland, G.R. (1975) The dentinal tubule and odontoblast process in the cat. *J. Anat.,* 120: 169–177.

Holland, G.R. (1976a) The extent of the odontoblast process in the cat. *J. Anat.,* 121: 133–149.

Holland, G.R. (1976b) An ultrastructural survey of cat dentinal tubules. *J. Anat.,* 122: 1–13.

Holland, G.R. (1985) The odontoblast process: form and function. *J. Dent. Res.,* 64: Spec. Iss. 499–514.

Holland, G.R., Matthews, B. and Robinson, P.P. (1987) An electrophysiological and morphological study of the innervation and reinnervation of cat dentine. *J. Physiol. (London),* 386: 31–43.

Horiuchi, H. and Matthews, B. (1973) In-vitro observations on fluid flow through human dentine caused by pain-producing stimuli. *Arch. Oral Biol.,* 18: 275–294.

Horiuchi, H. and Matthews, B. (1974) Evidence on the origin of impulses recorded from dentine in the cat. *J. Physiol. (London),* 243: 797–829.

Karnovsky, J.J. (1965) A formaldehyde-glutaraldehyde fixative of high osmolarity for use in electron microscopy. *J. Cell Biol.,* 27: 137–138.

Kelley, K.W., Bergenholtz, G. and Cox, C.F. (1981) The extent of the odontoblast process in Rhesus monkeys (*Macaca mulatta*) as observed by scanning electron microscopy. *Arch. Oral Biol.,* 26: 893–897.

LaFleche, R.G., Frank, R.M. and Steuer, P. (1985) The extent of the human odontoblast process as determined by transmission electron microscopy: the hypothesis of a retractable suspensor system. *J. Biol. Bucc.,* 13: 293–305.

Matthews, B. (1985) Peripheral and central aspects of trigeminal nociceptive systems. *Phil. Trans. R. Soc. London,* B 308: 313–324.

Murray, R.W. (1960) The response of the ampullae of Lorenzini of elasmobranchs to mechanical stimulation. *J. Exp. Biol.,* 37: 417–424.

Murray, R.W. (1974) The ampullae of Lorenzini. In: A. Fessard (Ed.), *Electroreceptors and Other Specialized Receptors in Lower Vertebrates, Handbook of Sensory Physiology, Vol. III/3,* Springer-Verlag, Berlin, pp. 123 – 146.

Paunio, K. and Nanto, V. (1965) Studies on the isolation and composition of interstitial fluid in swine dentine. *Acta Odont. Scand.,* 23: 411 – 421.

Sigal, M.J., Aubin, J.E., Ten Cate, A.R. and Pitaru, S. (1984a) The odontoblast process extends to the dentinoenamel junction: an immunocytochemical study of rat dentine. *J. Histochem. Cytochem.,* 32: 872 – 877.

Sigal, M.J., Pitari, S., Aubin, J.E. and Ten Cate, A.R. (1984b) A combined scanning electron microscopy and immunofluorescence study demonstrating that the odontoblast process extends to the dentino-enamel junction in human teeth. *Anat. Rec.,* 210: 453 – 462.

Stevenson, T.S. (1965) Fluid movement in human dentine. *Arch. Oral Biol.,* 10: 935 – 944.

Takuma, S. (1967) Ultrastructure of dentinogenesis. In: A.E.W. Miles (Ed.), *Structural and Chemical Organisation of Teeth, Vol. I,* Academic Press, London, pp. 325 – 370.

Thomas, H.F. (1979) The extent of the odontoblast process in human dentin. *J. Dent. Res.,* 58: 2207 – 2218.

Thomas, H.F. and Carella, P. (1984) Correlation of scanning and transmission electron microscopy of human dentinal tubules. *Arch. Oral Biol.,* 29: 641 – 646.

Thomas, H.F. and Payne, R.C. (1984) The ultrastructure of dentinal tubules from erupted human premolar teeth. *J. Dent. Res.,* 62: 532 – 536.

Tsatas, B.G. and Frank, R.M. (1972) Ultrastructure of dentinal tubules near the dentino-enamel junction. *Calc. Tiss. Res.,* 9: 238 – 242.

Warshawsky, H. and Josephsen, K. (1981) The behavior of substances labelled with ^{3}H-proline and ^{3}H-fucose in the cellular processes of odontoblasts and ameloblasts. *Anat. Rec.,* 200: 1 – 10.

W. Hamann and A. Iggo (Eds.)
Progress in Brain Research, Vol. 74
© 1988 Elsevier Science Publishers B.V. (Biomedical Division)

CHAPTER 10

Electrophysiological analysis of chemosensitive neurons within the area postrema of the rat

Akira Adachi and Motoi Kobashi

Department of Physiology, Okayama University Dental School, Shikata-cho, Okayama 700, Japan

Summary

The area postrema (AP) has proved to be a chemo-receptive trigger zone for the emetic response. Evidence indicating other functions of the AP especially in the rat has grown in abundance recently. The present study is an attempt to demonstrate chemosensitive neurons within the AP electrophysiologically. Two different techniques were employed for chemical stimulation of the AP neurons: (1) the floor of the exposed fourth ventricle was superfused with isotonic glucose solution, hypertonic or hypotonic Ringer solution, or LiCl Ringer solution; (2) these solutions were injected into the left carotid artery. To confirm vagal afferent influences on given AP neurons, single shock electrical stimulation was delivered to the cervical vagal trunks of both sides. Three types of chemosensitive neurons were identified: (1) glucose responsive neurons that may participate in the control of satiety, (2) sodium (osmotic pressure) responsive neurons that may contribute to salt preference or control of water balance, and (3) LiCl responsive neurons that may play a role in conditioned taste aversion. Some of these chemosensitive neurons were influenced by the vagal afferent inputs, suggesting a close relationship between chemoreceptor mechanisms of the AP and visceral afferents.

Introduction

In general the function of the area postrema (AP) has been elucidated as being a chemoreceptive trigger zone for the emetic response (Borison and Wang, 1953). Evidence that indicates other functions of this structure is gradually accumulating (Borison, 1974). Lesions destroying the AP cause changes in salt intake without deficits in gustatory function in the rat (Contreras and Stetson, 1981). Ablation of the AP causes exaggerated consumption of preferred foods in the rat (Edwards and Ritter, 1981). Based on these facts, the authors postulated chemoreceptor functions of the AP not only for the emetic response, but for ingestive behavior that could be important for homeostatic control. Our preliminary study has revealed the existence of glucose responsive neurons as well as sodium responsive ones within the AP in the rat (Adachi and Kobashi, 1985). Glucose responsive neurons induced a marked decrease in the discharge rate in response to topical application of glucose by means of microelectro-osmotic techniques. Two different types of sodium responsive neurons were also identified by means of topical iontophoretic application of sodium ions. The purpose of the present study is to extend our previous observation in order to confirm further the glucose as well as sodium responsive neurons within the

AP by use of different techniques for chemical stimulation of the AP. In addition, the AP plays a critical role in the formation of conditioned taste aversions by lithium chloride (Ritter et al., 1980). In this study, effects of chemical stimulation by LiCl on AP neurons were also examined to elucidate LiCl responsive neurons besides the glucose or sodium responsive ones.

Methods

A total of 49 male Sprague – Dawley rats (Charles River of Japan), weighing 300 – 400 g were used as subjects. Under urethane – chloralose anesthesia (urethane 0.8 g/kg, chloralose 65 mg/kg, i.p.), a catheter was inserted into the left carotid artery toward the heart as shown in Fig. 1B, in order to apply chemical stimuli to the AP through the blood vessel. The right carotid artery was ligated. To examine vagal afferent invasion in the AP, implanted stimulating electrodes were fixed on the cervical vagal trunks of both sides. In one case the celiac branch of the vagus was stimulated. Then the animals were mounted on a stereotaxic apparatus. To place the medulla oblongata in a horizontal position, the incisors were fixed 25 mm below the level of the auditory meatus. The occipital bone was removed with a dental drill, and the caudal part of the medulla was exposed. In this way, the surface of the AP was completely exposed without removing the cerebellum by suction. As illustrated in Fig. 1A, the surface of the AP was superfused with standard Ringer solution (Na 147 mEq, K 4 mEq, Ca 4.5 mEq, Cl 155.5 mEq). A glass pipette electrode filled with 0.5 M sodium acetate and 2% pontamine sky blue was used for recording unitary discharges. Under inspection through a dissecting microscope, the recording electrode was introduced into the AP by means of a micromanipulator until unit discharges were observed. Then single shock electrical stimulation was delivered to the cervical vagal trunks in order to confirm a vagal afferent supply to the AP. After this examination, superfusion with Ringer solution was switched to isotonic glucose solution (300

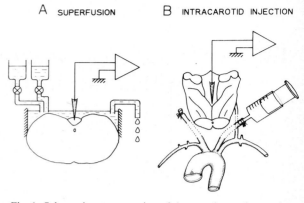

Fig. 1. Schematic representation of the experimental procedure. Two different techniques employed for chemical stimulation of the AP neurons are illustrated.

mM), hypertonic, hypotonic Ringer solution or LiCl (147 mM) containing Ringer solution respectively. Hypertonicity was achieved by the addition of 147 mM NaCl to the standard Ringer solution. Hypotonicity was achieved by decreasing the NaCl concentration by 74 mM in the standard Ringer solution. These test solutions were also applied through the carotid catheter to elucidate responses of the AP neurons to the chemical stimuli supplied through the fenestrated blood vessel. All records were stored on magnetic tape for later analysis. The number of impulses in each 5 s was plotted by means of a pulse-rate meter. Recording sites were marked by iontophoretic dye injection and examined afterward histologically.

Results

It is noticed that spontaneous discharges have been rarely observed within the AP in previous studies, due presumably to a sparse neuronal distribution in this structure. Therefore, responses have been infrequently obtained even when exploring within the AP by means of the microelectrode technique.

Figs. 2 and 3 show two different types of AP neurons in response to glucose. When superfusion of the exposed surface of the fourth ventricle with standard Ringer solution was switched to isotonic glucose solution (indicated by G), a marked decrease in discharge rate is seen (Fig. 2A$_a$). The decreased neuronal activity gradually returned to the control discharge rate when glucose solution was changed back to the Ringer solution. This response is characterized by a negative correlation between the discharge rate and glucose concentration. The superfusion of hypertonic Ringer solution containing 294 mM NaCl (indicated by S) induced no response in this neuron. Fig. 2A$_b$ shows responses of this glucose responsive neuron to single shock electrical stimulation (intensity 3 V, duration 3 ms) of the celiac branch of the vagus. The latency from the onset of single shock electrical stimulation until the unit discharge was evoked was approximately 160 ms. Because preceding spontaneous discharges did not cancel the evoked discharges by collision (see the second and third traces from the top), this neuron was activated by afferent invasion via the celiac branch of the vagus. It implies that some neurons within the AP are responsive to changes in glucose concentration of the cerebrospinal fluid (CSF) and also receive afferent signals from the abdominal organs. Fig. 2B$_a$ presents a response of this type of

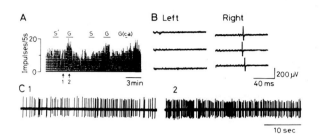

Fig. 3. (A) Effect of the superfusion with isotonic glucose solution (G), hypertonic (S) or hypotonic (S′) Ringer solution. Only glucose elicits marked increases in discharge rate. The intracarotid infusion of glucose indicated by G(ca) induces the same response. (B) Evoked response to single shock electrical stimulation of the right cervical vagal trunk. (C) Oscillograph records of unit discharges: (1) spontaneous discharges recorded from the time indicated by arrow 1 in A; (2) discharges responding to glucose recorded from the time indicated by arrow 2 in A. Note a marked difference in the discharge rate between C1 and C2.

glucose responsive neuron to the intracarotid infusion of isotonic glucose solution. This neuron rapidly responded to the glucose infusion (indicated by G), displaying a marked decrease in discharge rate followed by a return to the control discharge rate after cessation of the infusion. The same infusion with hypertonic Ringer solution (indicated by S) did not elicit any change in discharge rate. The response to the glucose infusion is similar to that of the superfusion with glucose solution. This unit did not respond to single shock electrical stimulation delivered to the celiac branch of the vagus as shown in Fig. 2B$_b$.

Opposite responses to glucose were observed in the other AP neuron. As presented in Fig. 3A, superfusion with glucose (indicated by G) markedly increased the discharge rate. Intracarotid infusion of the same solution also produced an increase in discharge rate as indicated by G(ca). However, no responses were observed when the superfusion with Ringer solution was switched to that with either hyper- or hypotonic Ringer solution (indicated by S and S′ respectively). This neuron responded to single shock electrical stimulation of the right cervical vagal trunk (same intensity and duration as in Fig. 2) but not to that of the left one

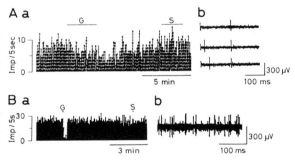

Fig. 2. Responses of two different glucose responsive AP neurons. Superfusion of the fourth ventricle with isotonic glucose solution (G) induced a marked decrease in discharge rate of an AP neuron (A$_a$). Note that hypertonic Ringer solution (S) is ineffective. (A$_b$) Responses to single shock electrical stimulation of the celiac branch of the vagus. Each oscillograph sweep is triggered by a stimulus pulse. Evoked unit discharge is seen in each trace. (B$_a$) Effect of intracarotid infusion of glucose on the other AP neuron. Note clear suppression by glucose (G) and no response to hypertonic Ringer solution (S). (B$_b$) Oscillograph record of discharges. Ten sweeps were superimposed. This neuron elicits no response to electrical stimulation of the celiac branch of the vagus.

as shown in Fig. 3B. Oscillographic records of the discharges are illustrated in Fig. $3C_1$ and C_2. Comparison of C_1 with C_2 also clearly indicates the increase in discharge rate in response to the superfusion with glucose.

Typical responses to hyper- and hypotonicity of

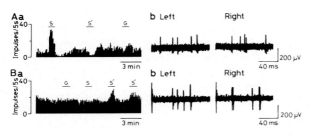

Fig. 4. (A_a) Response to the superfusion with hypertonic Ringer solution (S). Note a marked increase in discharge rate during a horizontal bar indicated by S followed by a decrease in discharge rate (after-effect). Hypotonic Ringer solution (S′) causes a decrease in discharge rate but glucose (G) does not. (A_b) Responses to electrical stimulation of the left and right vagus. Ten sweeps were superimposed. No response is elicited. (B_a) Response to the superfusion with hypotonic Ringer solution (S′). No response to superfusion with isotonic glucose (G) or hypertonic Ringer solution (S) is elicited. (B_b) The same oscillograph records as in A_b. No response is elicited.

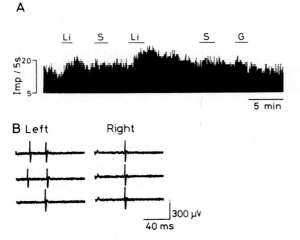

Fig. 5. (A) Response of an AP neuron to the superfusion with LiCl containing Ringer solution (Li). Note the lack of response to equiosmotic hypertonic Ringer solution (S). Glucose is also ineffective. (B) Oscillograph records of discharges elicited by electrical stimulation of the vagus of both sides.

some AP neurons are presented in Fig. 4A and B. When the superfusion with standard Ringer solution was switched to that with hypertonic Ringer solution (indicated by S), a marked increase in discharge rate was observed (Fig. $4A_a$). Immediately after switching back to standard Ringer solution, a suppression of neural response was recognized. This neuron shows an opposite response to hypotonic Ringer solution (indicated by S′), so a marked decrease in discharge rate is seen during a horizontal bar indicated by S′. No response is elicited by switching the superfusion to isotonic glucose solution (indicated by G). Single shock electrical stimulation of the cervical vagal trunk of both sides elicited no response in this neuron as shown in Fig. $4A_b$. Fig. $4B_a$ presents a response of the other AP neuron to hypotonicity. This neuron responded only to the hypotonic superfusion (indicated by S′) with a marked increase in discharge rate. Both isotonic glucose solution (G) and hypertonic Ringer solution (S) were ineffective. The same electrical stimulation of the vagus elicited no response as shown in Fig. $4B_b$. These neurons were not supplied by the vagal afferent inputs.

A specimen record from a lithium chloride responsive neuron within the AP is shown in Fig. 5. When the superfusion with standard Ringer solution was switched to that with LiCl containing Ringer solution (indicated by Li), an increase in discharge rate was observed. However, hypertonic Ringer solution that was equiosmotic to LiCl Ringer solution elicited no response (Fig. 5A). It indicates that the LiCl responsive neuron is insensitive to osmotic pressure as well as glucose. This neuron responded to electrical stimulation of the cervical vagal trunks of both sides. Fig. 5B presents evoked discharges by electrical stimulation of the left and right vagus (same intensity and duration as in Fig. 2). Latencies are approximately 46 ms.

A total of 46 neurons within the area postrema were examined. Among them, 25 neurons responded to electrical stimulation of the cervical vagal trunk. Four neurons decreased and one neuron increased the discharge rates in response to glucose.

Two neurons increased and two other neurons decreased the discharge rates in response to hypertonic Ringer solution. One neuron increased and one neuron decreased in response to hypotonic Ringer solution. Two LiCl responsive neurons were also observed. Some of these neurons responded only to chemical stimuli, others responded to both chemical and single shock electrical stimulation of the vagus. Thus, no correlation between the vagal afferent supplies and chemosensitivities of these AP neurons was recognized.

Discussion

The AP is a circumventricular organ of the fourth ventricle and lacks a blood – brain barrier. The existence of neural elements within this organ has been confirmed histologically (Leslie, 1986). These facts suggest various chemoreceptor mechanisms to detect blood- and CSF-borne chemical information not only for triggering the emetic response but also for homeostatic control. Many ablation experiments of the AP indicated other functions than the emetic response, for instance, control of satiety (Edwards and Ritter, 1981, 1986; Ritter and Edwards, 1984), control of sodium and water balance (Wise and Ganong, 1960; Contreras and Stetson, 1981; Edwards and Ritter, 1982), formation of conditioned taste aversion (Berger et al., 1973; Ritter et al., 1980) and cardiovascular control (Barnes et al., 1984). A postulate of AP chemoreceptors is common to these authors. The present study provides direct evidence for the existence of such chemoreceptor mechanisms which participate in these controls.

The glucose responsive neurons within the AP may play a role in the control of food intake. Oomura et al. (1969) were the first to reveal glucose responsive neurons in the hypothalamus by electrophysiological methods. Glucose responsive neurons were also found in the nucleus tractus solitarii (NTS) (Adachi et al., 1984; Mizuno and Oomura, 1984). Neural connections between the glucose responsive neurons in the central nervous system and a peripheral hepatic glucoreceptor (Niijima, 1969, 1982) was elucidated (Shimizu et al., 1983; Adachi et al., 1984). These neural networks suggest a hierarchical organization of glucose information in the body fluid processing by central and peripheral nervous systems (Oomura, 1983). The AP responsive neurons could be involved in this organization.

The possible function of the AP sodium (or osmo-) responsive neurons favors a similar conception to that of the glucose responsive ones in association with the control of sodium and water balance of the body fluid. Sodium (or osmo-) responsive neurons are located in the hypothalamus (Oomura et al., 1969) and the NTS as well (Kobashi and Adachi, 1985). Peripheral osmoreceptors exist in the liver (Adachi et al., 1976) and their afferent signals project to the caudal portion of the NTS (Adachi, 1981, 1984) and in turn to the hypothalamus via the parabrachial nucleus (PB) (Kobashi and Adachi, 1986). Convergence of the hepatic osmoreceptive signals onto the NTS sodium responsive neurons was also confirmed (Kobashi and Adachi, 1985). A survey of these previous reports strongly suggests involvement of the AP sodium responsive neurons in the neural control system for isosmosis and isovolemia of the body fluid.

Carpenter and Briggs (1986) recorded responses of neurons of the canine AP to iontophoretic application of insulin. They concluded that these responses provide further support for a critical role of the AP in triggering the emetic reflex. The existence of LiCl responsive neurons within the rat AP indicates that this brain region is involved in neural mechanisms inducing nausea, even though the emetic response is not easily elicited in the rat. In turn, such chemosensitive neurons may play a part in the formation of conditioned taste aversion. As many other chemicals such as scopolamine, amphetamine, hydroxytryptophan and so on induce conditioned taste aversion, it may be possible that the LiCl responsive neuron also responds to these chemicals.

A postulated scheme is presented in Fig. 6. Because some of the chemosensitive AP neurons

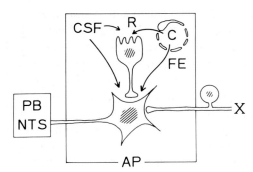

Fig. 6. Schematic diagram illustrating a possible neural connection of AP neurons. CSF, cerebrospinal fluid; R, chemoreceptor neuron; C, capillary; FE, fenestration; AP, area postrema; PB, parabrachial nucleus; NTS, nucleus tractus solitarii; X, vagus.

are excited by the vagal afferent but others are not, there can be a possibility that receptor-like neurons (R) are located in the AP. The former neurons themselves can also be chemosensitive, because convergence of the vagal afferent signals to chemosensitive neurons in the NTS has been ascertained (Adachi et al., 1984; Kobashi and Adachi, 1985). These neurons are responsive to either blood- or CSF-borne substances, because application of the chemical stimuli to both the fourth ventricle and the carotid artery elicited the neuronal responses. Close connections between the AP and the PB as well as the NTS have been clarified (Shapiro and Miselis, 1982). It is easily delineated that the internal chemical information detected in the AP may be transmitted to the other nuclei in the central nervous system, so that various reflexes including emesis can be induced. Certainly further studies should be necessary to elucidate such neural mechanisms.

Acknowledgements

This work was supported by Grant-in-Aid for General Scientific Research 62480378 from the Ministry of Education, Science and Culture in Japan and a Grant from the Society for Research on Umami Taste.

References

Adachi, A. (1981) Electrophysiological study of hepatic vagal projection to the medulla. *Neurosci. Lett.,* 24: 19–23.

Adachi, A. (1984) Projection of the hepatic vagal nerve in the medulla oblongata. *J. Auton. Nerv. Syst.,* 10: 287–293.

Adachi, A. and Kobashi, M. (1985) Chemosensitive neurons within the area postrema of the rat. *Neurosci. Lett.,* 55: 137–140.

Adachi, A., Niijima, A. and Jacobs, H.L. (1976) An hepatic osmoreceptor mechanism in the rat: electrophysiological and behavioral studies. *Am. J. Physiol.,* 231: 1043–1049.

Adachi, A., Shimizu, N., Oomura, Y. and Kobashi, M. (1984) Convergence of hepatoportal glucose-sensitive afferent signals to glucose-sensitive units within the nucleus of the solitary tract. *Neurosci. Lett.,* 46: 215–218.

Barnes, K.L., Ferrario, C.M., Chernicky, C.L. and Borosnihan, K.B. (1984) Participation of the area postrema in cardiovascular control in the dog. *Fed. Proc.,* 43: 2959–2962.

Berger, B.D., Wise, C.D. and Stein, L. (1973) Area postrema damage and bait shyness. *J. Comp. Physiol. Psychol.,* 83: 475–479.

Borison, H.L. (1974) Area postrema: chemoreceptor trigger zone for vomiting – is that all? *Life Sci.,* 14: 1807–1817.

Borison, H.L. and Wang, S.C. (1953) Physiology and pharmacology of vomiting. *Pharmacol. Rev.,* 5: 193–230.

Carpenter, D.O. and Briggs, D.B. (1986) Insulin excites neurons of the area postrema and causes emesis. *Neurosci. Lett.,* 68: 85–89.

Contreras, R.J. and Stetson, P.W. (1981) Changes in salt intake after lesions of the area postrema and the nucleus of the solitary tract in rats. *Brain Res.,* 211: 355–366.

Edwards, G.L. and Ritter, R.C. (1981) Ablation of the area postrema causes exaggerated consumption of preferred foods in the rat. *Brain Res.,* 216: 276.

Edwards, G.L and Ritter, R.C. (1982) Area postrema lesions increase drinking to angiotensin and extracellular dehydration. *Physiol. Behav.,* 29: 943–947.

Edwards, G.L. and Ritter, R.C. (1986) Area postrema lesions: cause of overingestion is not altered visceral nerve function. *Am. J. Physiol.,* 251: R575–R581.

Kobashi, M. and Adachi, A. (1985) Convergence of hepatic osmoreceptive inputs on sodium-responsive units within the nucleus of the solitary tract of the rat. *J. Neurophysiol.,* 54: 212–219.

Kobashi, M. and Adachi, A. (1986) Projection of nucleus tractus solitarius units influenced by hepatoportal afferent signal to parabrachial nucleus. *J. Auton. Nerv. Syst.,* 16: 153–158.

Leslie, R.A. (1986) Comparative aspects of the area postrema: fine-structural considerations help to determine its function. *Cell. Mol. Neurobiol.,* 6: 95–120.

Mizuno, Y. and Oomura, Y. (1984) Glucose responding neurons in the nucleus tractus solitarius of the rat: in vitro study. *Brain Res.,* 307: 109–116.

Niijima, A. (1969) Afferent impulse discharges from gluco-receptors in the liver of the guinea pig. *Ann. N.Y. Acad. Sci.,* 157: 690 – 700.

Niijima, A. (1982) Glucose-sensitive afferent nerve fibers in the hepatic branch of the vagus nerve in the guinea-pig. *J. Physiol. (London),* 332: 315 – 323.

Oomura, Y. (1983) Glucose as a regulator of neuronal activity. In: A.J. Szabo (Ed.), *Advances in Metabolic Disorders, Vol. 7,* Academic Press, New York, pp. 31 – 65.

Oomura, Y., Ono, T., Ooyama, H. and Wayner, M.J. (1969) Glucose and osmosensitive neurons of the rat hypothalamus. *Nature (London),* 222: 282 – 284.

Ritter, R.C. and Edwards, G.L. (1984) Area postrema lesion cause overconsumption of palatable foods but not calories. *Physiol. Behav.,* 32: 923 – 927.

Ritter, S., McGlone, J.J. and Kelley, K.W. (1980) Absence of lithium-induced taste aversion after area postrema lesion. *Brain Res.,* 201: 501 – 506.

Shapiro, R.E. and Miselis, R.R. (1982) An efferent projection from the area postrema and the caudal medial nucleus of the solitary tract to the parabrachial nucleus in rat. *Proc. Soc. Neurosci.,* 8: 269.

Wise, B.L. and Ganong, W.F. (1960) Effect of brain-stem stimulation of renal function. *Am. J. Physiol.,* 198: 1291 – 1295.

W. Hamann and A. Iggo (Eds.)
Progress in Brain Research, Vol. 74
© 1988 Elsevier Science Publishers B.V. (Biomedical Division)

CHAPTER 11

Responses of muscle spindles depend on their history of activation and movement

J.E. Gregory, D.L. Morgan and U. Proske

Departments of Physiology and of Electrical Engineering, Monash University, Clayton, Vic., Australia

Introduction

After-effects, defined here as variations in the responsiveness of muscle spindles resulting from preceding activity and movement of the muscle, have long been known to exist (Hunt and Kuffler, 1951). They are commonly encountered as the 'stuck' spindle where the resting discharge in the passive muscle may undergo large 'spontaneous' changes in rate (Eldred et al., 1976). However, the resting discharge is only one of several aspects of a spindle's response that may be altered by the preceding history. Others include the 'initial burst' of impulses at the onset of a ramp stretch (Brown et al., 1969), the response to a tendon tap (Gregory et al., 1987) and the response to fusimotor stimulation (Emonet-Denand et al., 1985a,b).

Emonet-Denand et al. have shown that the response of a spindle to dynamic fusimotor stimulation during a slow stretch can be large or small depending on whether or not this is preceded by a conditioning period of rapid movements or fusimotor stimulation. The test used in their experiments was a brief fusimotor tetanus and the measure of the after-effect was the amplitude of the resulting burst of afferent impulses. A limitation of this test is its binary nature, signalling the presence of an after-effect simply by whether the burst is large or small. Another quite different problem is that the slow stretch during which the test tetanus is applied in one sequence may act to condition the test response recorded in the next sequence. In other words, the persistent nature of after-effects makes it necessary to carefully define the unconditioned state. Because of this, in our own experiments we have chosen to always condition the muscle by a defined procedure, and to avoid any 'unconditioned state'. Rather than using a brief fusimotor tetanus for the test we have preferred to use tetani of longer duration. This converts a large or small afferent burst into a change in delay of onset of a sustained afferent response (Morgan et al., 1984). The advantage of such a test is that it allows after-effects to be quantified.

After trying a variety of different conditioning and test procedures to show up after-effects we have concluded that the underlying cause lies in the mechanical properties of the intrafusal fibres. Depending on their previous history of activation and length changes they may or may not be able to shorten themselves, when a shortening is imposed on the whole muscle. If not, they may fall slack. The presence of any intrafusal slack is signalled by a delay in onset of the afferent response to an intrafusal contraction, representing the time required for the shortening fibre to take up the slack. (A small afferent burst in response to a brief tetanus simply means that the intrafusal contraction did not last long enough to do more than just take up the slack and produce a small modulation of the afferent discharge, Fig. 1.) Procedures which, we believe, introduce slack in the intrafusal bundle include stretching the muscle and holding it stretched for some seconds before returning it to the length at which the fusimotor test is to be applied. Here it is immediately apparent that if the test procedure itself involves a slow stretch then this will act to condition any subsequent test. Procedures which remove existing intrafusal slack include whole muscle contraction or fusimotor stimulation at the test length, or a series of rapid lengthening and shortening movements ending at the test length. Stimulation at a length longer than the test length but immediately followed by shortening to the test length also prevents development of any slack. We propose that the time required for development of slack represents the slow rate of formation of long-lasting cross-bridges (Hill, 1968) between actin and myosin of intrafusal fibres. It is these cross-bridges which are thought to give muscle its 'stiction' or thixotropic property (Hagbarth et al., 1985). Similarly, the short-range elasticity of intrafusal fibres is thought to give rise to the initial burst in the response of the spindle during a ramp stretch (Brown et al., 1969).

We report here two experiments designed to test our hypothesis for development of slack in intrafusal fibres. The first considers the effect of altering the amount by which conditioning and test lengths differ. If the muscle is contracted at a length longer than the test length, held there for several seconds and then brought back to the test length, the amount of intrafusal slack developed and hence the size of the delay in onset of the response to a test fusimotor tetanus should increase as the length difference is made bigger. However, when the conditioning length is shorter than the test length, any pre-existing slack in intrafusal fibres should be taken up during the stretch required to return the muscle to the test length.

Methods and results

The preparation used in these experiments is essentially the same as that described in our previous reports on this subject (Gregory et al., 1986, 1987). We have used the cat soleus muscle and recorded from identified primary afferents of spindles in dorsal root filaments. Muscle length was related to the maximum in the body (L_{max}). The test length was chosen to correspond approximately to the optimum for a muscle contraction. For the results presented here, the conditioning procedure involved stretching or releasing from the test length at a rate of 10 mm/s, holding the muscle there, and then stimulating the muscle nerve at 30 pulses/s with a stimulus strength sufficient to engage fusimotor fibres. After stimulation the muscle was kept still for a further 5 s and then returned to the test length. The testing procedure consisted of measuring the delay in onset of the afferent response to tetanic stimulation (500 ms tetanus at 50 pulses/s) of an identified dynamic fusimotor fibre supplying the test spindle. The fusimotor tetanus was given 1 s after commencement of a slow stretch (1 mm/s), the stretch being initiated 3 s after return to the test length (see Fig. 1). The delay or latency was measured as the time from delivery of the stimulating pulses to 50% of the peak of the spindle response. Measurement of latency had a resolution of 5 ms and reproducibility of 5 – 10 ms. For all five spindle and dynamic fusimotor pairs studied, the afferent response to stimulation rose sufficiently rapidly for the choice of point of measurement not to be critical.

The entire testing sequence is shown in Fig. 1. When conditioning involved stretching to a length longer than the test length (LONG), the subsequent test response was identified as 'LONG'. When conditioning was at a shorter length than the test length this was identified by 'SHORT'. The afferent discharge is shown as an instantaneous frequency display and the test response to the fusimotor tetanus is indicated by an arrow. Here, for the sake of illustration, we have used a brief test tetanus, one which shows the effect of conditioning as a change in size of the afferent burst. In all subsequent figures a longer tetanus was used, long enough to measure a delay in onset of afferent response (see Fig. 2).

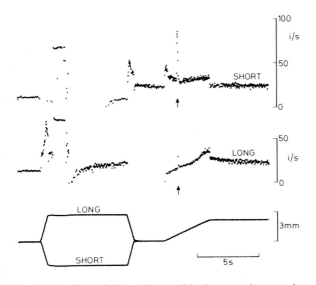

Fig. 1. The effect of alternative conditioning procedures on the response of the primary ending of a soleus muscle spindle to a brief dynamic fusimotor tetanus applied during a slow stretch. In the lower part of the figure are shown two superimposed traces of muscle length, while the upper part shows the corresponding traces of spindle discharge as instantaneous frequency (reciprocal of interval between successive impulses). The muscle was initially at a length 11 mm shorter than maximum length in the body and was then either stretched (long) or shortened (short) by 3 mm, following which the muscle nerve was stimulated at a rate of 30 s^{-1} for 1 s. The muscle was then held at the long or short conditioning length for a further 5 s before being returned to the mean test length. After a short pause, the test dynamic fusimotor tetanus (100 s^{-1}, 60 ms duration) was delivered during a slow stretch. The response (indicated by arrow) is of smaller amplitude following conditioning at the long length than after conditioning at the short length.

In Fig. 2 is shown the lack of any change in latency when the test is preceded by a conditioning contraction at a length 0.5 mm longer or shorter than the test length (A). However, a large latency shift becomes apparent when the conditioning length is increased to 3 mm longer or shorter than the test length. This result is in accord with our predictions. For conditioning at lengths shorter than or equal to the test length (negative length differences), no intrafusal slack develops and the measured latency is small and constant. For positive length differences where now the condi-

tioning length is longer than the test length a latency difference between the 'LONG' and 'SHORT' condition becomes apparent, but only if the conditioning length exceeds the test length by a sufficient amount. For example in Fig. 2, 0.5 mm is clearly not sufficient. Making the conditioning length longer results in development of a latency difference which gets bigger with further length increases but which reaches a plateau value depending on the muscle length at which the test measurements are made. When the test length is long ($L_{max} - 6$) the maximum latency difference (130 ms) is measured with a conditioning length 2 mm longer than the test length. When the test

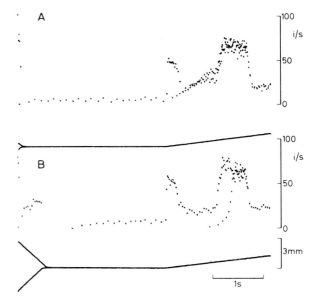

Fig. 2. Effect of size of conditioning length step on latency of response to test dynamic fusimotor stimulation. Both A and B show two superimposed spindle responses above two superimposed length traces in which the length changes from long or short conditioning lengths to the test, mean length can be seen to the left. Interval between the end of conditioning whole muscle tetanus and start of return to test length is 10 s. (A) Conditioning at lengths 0.5 mm longer and shorter than the test length produces no difference in the latency of the responses to test dynamic fusimotor stimulation at 50 s^{-1} for 0.5 s. (B) The latency of the response following conditioning at a length 3 mm longer than the test length is 0.28 s longer than after conditioning at the short length. Mean muscle length 11 mm shorter than maximum length in the body ($L_{max} - 11$).

length is shorter ($L_{max} - 11$) a maximum latency difference of 250 ms is measured for a 4 mm difference between conditioning and test lengths (Fig. 3). The shorter latency measured at longer muscle lengths suggests that some of the intrafusal slack introduced by conditioning is 'spontaneously' taken up as a result of the greater passive tension in the muscle. The fact that latency has already reached a plateau with a length difference of 2 mm suggests that at these longer lengths intrafusal fibres will not develop more than a limited amount of slack. Perhaps slack beyond a certain point is again taken up 'spontaneously' as lateral compressive forces from the intrafusal fibre's immediate extrafusal surroundings and the fibre's own passive resistance to bending reach sufficient levels to lead to detachment of some of the long-lasting cross-bridges, and their reformation after some fibre shortening. Notice too in Fig. 3 that at longer test lengths the minimal length difference for a latency shift is $1 - 2$ mm. At the shorter test length, a 1 mm difference already gives a latency shift of nearly 200 ms. This again suggests that in the face of a greater passive tension a larger shortening step must be used to introduce measurable slack.

The second experiment described here considers the effect of varying the time for which the muscle is held at the conditioning length before being returned to the test length. Our theory predicts that this hold time must be long enough to allow sufficient numbers of stable cross-bridges to form, following muscle contraction, to stiffen the intrafusal fibres enough for them not to shorten but to fall slack when the whole muscle is shortened. As muscle fibre shortening is brought about by passive forces, these would be expected to be greater at longer mean muscle lengths so that the amount by which an intrafusal fibre must be stiffened to prevent it from shortening would be expected to be greater at longer lengths, implying a longer necessary hold time.

The result of an experiment exploring this point is shown in Fig. 4. Here the conditioning length was always made either 3 mm longer or shorter

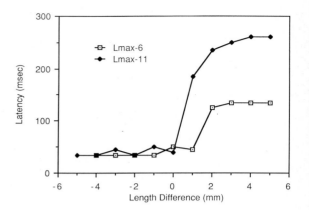

Fig. 3. For one spindle, plots of difference between conditioning and test lengths against latency of responses to dynamic fusimotor stimulation, at two test lengths. Details of stimulation etc. as in Fig. 2, which shows examples of records from which values plotted were read. Latency is the same for all conditioning lengths shorter than the test length, but increases progressively when the conditioning length is made longer than the test length. When muscle mean length is increased, the latency reaches a lower maximum.

than the test length. When the muscle contraction at the conditioning length was followed by immediate return to the test length (0 s, Fig. 4) no latency difference developed. When, however, the muscle was held at the conditioning length for 20 s after the contraction a large latency difference between the 'long' and the 'short' condition developed (20 s, Fig. 4).

This experiment was repeated at a number of different muscle lengths for a range of different hold times of between 0.1 s and 100 s (Fig. 5). As predicted, the hold time required to achieve the same latency shift was found to be longer at longer mean muscle lengths. Notice that at $L_{max} - 2$ mm the latency shift was small, $40 - 50$ ms, and needed a hold time of at least 10 s to become apparent. Once again the conclusion is that some 'spontaneous' intrafusal shortening can occur following development of slack and this becomes progressively more pronounced at longer muscle lengths. Here presumably there is slippage in some sarcomeres, or part of the muscle, and sticking in other parts. Partial shortening, uniformly distributed along the whole length of the intrafusal fibre, seems unlikely as once the cross-bridges of a sarcomere are broken the sarcomere would be expected to continue shortening until there remained little or no passive tension within it.

Another feature of Fig. 5 is that intrafusal fibres continue to become more firmly stuck over hold intervals of 20 s or more. There is a progressive increase in latency over this whole period. Such behaviour is consistent with the known properties of stable cross-bridges (Hill, 1968).

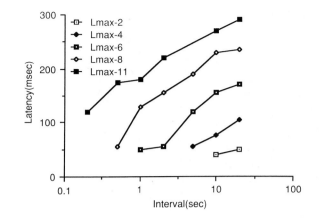

Fig. 5. For one spindle, plots of duration of periods of holding muscle at conditioning length after whole muscle contraction (Interval) against latency of response to test dynamic fusimotor stimulation, at five different mean muscle lengths. Values read from records similar to those shown in Fig. 4. Latency increases with increased interval. As the muscle length is increased, a larger interval is required to achieve the same latency. Note the logarithmic time scale.

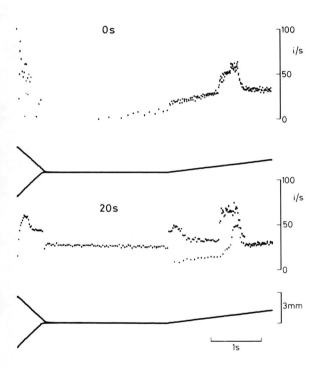

Fig. 4. Effect of changing the interval during which the muscle is held at the long or short length after the conditioning whole muscle contraction. Two length traces and two records of spindle discharge are superimposed in each panel. Details of muscle and fusimotor stimulation as in Fig. 2. In the upper part of the figure, when the interval is zero (i.e., immediately after the end of contraction, shortening to the test length begins), there is no difference in latency between conditioning at lengths longer and shorter than the test length. With an interval of 20 s, the response to fusimotor stimulation following conditioning at the long length is delayed by 0.25 s. Mean muscle length $L_{max} - 11$.

Conclusion

To conclude, we believe the experiments described here support our explanation of after-effects and are difficult to explain in any other way. The general proposition is that a spindle will develop depression of its responsiveness if it is held passive for a sufficient period and is then shortened. The time necessary for development of this depression is greater at longer muscle lengths, ranging from seconds to tens or even hundreds of seconds. According to our explanation this time is required for 'permanent' or 'slow-turnover' cross-bridges to form in sufficient numbers to resist the passive forces imposed on sacromeres by elastic tissue during muscle shortening. Anything that leads to detachment of these bridges during their period of formation will tend to reduce spindle depression by allowing intrafusal fibres to subsequently shorten along with the whole muscle, thereby reducing the likelihood of development of any slack.

References

Brown, M.C., Goodwin, G.M. and Matthews, P.B.C. (1969) After effects of fusimotor stimulation on the response of muscle spindle primary afferent endings. *J. Physiol. (London),* 205: 677–694.

Eldred, E., Hutton, R.S. and Smith, J.L. (1976) Nature of the persisting changes in afferent discharge from muscle following its contraction. In: S. Homma (Ed.), *'Understanding The Stretch Reflex, Progress in Brain Research,* Vol. 44, Elsevier, Amsterdam, pp. 157–170.

Emonet-Denand, F., Hunt, C.C. and Laporte, Y. (1985a) Fusimotor after-effects on response of primary endings to test dynamic stimuli in cat muscle spindles. *J. Physiol. (London),* 360: 187–200.

Emonet-Denand, F., Hunt, C.C. and Laporte, Y. (1985b) Effects of stretch on dynamic fusimotor after-effects in cat muscle spindles. *J. Physiol. (London),* 360: 201–213.

Gregory, J.E., Morgan, D.L. and Proske, U. (1986) After-effects in the responses of cat muscle spindles. *J. Neurophysiol.,* 56: 451–461.

Gregory, J.E., Morgan, D.L. and Proske, U. (1987) Changes in the size of the stretch reflex of cat and man attributed to after-effects in muscle spindles. *J. Neurophysiol.,* in press.

Hagbarth, K.E., Hagglund, J.V., Nordin, M. and Wallin, E.U. (1985) Thixotropic behaviour of human finger flexor muscles with accompanying changes in spindle and reflex responses to stretch. *J. Physiol. (London),* 368: 323–342.

Hill, D.K. (1968) Tension due to interaction between the sliding filaments in resting striated muscle. The effect of stimulation. *J. Physiol. (London),* 199: 637–684.

Hunt, C.C. and Kuffler, S.W. (1951) Further study of efferent small-nerve fibres to mammalian muscle spindles. Multiple spindle innervation and activity during contraction. *J. Physiol. (London),* 113: 283–297.

Morgan, D.L., Prochazka, A. and Proske, U. (1984) The after-effects of stretch and fusimotor stimulation on the responses of primary endings of cat muscle spindles. *J. Physiol. (London),* 356: 465–477.

W. Hamann and A. Iggo (Eds.)
Progress in Brain Research, Vol. 74
© 1988 Elsevier Science Publishers B.V. (Biomedical Division)

CHAPTER 12

Influence of adrenaline and hypoxia on rat muscle receptors in vitro

J. Kieschke, S. Mense and N.R. Prabhakar[a]

Anatomisches Institut III, Universität Heidelberg, Im Neuenheimer Feld 307, D-6900 Heidelberg, FRG

Summary

The effects of sympathetic efferent activity on sensory nerve endings are difficult to interpret, since in vivo direct chemical influences cannot be separated from indirect ones, e.g., those due to ischaemia. In the present study, a rat hemidiaphragm – phrenic nerve preparation in vitro was used to study the effects of hypoxia and increased concentrations of adrenaline on single diaphragmatic receptors. The main influence of adrenaline 100 μg/l or 1 mg/l on muscle spindles was a depression, while slowly conducting afferent units (group III and IV receptors) were often activated, particularly the nociceptive ones. Hypoxia abolished the impulse activity in most of the muscle spindles, whereas the majority of the group III and IV receptors were excited.

Introduction

The question of an efferent sympathetic control of sensory nerve endings has been studied by various groups of workers in different receptor types such as carotid baroreceptors and chemoreceptors

(Eyzaguirre and Lewin, 1961; Koizumi and Sato, 1969; Aars, 1971), mechanoreceptors (Loewenstein, 1956; Akoev, 1981; Cash and Linden, 1982; Passatore and Filippi, 1983; Barasi and Lynn, 1986) and cold receptors (Spray, 1974; Davies, 1985). With regard to muscle receptors a sympathetic influence has been discussed mainly for muscle spindles (Paintal, 1959; Eldred et al., 1960; Hunt, 1960; Hunt et al., 1982; Passatore and Filippi, 1982) since anatomical studies had yielded data indicating that they receive a sympathetic innervation (Santini and Ibata, 1971; Barker and Saito, 1981).

Up to now, no studies dealing with possible effects of sympathetic activity on muscle receptors with slowly conducting afferent fibres (below 30 m/s) have been performed. These receptors contain different types of nociceptive and non-nociceptive units (Mense and Meyer, 1985); particularly the former might be involved in the production of deep pain which accompanies some forms of sympathetic reflex dystrophies (Nathan, 1983; Jänig, 1985).

When studying the effects of efferent sympathetic fibres (or their transmitters) on sensory nerve endings in vivo one has to cope with the problem that it is difficult to differentiate between a direct chemical influence of the transmitter(s) on the endings and an indirect effect due to vasoconstriction and ensuing ischaemia. Thus, the same effect, namely an increase in the discharge rate of muscle spindles following stimulation of the sympathetic trunk, has been attributed to a direct action by Hunt (1960) while Eldred et al. (1960) considered it to be due to vasoconstriction.

In the present study a rat hemidiaphragm – phrenic nerve preparation in vitro has been used to examine the effects of adrenaline and hypoxia on single receptors of the diaphragm.

Methods

The experiments were performed on Wistar rats (100 – 200 g body weight) of both sexes. The animals were first anaesthetised by inhalation of halothane vapor and then killed by cutting both carotid arteries. The phrenic nerve of one side was quickly removed together with the corresponding hemidiaphragm and mounted in a lucite chamber containing an organ bath for the muscle and an oil pool for the nerve (Fig. 1). The temperature of the chamber and its contents was kept at 32°C by circulating warm water through a water jacket around the chamber. Hubbard tyrode solution was used for perfusion of the organ bath (6 ml/min), it was gassed with carbogen (95% O_2 plus 5% CO_2, pH 7.2). Before entering the organ bath the perfusion solution passed through a heating coil in the water jacket.

With the use of sharpened watchmaker's forceps

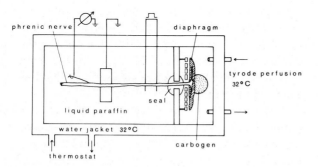

Fig. 1. Experimental set-up, view from above. The hemidiaphragm is mounted vertically on a perforated lucite plate in the organ bath. The phrenic nerve runs into a neighbouring oil pool where the impulse activity of single fibres is recorded from small filaments of the nerve. The preparation is kept at 32°C.

small filaments were split from the phrenic nerve in the oil pool and put over the recording electrode. The conduction velocity of the fibres under study was determined by stimulating the nerve electrically close to the organ bath. The nomenclature by Lloyd (1943) – which was developed for the cat – was used for classifying slowly conducting units as group IV if they conducted at less than 2.5 m/s and as group III if their conduction velocity was between 2.5 and 30 m/s. The Q_{10} value of the conduction velocity was determined to be 1.6 in three slowly conducting fibres; this value was used for calculating the velocity at 37°C. Since the short conduction distance did not allow us to determine accurately the conduction velocity of fast fibres, the identification of these units relied on their response behaviour. Receptors were classified as primary endings of muscle spindles (Ia) if they displayed a resting activity and had a marked differential response behaviour upon slightly stretching the muscle; secondary endings (group II) lacked this dynamic behaviour. If favourably situated in the diaphragm, both receptors showed a short period of depression during a muscle twitch. Receptors behaving like Golgi tendon organs (no resting activity, activation by muscle twitch) were rarely encountered and are not included in the evaluation.

Mechanical stimulation of the receptive endings in the diaphragm was performed using an artist's brush and a set of von Frey hairs which had been calibrated with an analytic scale. Group III and IV units were classified as low-threshold mechanosensitive (LTM) if they were clearly excited by touching or slightly stroking the diaphragm with the artist's brush, and as nociceptive if they required firm pressure with the handle of the brush or 'stabbing' with the brush to be activated. The borderline between LTM and nociceptive receptors corresponded to a von Frey threshold of approximately 0.7 p, but this value was not used for classification purposes. In order to be able to differentiate between nociceptors and thermosensitive receptors which likewise are present in skeletal muscle and respond to noxious pressure (Mense and Meyer, 1985), thermal stimulation of the receptors was performed by injecting cold or warm water into the organ bath.

For application of adrenaline or other test substances the perfusion system was switched to a Hubbard solution containing the desired concentration of the substance. In the organ bath, hypoxia could be induced by gassing it with 95% N_2 and 5% CO_2 (resulting in a pO_2 of about 20 mm Hg). When gassed with carbogen, the organ bath had a pO_2 of about 390 mm Hg.

Results

Muscle spindles

Since all the spindles studied had a resting dis-charge, both depressions and activations could be evaluated. The most frequent reaction of muscle spindles to adrenaline (100 μg/l or 1 mg/l) was a weak and transient depression in discharge frequency (Fig. 2A). An adrenaline-induced activation was observed in only one spindle (out of 17 tested). Although the depression was usually clear-cut in onset and duration, it was badly reproducible and not well graded if increasing concentrations of adrenaline were applied. In some units the direction of the adrenaline effect appeared to depend on the initial discharge frequency, spindles with a lower frequency showing an increase rather than a decrease in activity under the influence of adrenaline. It is not known whether a previous lesion to the ending (e.g., by hypoxia as shown in Fig. 2B) is a prerequisite for this behaviour.

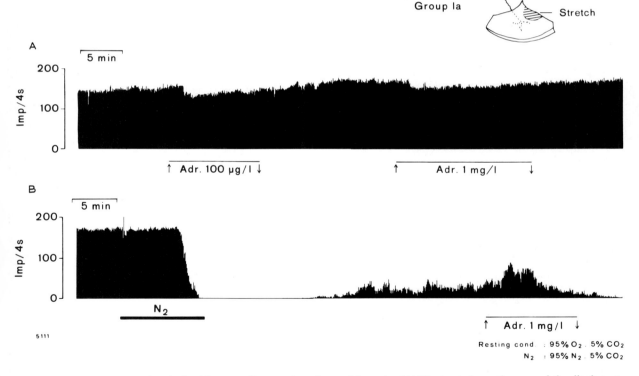

Fig. 2. Responses of a muscle spindle primary ending to adrenaline and hypoxia. (A) The inset shows the area of the diaphragm from which the receptor could be activated by stretch. The double curved line respresents the lower ribs which were left attached to the diaphragm. Perfusion of the organ bath with Tyrode solution containing adrenaline (Adr.) 100 μg/l or 1 mg/l is indicated by the line underneath the histogram of the fibre activity. (B) The period of gassing the organ bath with 95% N_2 and 5% CO_2 (N_2) for inducing hypoxia is marked by the thick bar underneath the histogram.

The responses of muscle spindles to hypoxia were usually much greater than those to adrenaline and had the form of a depression which usually resulted in total silence of the unit after several minutes of hypoxia (Fig. 2B). Switching back to gassing with carbogen in most cases restituted the initial degree of resting activity, but there were also units – such as that shown in Fig. 2B – which did not recover fully during the recording period. In eight of the 13 muscle spindles tested, hypoxia abolished the resting discharge completely; the remaining ones were either not affected or showed a weak activation. In Fig. 3, only data from those units are included which were tested with both adrenaline and hypoxia. It is apparent that the main effect of hypoxia on muscle spindles is a decrease in discharge frequency, which is combined with either a depressing or a missing action of adrenaline. Thus, increased tissue concentrations of adrenaline such as used in the present study influence muscle spindles in the same direction as hypoxia does, but the depressing effect of adrenaline is weaker and the proportion of affected receptors smaller.

Response Combinations to Adrenaline and Hypoxia

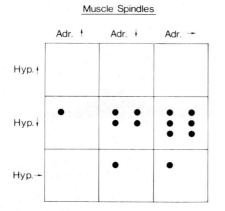

Fig. 3. Response combinations of muscle spindle afferent fibres that were tested with both adrenaline (Adr.) 100 μg/l or 1 mg/l and hypoxia (Hyp.).

Group III and IV receptors

Adrenaline in the concentrations used (100 μg/l and 1 mg/l) had predominantly excitatory effects on receptors with slowly conducting afferent fibres; a depression of resting activity was observed in two endings only (of 30 units tested). Relatively clear responses were obtained from nociceptors (Fig. 4B); these endings were never depressed by adrenaline. The unit shown in Fig. 4 was exceptional in that it reacted to thermal stimulation. It was not considered to be a thermoreceptor, though, since it did not exhibit a differential behaviour during fast temperature changes and responded only weakly to strong thermal stimuli. The response magnitude to adrenaline of nociceptive units was particularly great if their mechanosensitive receptive fields were under the continuous influence of a mechanical stimulus, e.g., of a weight pressing on the diaphragm. In some nociceptors, which did not react to an initial application of adrenaline, a clear response to this substance could be produced during mechanical irritation of the receptive field. In the unit shown in Fig. 4, prolonged hypoxia – 30 min of gassing with 95% N_2 or 75% N_2 plus 20% O_2 – did not elicit a clear response. Such a behaviour was the exception rather than the rule, since most of the group III and IV receptors were activated by a lowered pO_2 irrespective of their mechanical threshold.

The response combinations of units which were tested with both adrenaline and hypoxia are shown in Fig. 5. It is apparent that the main effect of adrenaline consists of an activation of both LTM and nociceptive units. For group III and IV receptors hypoxia is a weaker stimulus than for muscle spindles; again the main effect is excitatory.

Discussion

The results show that adrenaline in concentrations of 100 μg/l or 1 mg/l and hypoxia of a pO_2 of about 20 mm Hg are effective stimuli for a considerable proportion of diaphragmatic receptors.

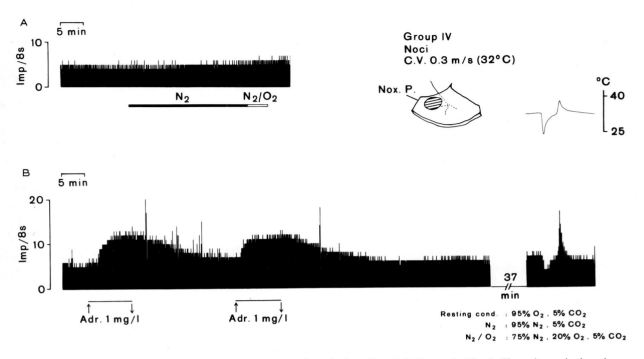

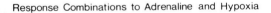

Fig. 4. Reaction of a nociceptive group IV receptor to hypoxia and adrenaline. Labelling as in Fig. 2. The unit required noxious stimulation of its receptive field (hatched) with local pressure Nox.P.) to be activated. The effect of hypoxia of long duration is questionable (A) while two applications of adrenaline 1 mg/l el cited clear responses of decreasing magnitude (B). Thermal stimulation in B (cooling to 24°C and warming to 38°C) showed that the unit was influenced by temperature changes but did not behave like a thermoreceptor.

Response Combinations to Adrenaline and Hypoxia

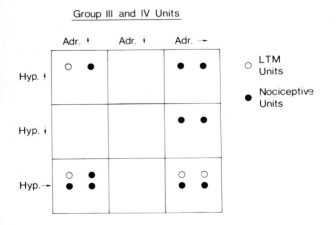

Fig. 5. Response combinations to adrenaline (Adr.) and hypoxia (Hyp.) of group III and IV receptors.

As to the strength of the stimuli used, adrenaline was applied in concentrations of about $5 \times 10^{-7} - 5 \times 10^{-6}$ mol/l which correspond to the values reported by Loewenstein (1956) and Akoev (1981) as necessary for producing effects on vertebrate mechanoreceptors. The hypoxia of 20 mm Hg pO_2 induced in the organ bath by gassing it with 5% CO_2 in N_2 appears not to be too severe if compared with pO_2 values in normal tissues. The mean pO_2 in the gastrocnemius soleus muscle of rats has been reported to be close to 22 mm Hg under normal conditions; it drops to zero within about 1 min after occlusion of the femoral artery (Angersbach et al., 1981). It has to be kept in mind, though, that in the present study the pO_2 was measured in the organ bath and not within the diaphragm. At the receptor site the pO_2 is probably lower. The fact that most of the muscle spindles reacted readily to the hypoxia indicates that it was sufficiently severe to be used as a test stimulus.

The responses of muscle spindles to electrical stimulation of sympathetic efferent fibres have been reported to be characterised by an initial increase in discharge frequency followed by a decrease or an abolition of the activity if the stimulation is intense and long enough (Eldred et al., 1960; Hunt, 1960). In the present study, such a response was often observed during hypoxia but rarely under the influence of adrenaline. Unless it is assumed that electrical stimulation of sympathetic fibres in vivo produces much higher local concentrations of adrenaline than those used in our experiments, it is likely that the effects described by Eldred et al. (1960) and Hunt (1960) are mainly due to the hypoxia and not to the direct influence of catecholamines on the nerve ending. A physiological function for the behaviour of muscle spindles under hypoxia and adrenaline is not known. While the abolition of resting activity during hypoxia might simply reflect a damage of the ending which is no longer capable of maintaining a high level of activity, the depression produced by adrenaline is not easy to understand. It is possible that the weak activation that sometimes precedes the depression under both hypoxia and adrenaline is the main effect occurring under physiological conditons. Thus, an increased activity in sympathetic efferent fibres during stress could produce a higher frequency in muscle spindle afferents which could increase the muscle tone (Passatore et al., 1985).

The excitatory action of adrenaline on many of the group III and IV nociceptors of the present experiments is at variance with recent studies reporting a lack of effect of sympathetic stimulation on the response behaviour of cutaneous nociceptors in the rabbit (Shea and Perl, 1985; Barasi and Lynn, 1986) and cat (Roberts and Elardo, 1985). A possible explanation for this discrepancy could be that diaphragmatic nociceptors are different from cutaneous nociceptors. Another explanation could be that some of the nociceptors in vitro display an altered responsiveness because of the in vitro condition. Although the diaphragmatic receptors in vitro behaved similarly to receptors of the skeletal muscle of the cat in vivo (Mense and Meyer, 1985), it cannot be excluded that at least some of the endings have developed an increased sensitivity to catecholamines due to an irritation produced by the excision of the diaphragm and/or handling in a recording chamber. The vigorous responses to adrenaline obtained from nociceptors under continuous mechanical pressure are consistent with such an assumption. In this context, it is interesting to note that nociceptors have been reported to be activated by sympathetic stimulation after they had been sensitised by noxious heating of their receptive fields (Roberts and Elardo, 1985). Possibly, a damage to the nociceptive endings or their environment is a prerequisite for the development of an adrenaline sensitivity which under special conditions might lead to chronic pain (Coderre et al., 1984).

The responses of group III and IV receptors to hypoxia were quite uniform; about half of the low-threshold mechanosensitive and the nociceptive endings were activated by this stimulus. Under the conditions of the present study the latencies of the hypoxia-induced activations were long (about 15 min) relative to the short latencies of the depressions in muscle spindles under hypoxia (1 – 6 min). The long latency of the response to hypoxia in group III and IV units might be indicative of an unspecific lesion of the ending or even the axon. Lehmann (1937) has shown long ago that A fibres of mammalian nerves in vitro become spontaneously active after about 8 min of anoxia.

In conclusion, the results show that the main effect of an increased tissue concentration of adrenaline is a decrease in discharge frequency in muscle spindle afferents combined with an increase in the activity of group III and IV afferent fibres, predominantly nociceptive ones. Hypoxia produces a similar effect, but under the conditions of the present study this stimulus appeared to be stronger, since most of the spindles fell totally silent and a greater proportion of both low-threshold mechanosensitive and nociceptive group III and IV receptors were activated.

References

Aars, H. (1971) Effects of noradrenaline on activity in single aortic baroreceptor fibers. *Acta Physiol. Scand.*, 83: 335 – 343.

Akoev, G.N. (1981) Catecholamines, acetylcholine and excitability of mechanoreceptors. *Progr. Neurobiol.*, 15: 269 – 294.

Angersbach, D., Ochlich, P. and Wilke, R. (1981) Changes of tissue pO_2 and aortic blood flow after ischaemia in the rat. *Bibl. Anat.*, 20: 389 – 394.

Barasi, S. and Lynn, B. (1986) Effects of sympathetic stimulation on mechanoreceptive and nociceptive afferent units from the rabbit pinna. *Brain Res.*, 378: 21 – 27.

Barker, D. and Saito, M. (1981) Autonomic innervation of receptors and muscle fibres in cat skeletal muscle. *Proc. R. Soc. London B*, 212: 317 – 332.

Cash, R.M. and Linden, R.W.A. (1982) Effects of sympathetic nerve stimulation on intra-oral mechanoreceptor activity in the cat. *J. Physiol. (London)*, 329: 451 – 463.

Coderre, T.J., Abbott, F.V. and Melzack, R. (1984) Effects of peripheral antisympathetic treatments in the tail-flick, formalin and autotomy tests. *Pain*, 18: 13 – 23.

Davies, S.N. (1985) Sympathetic modulation of cold-receptive neurones in the trigeminal system of the rat. *J. Physiol. (London)*, 366: 315 – 329.

Eldred, E., Schnitzlein, H.N. and Buchwald, J. (1960) Response of muscle spindles to stimulation of the sympathetic trunk. *Exp. Neurol.*, 2: 13 – 25.

Eyzaguirre, C. and Lewin, J. (1961) The effect of sympathetic stimulation on carotid nerve activity. *J. Physiol. (London)*, 159: 251 – 267.

Hunt, C.C. (1960) The effect of sympathetic stimulation on mammalian muscle spindles. *J. Physiol. (London)*, 151: 332 – 341.

Hunt, C.C., Jami, L. and Laporte, Y. (1982) Effects of stimulating the lumbar sympathetic trunk on cat hindlimb muscle spindles. *Arch. Ital. Biol.*, 120: 371 – 384.

Jänig, W. (1985) Causalgia and reflex sympathetic dystrophy: in which way is the sympathetic nervous system involved? *Trends Neurosci.*, 8: 1 – 7.

Koizumi, K. and Sato, A. (1969) Influence of sympathetic innervation on carotid sinus baroreceptor activity. *Am. J. Physiol.*, 216: 321 – 329.

Lehmann, J.E. (1937) The effect of asphyxia on mammalian A nerve fibers. *Am. J. Physiol.*, 119: 111 – 120.

Lloyd, D.P.C. (1943) Neuron patterns controlling transmission of ipsilateral hindlimb reflexes in cat. *J. Neurophysiol.*, 6: 239 – 315.

Loewenstein, W.R. (1956) Modulation of cutaneous mechanoreceptors by sympathetic stimulation. *J. Physiol. (London)*, 132: 40 – 60.

Mense, S. and Meyer, H. (1985) Different types of slowly conducting afferent units in cat skeletal muscle and tendon. *J. Physiol. (London)*, 363: 403 – 417.

Nathan, P.W. (1983) Pain and the sympathetic system. *J. Auton. Nerv. Syst.*, 7: 363 – 370.

Paintal, A.S. (1959) Facilitation and depression of muscle stretch receptors by repetitive antidromic stimulation, adrenaline and asphyxia. *J. Physiol. (London)*, 148: 252 – 266.

Passatore, M. and Filippi, G.M. (1982) A dual effect of sympathetic nerve stimulation on jaw muscle spindles. *J. Auton. Nerv. Syst.*, 6: 347 – 361.

Passatore, M. and Filippi, G.M. (1983) Sympathetic modulation of periodontal mechanoreceptors. *Arch. Ital. Biol.*, 121: 55 – 65.

Passatore, M., Grassi, C. and Filippi, G.M. (1985) Sympathetically-induced development of tension in jaw muscles: the possible contraction of intrafusal muscle fibres. *Pflüger's Arch.*, 405: 297 – 304.

Roberts, W.J. and Elardo, S.M. (1985) Sympathetic activation of A-delta nociceptors. *Somatosens. Res.*, 3: 33 – 44.

Santini, M. and Ibata, Y. (1971) The fine structure of thin unmyelinated axons within muscle spindles. *Brain Res.*, 33: 289 – 302.

Shea, V.K. and Perl, E.R. (1985) Failure of sympathetic stimulation to affect responsiveness of rabbit polymodal nociceptors. *J. Neurophysiol.*, 54: 513 – 519.

Spray, D.C. (1974) Characteristics, specificity and efferent control of frog cutaneous cold receptors. *J. Physiol. (London)*, 237: 15 – 38.

W. Hamann and A. Iggo (Eds.)
Progress in Brain Research, Vol. 74
© 1988 Elsevier Science Publishers B.V. (Biomedical Division)

CHAPTER 13

Dynamic response characteristics of the ampullae of Lorenzini to thermal and electrical stimuli

Heimo Wissing[a], Hans A. Braun[a] and Klaus Schäfer[b]

[a] *Physiologisches Institut, Universität Marburg, D-3550 Marburg, FRG and* [b] *Institut für Zoophysiologie, Universität Hohenheim, D-7000 Stuttgart 70, FRG*

Summary

The ampullae of Lorenzini are a multimodal secondary sensory system of elasmobranchs which responds to electrical and thermal stimuli. The stationary discharge rate depends on the actual temperature but is not affected by constant currents. Both types of stimuli, however, induce strong dynamic responses.

Step-like electrical stimuli induced dynamic frequency changes followed by gradual adaptation. The frequency responses on ramp-shaped electrical stimuli were uniformly characterised by fast frequency changes at the beginning of the ramps and gradual adaptation after the end of the ramps, whereas the frequency changes during ongoing current ramps were quite different in different fibres and at different stimulus conditions.

We assume that the broad variety of response characteristics during ongoing ramps results from a superposition of stimulating effects on the current change and adaptation effect of the transduction processes which may be of variable amount, depending on the individual fibre and on stimulus conditions. The uniformity of the response characteristics at the beginning and the end of the ramps may be due to the fact that only one of these components, stimulation or adaptation, is present.

Step-like temperature changes or fast temperature ramps often induced biphasic dynamic responses: the initial dynamic frequency changes were followed by second dynamic components of inverse direction. On slow temperature ramps, the two dynamic components were separated by a phase of gradual adaptation to the linearly changing value of the actual temperature. The onset of the second dynamic component thereby exactly coincided with the end of the ramp.

These results suggest that the dynamic frequency responses on temperature stimulation are mainly induced by the onset and offset of the temperature change and not by the temperature change itself.

Generally, the most effective parameter of an electrical stimulus seems to be the current change (dI/dt), whereas the effects of the temperature change (dT/dt) seemed to be almost negligible compared to the effects of the onset and offset of the temperature change (d^2T/dt^2). These suggestions also explain the biphasic response characteristics to fast temperature changes and why they were not observed on electrical stimulation.

Discharge pattern analysis revealed additional evidence for different receptor processes involved in the transduction of thermal and electrical signals and promises further insight in the transduction mechanisms of the ampullae of Lorenzini.

Introduction

Fishes of the class elasmobranchii possess a secondary sensory system, the ampullae of Lorenzini. The impulse activity of single afferent fibres is modulated by synaptic input of a high number of receptive cells, which are located in the ampullary wall (Waltman, 1966). It responds very sensitively to mechanical, chemical, thermal, electrical and magnetic stimulation (Hensel, 1955; Murray, 1957, 1962; Bromm et al., 1976; Akoev et al., 1976, 1980).

The present study is confined to the comparison of electrically and thermally induced frequency responses. Cathodal currents and fast cooling induce a dynamic increase of the discharge rate (frequency overshoot), while anodal currents and fast warming lead to a transient inhibition of the impulse activity (frequency undershoot). On electrical stimulation, the impulse frequency adapts to a steady state which is generally identical with the pre-stimulus value. In contrast, on thermal stimulation, the impulse frequency reaches a new steady state, which depends on the absolute temperature. Moreover, the initial dynamic frequency change is often followed by a second dynamic component of inverse direction.

These results indicate complex transfer characteristics of the ampullae of Lorenzini especially on thermal stimuli. In our experiments we therefore used ramp-shaped rather than step-like stimuli, thereby expecting further insight into the principles, similarities and differences of thermally and electrically induced responses.

Methods

The experiments were performed on isolated mandibular groups of the ampullae of Lorenzini of adult dogfish (*Scyliorhinus canicula*). Single ampullary capsulae, each containing about 5 – 7 ampullae, were dissected (Fig. 1). The ampullary canals were cut at a length of about 5 mm. The lengths of the afferent nerves were about 3 – 4 cm. The ampullary capsula was left intact. This preparation was placed on a thermode and continuously superfused with saline solution of a composition appropriate for selachians.

The thermode was circulated by water of constant low temperature (− 5°C). The desired

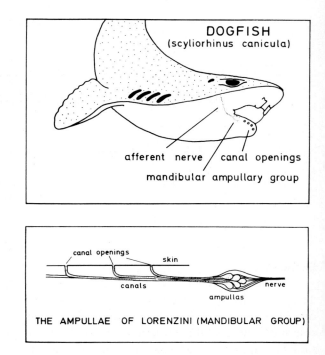

Fig. 1. Schematic drawings of the location and structure of the mandibular group of the ampullae of Lorenzini in the dogfish.

temperatures were obtained by an electric current (DC) passing a heating coil. The stimulus temperature was measured by a thermocouple and regulated by a negative feedback system according to the control voltage which was delivered by a ramp generator (Fig. 2). This arrangement allowed preselection of amplitude and slope of the temperature ramps in a range of 0 − 65°C and 0.001 − 10°C/s, respectively.

Electric currents were applied by large diameter glass micropipettes which were inserted in the ampullary canal. The micropipettes were filled with saline solution and connected to the current source by a platinum wire. For the current controlled stimulation, the voltage at a high series resistance was measured and fed back to a PID controller. The stimulus function was likewise provided by a ramp generator (Fig. 2).

Conventional methods of microdissection were used for extracellular recordings of the impulse activity of single afferent fibres which were placed on a platinum wire. After amplification, a spike level discriminator transformed the action potentials in-

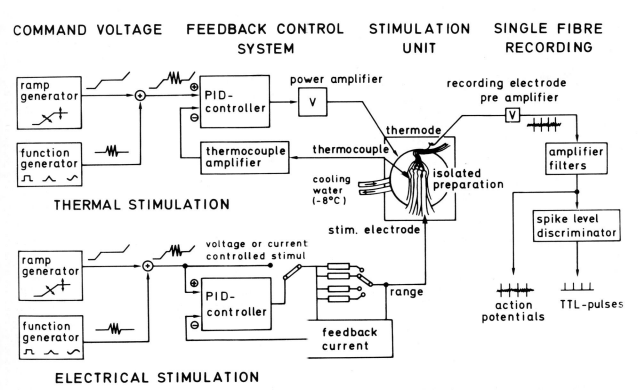

COMMAND VOLTAGE   FEEDBACK CONTROL   STIMULATION   SINGLE FIBRE
                        SYSTEM   UNIT   RECORDING

THERMAL STIMULATION

ELECTRICAL STIMULATION

Fig. 2. Schematic diagram of the experimental arrangement for thermal and electrical stimulation and single fibre recording.

to TTL pulses, which were used for further data analysis. Original recordings. TTL pulses and stimulus parameters were stored on magnetic tape. An audio channel served for documentation. The peri-stimulus–time histograms (given by an impulse counter) and the stimulus parameters were additionally documented by a pen recorder. Furthermore, the stimulus parameters and the interspike intervals were digitised and stored in a microcomputer. Computer aided data analysis included conventional methods (such as interval histograms) as well as special algorithms for identification and quantitation of periodic impulse activity.

Results

Isolated mandibular groups of the ampullae of

Lorenzini were obtained from 18 adult dogfish of a length of about 50–70 cm. Thirty-one single fibres were studied on both electrical and thermal stimulation. Typical frequency responses to current steps and fast temperature changes are illustrated in Fig. 3: frequency overshoot on cathodal currents and cooling, frequency undershoot on anodal currents and warming. On electrical stimulation the impulse frequency gradually approaches its steady state (Fig. 3A, B), whereas a biphasic response characteristic was found on thermal stimulation: the initial overshoot on cooling was followed by an undershoot (Fig. 3C), the initial undershoot on warming was followed by an overshoot (Fig. 3D). Maintained currents did not affect the discharge rate, while the afferent activity was markedly dependent on the actual temperature.

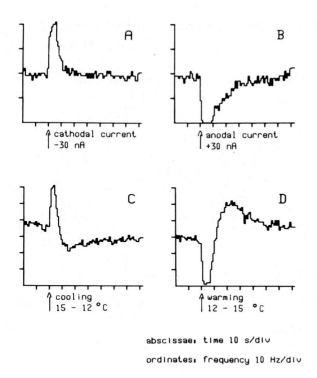

Fig. 3. Characteristic frequency responses of single fibres to step-like electrical stimuli (A, B) and fast temperature changes (C, D).

Frequency responses to ramp-shaped electrical stimuli

The most common types of frequency response characteristics to ramp-shaped electrical stimuli are summarised in Fig. 4. Considering first the four examples of a dynamic frequency increase on cathodal currents (Fig. 4A – D), the dynamic response characteristics appeared to be quite different from each other.

In the first example (Fig. 4A), an initial frequency increase at the beginning of the ramp was immediately followed by adaptation, approaching the steady state. A similar response characteristic is illustrated in Fig. 4B. There was again an initial frequency increase, followed by adaptation. Up to the end of the ramp, however, the impulse frequency remained somewhat higher than the steady state value. In other fibres, as in Fig. 4C, the cur-

rent ramp induced a frequency offset without marked frequency changes during the ongoing ramp. Finally, there were frequency responses, which were characterised by an increasing frequency during the ongoing ramp (Fig. 4D).

The frequency response characteristics to anodal current ramps are illustrated in Fig. 4E and 4F and looked like the counterparts of those of Fig. 4C and 4D. The onset of anodal current ramps induced an initial frequency decrease. During the ongoing ramp the impulse frequency sometimes remained almost constant (Fig. 4E) and sometimes it was further reduced (Fig. 4F). When, as in the example in Fig. 4F, the fibre became competely silent during the ongoing ramp, the impulse activity recovered at the very moment the ramp stopped. Then, as in example 4E, the discharge rate gradually approached its steady state. On anodal currents an inversion of the initial frequency change, a frequency increase during the ongoing ramp, was not observed.

Common characteristics of electrically induced frequency responses were associated with the beginning and the end of the ramps: (1) the onset of a cathodal or anodal current ramp induced a relatively fast frequency increase or decrease, and (2) the end of a current ramp gradually reinstated the original impulse frequency.

The differences of the response characteristics concerned mainly the frequency changes during the ongoing ramps. Qualitatively, almost all types of frequency changes were found. The differences were not only observed in different fibres but also in the same fibre when the slope of the current ramp was changed. For example, the recordings in Fig. 4C and 4D are from the same fibre and all stimulus parameters, except of the slope of the current ramp, were the same. During a current ramp of 0.5 nA/s the impulse frequency remained almost constant (Fig. 4C), whereas a current ramp of 1 nA/s induced a further frequency increase (Fig. 4D).

Frequency responses to ramp-shaped thermal stimuli

Compared to electrical stimulation, the dynamic response characteristics to ramp-shaped thermal stimulation were more complex, but nevertheless rather uniform. The essential principles of the frequency response characteristics to slow cooling and warming ramps are illustrated in Fig. 5A, B. Slow cooling induced a frequency increase at the beginning of the ramp and slow warming led to a frequency decrease. These initial effects were followed by adaptation.

The most interesting effects, however, occurred at the end of the ramps. There was not a gradual transition to the steady state like on electrical stimulation, but there was a second dynamic response which was of inverse direction compared to that at the beginning of the ramp: the end of a cooling ramp induced a dynamic frequency decrease, whereas the end of a warming ramp induced a dynamic frequency increase.

When the steepness of the temperature ramps was enhanced, as illustrated in Fig. 5C, D, the dynamic response characteristics resembled those to step-like temperature stimuli: a first dynamic frequency increase or decrease changes to a second dynamic component of inverse direction. Ramp-

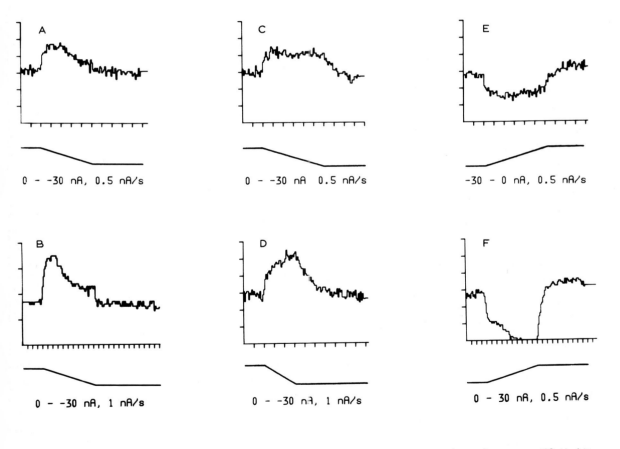

abscissae: time 10 s/div   ordinates: frequency 10 Hz/div

Fig. 4. Different types of dynamic frequency responses of single fibres to ramp-shaped electrical stimulation. A – D: cathodal currents; E,F: anodal currents.

104

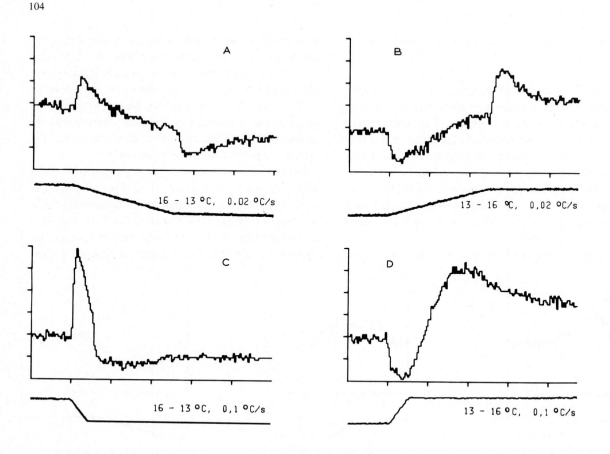

abscissae: time 1 min/div   ordinates: frequency 10 Hz/div

Fig. 5. Frequency response characteristics of a single fibre to slow (A, B) and fast (C, D) ramp-shaped thermal stimulation.

shaped stimulation, however, revealed that the onset of the second dynamic component was again correlated with the end of the stimulus: the frequency decrease was accelerated exactly at the end of a cooling ramp, and a sudden frequency increase occurred exactly at the end of a warming ramp.

Discussion

The dynamic frequency responses of the ampullae of Lorenzini are usually described as frequency overshoot or undershoot followed by adaptation. In contrast to these rather uniform characterisations, ramp-shaped stimulation revealed a broad variety of different response characteristics dependent on the individual fibres as well as on stimulus parameters. Nevertheless, common principles of electrically induced frequency responses on the one hand and thermally induced frequency responses on the other hand could be found. But these experiments also revealed essential qualitative differences in electrically and thermally induced frequency responses.

Considering first the dynamic frequency responses to electrical stimulation the common properties were uniquely related to the beginning and the end of the current ramps. There was (1) a sudden initial frequency change at the beginning of the ramps and (2) a gradual frequency adaptation to the steady state value at the end of the ramps. In contrast, the frequency changes during ongoing ramps were different between different fibres and under different stimulating conditions. Nevertheless, the different frequency responses during ongoing ramps may be ascribed to the same mechanisms that may be responsible for the uniform frequency responses at the beginning and at the end of the ramps: the effects of stimulation and adaptation.

Without discussing the possible underlying receptor mechanisms, the fast frequency change at the beginning of an electrical ramp can be ascribed exclusively to the stimulating effect of the current change. At this moment adaptation is not present, because adaptation, by definition, needs the frequency change to be induced. The opposite is found after the end of an electrical ramp: there is no current change and therefore no stimulating effect, but only adaptation. By these suggestions, it can be expected that the frequency changes at the beginning and the end of the ramps are rather uniform, because only one of the two components, stimulation or adaptation, is involved in the transduction processes.

In contrast, during ongoing current ramps both effects are present. Stimulation and adaptation superpose. The time course of the discharge frequency now depends on which of these effects is the stronger. This again depends on the transduction characteristics of the individual receptors as well as on the stimulus conditions. Therefore a broad variety of frequency changes can be expected. Remembering, for example, the recordings in Fig. 3C, D, it can of course be expected that a current change of 1 nA/s induces a stronger stimulation effect (frequency increase) than a current change of only 0.5 nA/s (constant frequency offset).

On thermal stimulation the situation is more complex. During ongoing temperature ramps not only the stimulating effects of the temperature changes must be considered, but also those of the absolute temperature. As the frequency changes tend to follow the temperature curve, it seems that the effects of adaptation to the actual temperature value are much more pronounced than the stimulating effects of the temperature change.

The second dynamic components at the end of slow temperature ramps demand particular interest. These components can in no way be explained by effects of the temperature change (dT/dt), but uniquely demonstrate that the transition from temperature change to constant temperature (d^2T/dt^2) essentially contributes to the dynamic frequency response. As the effects of an ongoing temperature change seem to be almost negligible, it can correspondingly be assumed that the first dynamic component is primarily caused by the onset of the temperature change and not by the temperature change itself.

These suggestions explain the occurrence of two dynamic frequency components which are exactly correlated with the beginning and the end of slow temperature ramps and which are necessarily of inverse direction. At fast temperature ramps or step-like temperature changes, the time delay between onset and offset of the temperature change is shortened, and it must therefore be expected that the two dynamic components overlap and finally change to a smooth biphasic response.

In this context, it may be of interest that biphasic frequency responses on temperature stimulation were not only induced in the ampullae of Lorenzini, but sometimes also in specific cold and warm receptors (Hellon et al., 1975; Duclaux et al., 1980). We therefore assume that similar effects as described for the ampullae of Lorenzini could be involved in the transduction processes of cold and warm receptors, too, but no results from ramp-shaped stimulation of these receptors are so far available.

Further insight into the transduction processes may be achieved by the methods of impulse pattern analysis. From the analysis of stationary impulse patterns, we know that the impulse activity of the ampullae of Lorenzini is governed by oscillating receptor processes. This corresponds to findings from other thermosensitive receptors (Braun et al., 1984a,b) and can be postulated from interval distributions as in Fig. 6A, B: the interspike intervals are not randomly distributed but concentrated at values which are about integer multiples of a basic discharge period. This implies the existence of an oscillating receptor process which sometimes fails to reach the spike triggering threshold (illustrated by an analogue computer simulation in Fig. 6C). The discharge rate thereby depends on (1) the oscillation period and (2) the probability of spike triggering.

Preliminary results from discharge pattern analysis during dynamic responses indicate that the frequency changes on electrical stimulation were almost exclusively produced by a changed probability of spike triggering, whereas thermal stimulation additionally influenced the oscillation period. According to these results and because of the high synaptic convergence of receptive cells to single afferent fibres, it may be suggested that (1) the oscillating receptor process is located in the afferent nerve terminals and only influenced by tem-perature stimuli, whereas (2) the probability of spike triggering is modulated by synaptic transmission and influenced by both thermal and electrical stimuli.

These suggestions can again be correlated to results reported by Akoev and Andrianov (1980), where a blocking of the synaptic transmission reduced and inverted the frequency responses to thermal stimulation, but completely abolished the frequency responses to electrical stimulation. A combination of these different methodological approaches, including reliable stimulation procedures, experimental manipulation of the synaptic transmission as well as discharge pattern analysis, therefore promises an excellent tool for further elucidation of the transduction processes of this multimodal, secondary sensory system.

Acknowledgements

This work was supported by the Deutsche Forschungsgemeinschaft and the Biologische Anstalt Helgoland.

References

Akoev, G.N. and Andrianov, G.N. (1981) The action of divalent drugs on thermal and electric sensitivity of the ampullae of Lorenzini. In: T. Szabo and G. Gzeh (Eds.), *Sensory Physiology of Aquatic Lower Vertebrates, Advances in Physiological Science,* Vol. 31, Akadémiaí Kiadó, Budapest, pp. 57 – 73.

Akoev, G.N., Ilyinski, O.B. and Zadan, P.M. (1976) Response of electroreceptors (ampullae of Lorenzini) of skates to electric and magnetic fields. *J. Comp. Physiol. A,* 106: 127 – 136.

Akoev, G.N., Volpe, N.O. and Zhadan, G.G. (1980) Analysis of the effects of chemical and thermal stimuli on the ampullae of Lorenzini of the skates. *Comp. Biochem. Physiol.,* 65A: 193 – 201.

Braun, H.A., Schäfer, K. and Wissing, H. (1984a) Theorien und Modelle zum Übertragungsverhalten thermosensitiver Rezeptoren. *Funkt. Biol. Med.,* 3: 26 – 36.

Braun, H.A., Schäfer, K., Wissing, H. and Hensel, H. (1984b) Periodic transduction processes in thermosensitive receptors. In: W. Hamann and A. Iggo (Eds.), *Sensory Receptor Mechanisms,* World Science Publishing Corp., Singapore, pp. 147 – 156.

Bromm, B., Hensel, H. and Tagmut, A.T. (1976) The elec-

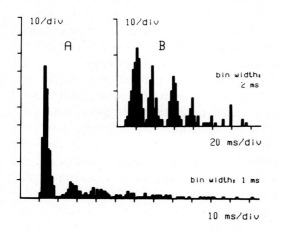

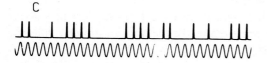

Fig. 6. Multimodal interval distributions of stationary impulse sequences of single fibres (A, B). Analogue computer simulation illustrating the possible transduction mechanisms causing the multimodal interval distribution: spike triggering oscillation superposed by stochastic components (C).

trosensitivity of the isolated ampullae of Lorenzini in the crayfish. *J. Comp. Physiol.,* 111: 127 – 136.

Duclaux, R., Schäfer, K. and Hensel, H. (1980) Response of cold receptors to low skin temperatures in the nose of the cat. *J. Neurophysiol.,* 43: 1571 – 1577.

Hellon, R.F., Hensel, H. and Schäfer, K. (1975) Thermal receptors in the scrotum of the rat. *J. Physiol. (London),* 248: 349 – 375.

Hensel, H. (1955) Quantitative Beziehungen zwischen Temperaturreiz und Aktionspotentialen der Lorenzinischen Ampullen. *Z. Vergl. Physiol.,* 37: 509 – 526.

Murray, R.W. (1957) Evidence for a mechanoreceptive function of the ampullae of Lorenzini. *Nature (London),* 179: 106 – 107.

Murray, R.W. (1962) The response of the ampullae of Lorenzini of the elasmobranchs to electrical stimulation. *J. Exp. Biol.,* 39: 119 – 128.

Waltmann, B. (1966) Electrical properties and fine structure of the ampullary canals of Lorenzini. *Acta Physiol. Scand.,* 66 Suppl. 264: 1 – 60.

W. Hamann and A. Iggo (Eds.)
Progress in Brain Research, Vol. 74
© 1988 Elsevier Science Publishers B.V. (Biomedical Division)

Mechanisms of Transduction II: Summary

W. Hamann

This session started with a paper introducing new approaches to the question of how Merkel cell receptors are organised. The known effects of Ca^{2+} channel blockers on frog type 1 (Ft1) and frog type 2 (Ft2) receptors were reinvestigated in combination with transcutaneous electrical stimulation. Evidence was presented that the latter type of stimulation can reproduce response patterns caused by natural stimulation. However, in Ft1 receptors it was not possible to evoke response patterns attributable to stimulation of primary afferent terminals, thus providing proof of synaptic delay. Ca^{2+} channel blockers were able to reproduce nervous responses caused by mechanical as well as electrical stimulation. A lively discussion developed about the significance of extracellular electrical stimulation. This mode of stimulation is thought to elicit impulses at the first node of Ranvier. It may therefore not provide results relevant to stimulus transduction. Additionally, interpretation of results is not facilitated by the uncertain distribution of transcutaneous current flow. Results were also presented using the presynaptic Ca^{2+} blocker ω-conotoxin. Use of this substance offers a new approach to the still uncertain question whether there is a chemical synapse between Merkel cells and afferent nerve terminals. Experiments with this substance on a primary sensory receptor will considerably enhance the significance of these findings. The original data presented, in a way, put emphasis on the point that full understanding of Merkel cell receptors has to await the development of techniques allowing direct measurements from Merkel cells.

Progress was evident in the knowledge about the ultrastructure of sensory receptors in the pulp and dentine. However, there still remains uncertainty about the function of these receptors. Morphologically, similarity was pointed out between receptor endings in pulp and dentine and the sensitive ending of insect joint receptors. To date it is still not clear why pulp and dentine should have such rich sensory innervation. The rigidity and thermal conductivity of teeth will not permit sensory discrimination to the degree of precision suggested by the density of innervation of dentinal and pulpal tissue. Dr Kruger proposed a dual sensory-effector role for these nerve endings giving them a control function in the Ca^{2+} metabolism of teeth. This hypothesis was supported by the finding of high concentrations of calcitonin gene related peptide in dentinal and pulpal nerve terminals.

Epiphenomena affecting responsiveness may obscure the input – output relationship of transducers in sensory receptors. Especially in mechanoreceptors this may cause difficulties in experiments requiring repetitive stimulation with standard stimuli at relatively short intervals. In muscle spindle a possible mechanism for such an epiphenomenon is the development of stable cross-bridges during contraction of intrafusal muscle fibres. Results were reported in support of this concept in cat soleus muscle. The discussion centred around possible alternative explanations of the experimental findings and on alternative experimental designs. The author suggested the use of hypertonic solutions. The results should also show temperature dependence, as the number of fixed cross-bridges is the function of the temperature. The present findings cannot be explained in terms of rearrangement of extramuscular tissue, because of greater passive tension after conditioning.

Neurones in the area postrema of the rat were found to have properties of chemo- or osmo-receptors. A variety of substances, many of them naturally occurring in the body, were applied, iontophoretically with microelectrodes as well as in gross application, either topically or into the carotid artery. Solutions with high or low osmolarity were also employed. Lithium chloride Ringer was used because of its known effect as an emetic. In view of the multiple effects lithium has on cellular function, it would be useful to know how lithium produces this effect.

The fifth presentation during this session dealt with the question of sensitivity of somatosensory receptors to catecholamines and hypoxia. The topic assumes particular importance with the increasing awareness of the involvement of the autonomic nervous system in many conditions of chronic pain. Eight out of 14 small afferent fibres were excited either by adrenaline or by hypoxia or by both. This is at variance with in vivo investigations on cutaneous nociceptors, which are not normally excited by efferent sympathetic stimulation. The authors offered as an explanation the possibility of previous damage caused by transient hypoxia during dissection of this in vitro preparation. Similarly some joint nociceptors require preconditioning with inflammation to be activated. In more general terms this raises the question of the nature of adequate stimuli for many nociceptors.

The session concluded with an investigation into transduction characteristics of the ampullae of Lorenzini in the dogfish. Sensory receptors in the ampulla are of the secondary type and may be excited by thermal as well as by electric field stimuli. An attractive hypothesis was presented for the organisation of these receptors. Impulses in primary afferent fibres were found to be distributed in intervals representing multiples of standard time units. It was therefore assumed that primary afferent terminals in these receptors function as oscillators (frequency of 50 Hz in the example given), with electrical stimuli influencing the probability of firing and thermal stimuli additionally controlling the oscillation period. In the discussion the terminal branching pattern was offered as an explanation for the irregular firing pattern. The author did not agree with the idea that changing ion composition of the jelly overlying the receptor cells was an important parameter affecting stimulus transduction.

Visceral Receptors, Chemoreception and Molecular Aspects of Receptor Function

W. Hamann and A. Iggo (Eds.)
Progress in Brain Research, Vol. 74
© 1988 Elsevier Science Publishers B.V. (Biomedical Division)

CHAPTER 14

Comparative anatomy of vertebrate electroreceptors

K.H. Andres and M. von Düring

Ruhr-Universität Bochum, Abteilung für Neuroanatomie, Postfach 102148, 4630 Bochum, FRG

Introduction

Electrosensitivity plays an important role in the biological activities of fish and amphibia for prey detection, feeding behaviour and social communication (for review see Bullock, 1982; Bullock and Heiligenberg, 1986), and its significance is reflected in the number of sensory cells and the amount of nerve supply which ranks in the order of other sensory systems. In elasmobranchs the ampullae of Lorenzini are electrosensitive receptors (Murray, 1960, 1962, 1974; Dijkgraaf and Kalmijn, 1963; Bennett and Clusin, 1978) with a known morphological structure and innervation (Retzius, 1898; Metcalf, 1916; Dotterweich, 1932; Waltman, 1966; Derbin, 1970; Szabo et al., 1972; Murray, 1974). Two types of electroreceptors are characteristic in teleost as well as non-teleost fishes and in some amphibia: the ampullary and the tuberous receptor organs (for review see Szabo, 1974; Zakon, 1986). Ampullary receptors occur in most non-teleosts, in Siluriformes (Mullinger, 1964; Sato and Katagiri, 1969; Wachtel and Szamier, 1969; Srivastava and Seal, 1980), Mormyriformes (Derbin, 1974; Szamier and Bennett 1974), Gymnotiformes (Szamier and Wachtel 1970; Derbin and Denizot, 1971), in a subfamily of the Osteoglossomorpha, in Xenomystinae (Jörgensen and Bullock, 1987) and in some amphibians as in aquatic urodela (Bullock et al., 1983; Fritzsch and Wahnschaffe, 1983). Tuberous receptors however, are only observed in Gymnotiformes (Wachtel and Szamier, 1964; Szamier and

Wachtel, 1970) and Mormyriformes (Derbin and Szabo, 1968). Recently, a type of tuberous receptor was described in one species of Siluriformes, Pseudocetopsis sp. (Andres et al., 1988).

Recently, electrosensitivity was observed in the monotreme mammal *Ornithorhynchus anatinus* (Scheich and Langer, 1986) by evoked cortical potentials using artificial electric fields. Direct electrical stimulation of spots of the lateral bill skin in platypus established that the electroreceptors are located in the bill (Gregory et al., 1986). The presumed electroreceptors are associated with specialised cutaneous glands which contain the gland duct sensory receptors in platypus as well as in echidna (Andres and von Düring, 1984).

For comparison of this newly discovered sensory system in monotremes with the well-known electroreceptors in fish we first describe the structure of ampullae of Lorenzini in different chondrichthyes. In a second part we focus on electroreceptors in holocephali, which exhibit in addition to the ampullae of Lorenzini a type of microampullae in a characteristic arrangement together with specialised epidermal glands. In a third part, we present the unique structure of the sensory gland duct receptors of the platypus bill associated with special mucous and serous glands.

Ampullae of Lorenzini in chondrichthyes

The ampulla of Lorenzini consists of one or several alveoli at the blind end of a jelly-filled tube, which opens in a pore on the skin surface. The alveoli are

114

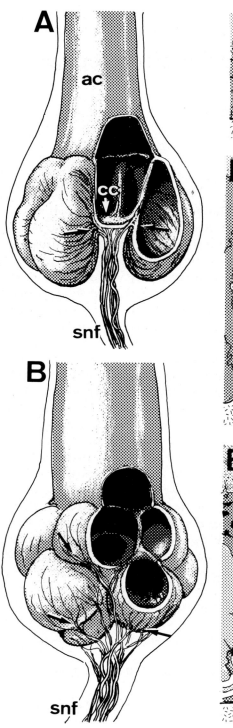

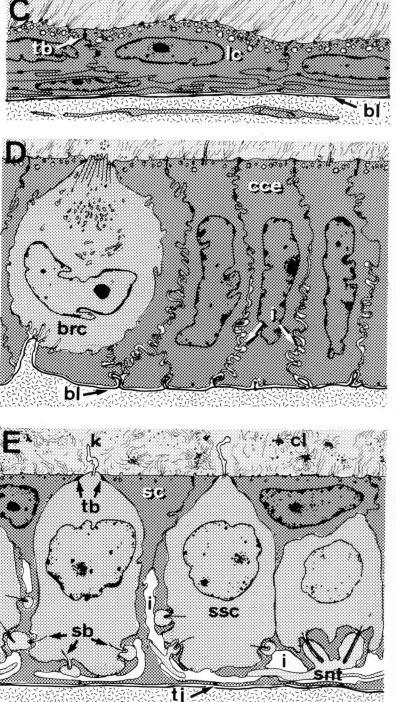

grouped in clusters mainly restricted to the skin of the head. The tubes may expand and open to many directions to the dorsal, lateral and ventral body surface in a species specific distribution pattern and the length may differ remarkably even in one species (Murray, 1960; Rashi, 1978; Chu and Meng, 1979; Bodznick and Schmidt, 1984; Fields, 1982; Bodznick and Boord, 1986). In rays and skates the canal length may extend up to half of the body size. The mini-ampullae of freshwater rays, however, exhibit very short canals of about 300 – 500 μm length (Szabo et al., 1972; Szamier and Bennett, 1980).

Raschi (1984) documented in 40 species of skates the topography, distribution and density of the ampullae. He found a correlation between his data and the territory, habitat and special feeding mode of the fish. In *Raja erinacea* which feeds mainly on benthic invertebrates the receptor density with about 1 pore/cm^2 is highest on the ventral body side in contrast to *Raja alba* as a predatory fish with only 0.04 pores/cm^2 on its ventral side. In *Manta birostris*, however, a fish with a filter-feeding behaviour, one small group of ampullae of Lorenzini occurs on each side of the head (Chu and Meng, 1979).

Three types of ampullae can be distinguished in chondrichthyes with regard to the length of the canal and the size and differentiation of the alveolus: macro-ampullae, micro-ampullae and mini-ampullae.

The macro-ampullae (known as the ampullae of Lorenzini) are macroscopically identified by large pores in the skin surface. They have long jelly-filled canals which lead to clustered alveoli in restricted skin regions of the head. Five groups of macro-ampullae are described in relation to the special topography of the head (Chu and Meng, 1979). They are the most common type (Fig. 1A). Mini-ampullae are only observed with the microscope due to the small alveoli, relatively short canals and small pores. Mini-ampullae of freshwater rays are distributed over the body surface. They are described in *Potamotrygon circularis* (Szabo et al., 1972; Szamier and Bennett, 1980). We also observe these mini-ampullae in *Potamotrygon motoro* and *Paratrygon laticeps*. The alveoli lie adjacent to the epidermal layer. Short twisted canals of about 450 μm length open into small pores. For a third group of ampullae of Lorenzini we propose the term micro-ampullae. Micro-ampullae occur in restricted areas of the maxillary and the mandibular processes of Holocephali (Fig. 1B) and Hexanchidae. The length of the canals varies from 1.5 mm to 10 mm depending on their location. They open into pores of varying diameter from 20 to 100 μm (Fig. 10).

Several types of ampullary alveoli are observed (Dotterweich, 1932; Chu and Meng, 1979). With regard to the alveolus arrangement we propose the following classification: (1) single alveolate type, (2) multi-alveolate type, (3) branched alveolate type, (4) centrum cap type, (5) club-shaped type. A special arrangement of bundled canals and a special of alveolus is described in the ampullae of Hexanchus (Dotterweich, 1932). In *Heptranchias*

Fig. 1. Semi-schematic representation of ampullae of Lorenzini with two types of alveoli: macro-ampulla of the centrum cap type (A) and micro-ampulla of a multi-alveolate type (B) and the epithelial differentiation of the ampullae (C, D, E). (A) Macro-ampulla of the centrum cap type of *Scyliorhynus canicula*. Section through the alveolus wall exhibits the interior with the rib-like extensions of the centrum cap (cc). Note the course of the unmyelinated axons from the base of the connective tissue papilla of the centrum cap and along the rib-like extensions between adjacent alveoli; entrance zone of the axons into the sensory epithelium (arrows); ampullary canal (ac); sensory nerve fibre bundle (snf). (B) Micro-ampulla of the multi-alveolate type of Callorhynchus with its nerve supply. Axons enter the sensory epithelium at different sites (arrows); sensory nerve fibre bundle (snf). (C) Lining epithelium of the ampullary canal. Lining cells (lc) with secretory granules; filamentous material attached to the surface; terminal bar (tb); narrow intercellular space with interdigitations; basement lamella (bl). (D) Segment of the centrum cap epithelium with the columnar epithelial cells (cce) and a kind of brush cell (brc); distinct intercellular space (i) with strands of basement lamella (bl). (E) Segment of the sensory epithelium with main structures of sensory cell (ssc), supporting cell (cs) and sensory nerve terminals (snt); kinocilium (k); synaptic bar (sb); corpuscular layer (cl); intercellular space (i); terminal bar (tb); tight junction (tj).

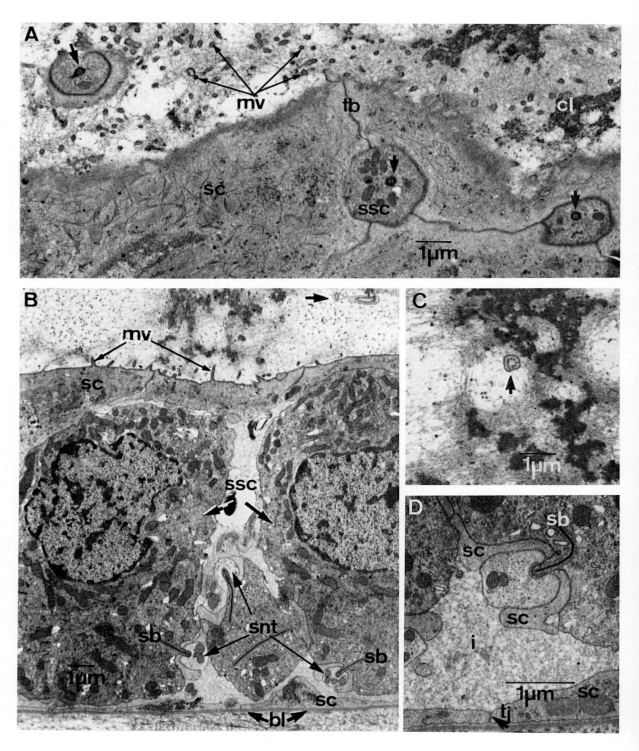

perlo we observe a similar arrangement of canals of micro-ampullae bundled up into three or six which open as groups in a small pit of about 200 – 300 μm. The alveoli, however, are of the multi-alveolate type.

Ultrastructure of the ampullae of Lorenzini (centrum cap type)

As a characteristic example of the structural organization of the ampullae of Lorenzini we focus on the ampullae of the dogfish *Scyliorhinus caniculus*. The macro-ampullae of Scyliorhinus are of the centrum cap type.

The centrum cap is composed of a connective tissue papilla invading the ampulla from its base. It separates the single alveoli from each other and extends between neighbouring alveoli in a rib-like fashion (Fig. 1A).

The epithelium of the centrum cap separates the sensory epithelia of the adjoining alveoli. It is a stratified columnar epithelium with large intercellular spaces and interdigitations to the neighbouring cells (Fig. 1D). Strands of basement lamella penetrate in the basal intercellular clefts. The apical part of the cell contains numerous granules with mucous secretion. The structure of the jelly-like material overlying the centrum cap epithelium exhibits the same filamentous structure as the contents in the granules. A type of brush cell is observed in the centrum cap epithelium at the border to the sensory epithelium. The cell is characterised by a decoration of stiff microvilli on its apical surface. The cytoplasm of the brush cell contains numerous profiles of rough and smooth endoplasmic reticulum. This type of brush cell

usually occurs in a comparable topography in the epithelium which borders the sensory epithelium of lateral line organs. Mitotic figures are regularly observed in the centrum cap epithelium at the border of the sensory epithelium. The sensory epithelium consists of sensory and supporting cells. It is covered with a special corpuscular layer of extracellular material (Fig. 1E).

The corpuscular layer varies from 2 to 12 μm in thickness in fixed material. It is composed of a filamentous material in a net-like arrangement containing large osmiophilic particles and profiles (Fig. 2A,B,C). It is restricted to the sensory epithelium.

The sensory epithelium borders with the cap epithelium and the epithelium of the marginal zone which is continuous to the lining cells of the canal (Fig. 1). The supporting cells extend from the basement lamella to the luminal surface. Some slender microvilli and one short kinocilium decorate the large surface area and project into the corpuscular layer. A terminal bar is observed throughout the epithelial surface of the ampulla (Fig. 2). An obvious wide intercellular space in the basal third of the sensory epithelium is filled with a filamentous material and contains the unmyelinated afferent axonal branches (Fig. 2D). Basal processes of the supporting cells, which are connected by tight junctions, form a complete sheath adjacent to the basement lamella. The sensory cell contacts the corpuscular layer with a small area of $3.5 - 4$ μm^2 and bears one short kinocilium of about 5 μm in length (Fig. 1E, 2A). In cross-sections near the base of the kinocilium nine double filaments arranged as $8 + 1$ are obvious, more distally the microtubules are arranged $9 + 0$. The exposed

---

Fig. 2. Sections of the sensory epithelium of the ampulla of Lorenzini of the dogfish *Scyliorhinus caniculus*. (A) Apical part of the sensory epithelium in tangential section with sensory cells (ssc) each containing a basal body (arrows) and supporting cells (sc) with a net of tonofilaments; terminal bar (tb); microvilli (mv) of the supporting cell project into the corpuscular layer (cl). (B) Arrangement of synapses at the basis of sensory cells (ssc) with sensory nerve terminals (snt); synaptic bar (sb); basement lamella (bl); microvilli (mv); supporting cell (sc); kinocilium (arrow). (C) Elements of the extracellular material of the corpuscular layer with one sensory kinocilium in cross-section (arrow). (D) Senso-neuronal synapse with a cuff of supporting cell cytoplasm (sc) inserted between the sensory cell and the afferent nerve fibre terminal; synaptic bar (sb); intercellular space (i) with filamentous material; tight junction (tj) between the basal supporting cell processes.

luminal area of the sensory cell is only 0.6% of the total cell surface. Neighbouring sensory cells are closely attached together. Gap junctions are not observed. At the lateral and basal parts of the sensory cells unmyelinated segments of myelinated axons are in synaptic contact with the sensory cells. Long synaptic bars (5 μm in length) covered with spherical vesicles occur opposite to the afferent nerve fibre terminals. They are located within ridge-like evaginations invading the axon profile (Waltman, 1966; Derbin, 1970; Szabo, 1972; Murray, 1974). The ridge-like evagination of the sensory cell is surrounded by a small cuff of supporting cell cytoplasm giving the impression of a cellular isolation of the senso-neuronal synapse (Fig. 2D). The nerve fibre terminals, however, are incompletely covered with supporting cell processes, thus being in direct contact with the large intercellular space. We observed 4 – 6 synapses per sensory cell.

The sensory epithelium of the ampullae is only innervated by myelinated nerve fibres. In the submandibular group, we regularly saw 16 myelinated axons (10 μm in diameter), supplying one ampulla with eight clustered alveoli. The nerve fibres lose the myelin sheath about 150 – 200 μm before they enter the sensory epithelium. The myelinated fibres split up into several unmyelinated branches. They traverse the connective tissue of the rib-like extensions of the centrum cap in bundles of up to 16 nerve fibres to enter the sensory epithelium from the medial to the most lateral part of the alveoli

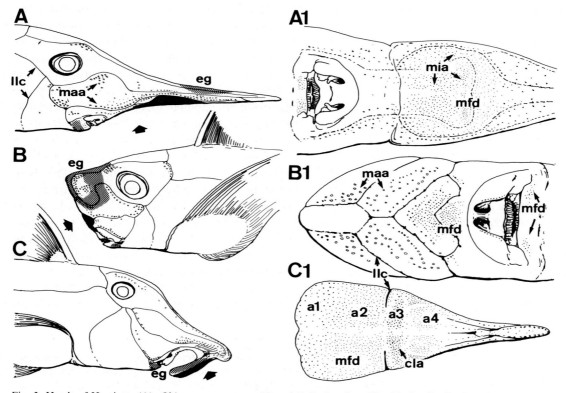

Fig. 3. Heads of Harriotta (A), *Chimaera monstrosa* (B) and Callorhynchus (C) with the distribution of cutaneous sensory organs. Pores of macro-ampullae (maa); fields of micro-ampullae (dark hatching); areas of epidermal glands (eg, light hatching); thick black arrows indicate views in $A_1 - C_1$. Lateral line channels (llc). Ventral view of the rostral processes of Harriotta (A_1), Chimaera (B_1) and Callorhynchus (C_1). Micro-ampullae (mia); fields of micro-ampullae (mfd); club-shaped ampullae (cla); pores of macro-ampullae (maa); the field of micro-ampullae in C_1 is divided into subareas (a1 – a4); channels of lateral line (llc).

(Fig. 1A). The axons arborise and spread in the enlarged intercellular space of the basal third of sensory epithelium partly covered with supporting cell processes. Waltman (1966), however, described the course of the unmyelinated axons in the ampullae of Lorenzini of rays in just the opposite direction from the border of the marginal zone.

The epithelium of the marginal zone between the alveoli and the canal is similar in structure to the epithelium of the centrum cap but is simple columnar. A continuous transition to the pseudo-stratified squamous canal lining cells with a basal cell layer containing bundles of tonofibrils occurs at the entrance of the canal. The intercellular space between these canal cells is narrow with interdigitations and desmosomes. The cells lining the lumen of the ampullary canal contain granules with mucous secretion (Fig. 1C). The jelly-like material in the canal exhibits fine structural arrangements and nets of filaments comparable to the material overlying the centrum cap epithelium.

Specialised electrosensitive ampullary fields of holocephali (Chimaera, Harriotta and Callorhynchus)

Generally, the differentiation of the rostral process in elasmobranchs is believed to depend on the development and distribution of ampullae of Lorenzini (Merkel, 1890, cited in Dotterweich, 1932). Among the holocephali, Callorhynchus shows an extraordinary differentiated rostral process which has been inverted at its distal segment and is formed into a kind of ploughshare. Harriotta with an elongated process and *Chimaera monstrosa* with a blunt rostral process seem less specialised (Fig. 3A – C). Pores of micro-ampullae in a special arrangement and density open into the surface of the rostral process. They are intermingled with pores of epidermal glands (Figs. $3A_1 - C_1$, 4). The density of ampullary pores in these special restricted areas varies between 0.3 and 1.3 pore/mm^2.

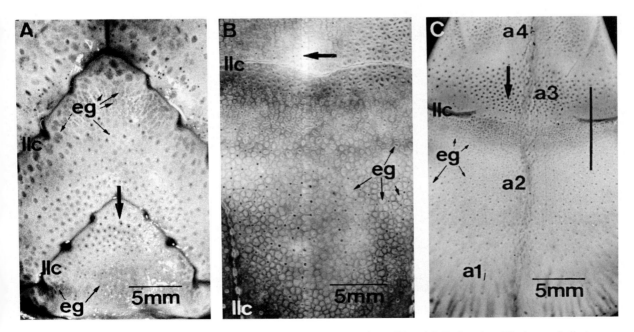

Fig. 4. Surface view of a part of the rostral processes of Chimaera (A), Harriotta (B) and Callorhynchus (C). Arrows indicate areas with the densest arrangement of pores of micro-ampullae; channels of lateral line (llc); a1 – a4 differentiate in their pore pattern in Callorhynchus; perpendicular bar in area 2/area 3 indicates the direction of section in Fig. 10; epidermal glands (eg).

The most differentiated pore pattern is obvious in the rostral process of Callorhynchus. The ventral side of the ploughshare facing to the ground shows four areas which differ in pore size and pore density (Figs. 3C$_1$, 4C). Area 1 is characterised by single pores (150 μm in diameter) and a density of 0.6 pore/mm^2. Area 2 exhibits an ampullary pore density of 1/mm^2. The pore diameter is about

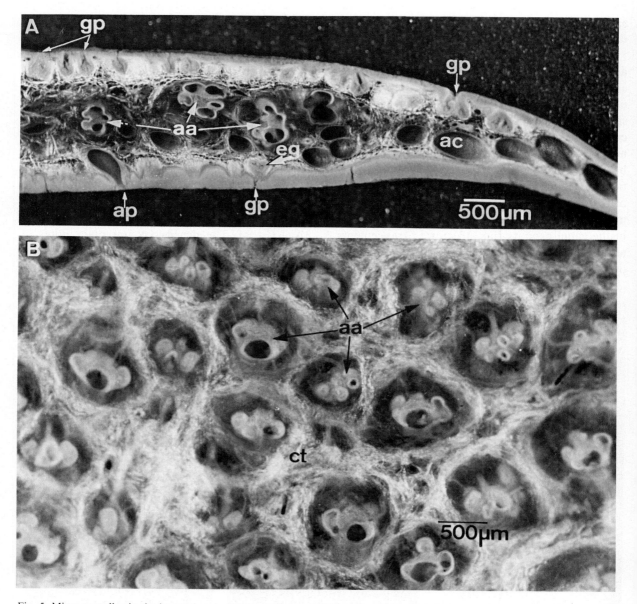

Fig. 5. Micro-ampullae in the inverted rostral process of area 1 (A) and area 2 (B) of Callorhynchus. (A) Sagittal section of area 1. Pores of the micro-ampullae (ap) open exclusively to the side facing the ground. Gland pores (gp) open into the ventral and dorsal side of the process; alveoli of the multi-alveolate type (aa) and their diagonal canals (ac) within the connective tissue; epidermal glands (eg). (B) Tangential section through the subepidermal layer of area 2 showing the dense arrangement of the alveoli of the micro-ampullae (aa) separated by densely arranged collagenous tissue (ct).

80 – 100 μm. Clustered pores of epidermal glands (20 – 50 μm) are intermingled (Figs. 5, 6). Area 3 shows small and large single pores (80 μm, 200 – 250 μm) with a density of up to 4/mm^2 (Fig. 9). Area 4 shows a pore pattern and pore density similar to area 2 (Figs. 3C$_1$, 4C). The single pores of the area 1 belong to micro-ampullae with oblique canals of 4 – 5 mm length. The straight canals of the micro-ampullae (multi-alveolate type) in area 2 are shorter, most of them 2 mm in length. Area 3 is characterised by micro-ampullae with two types of alveoli. Ampullae of a simple alveolate type with 2.6 mm long straight canals open into the small pores and ampullae of the club-shaped type and oblique tubes with 0.8 – 1 cm length open into the large pores (Fig. 10).

The epidermal glands show a special pattern of distribution in Chimaera, Harriotta and Callorhynchus. They occur together with the micro-ampullae on the rostral processes of the maxilla and on the mandibular processes. On the dorsal processes of the maxilla they also occur in isolated fields without micro-ampullae (Fig. 3A – C). The glands in all the fields are of a simple branched alveolar type. The alveoli protruding into the adjacent connective tissue layer are connected with short gland ducts. Three cell types are

observed, epidermal spinous cells, branched brush cells and lining cells with stereocilia (Figs. 7, 8). The epidermal cells contain bundles of tonofibrils. They are mainly located in the basal part of the alveoli. The branched brush cell extends from the basement lamella to the lumen of the gland. It contacts the lumen at several sites with a brush of short microvilli. Its basal cell membrane is densely infolded whereas interdigitations and desmosomes are numerous on the lateral sides. The lining cells mainly cover the surface of the alveoli. They exhibit large granules in their apical cytoplasm. The stereocilia of the lining cells with a distinct coat of filamentous material are short in the alveoli and their length increases in the gland duct to about 16 μm (Figs. 7, 8B). The luminal side of the gland is sealed by a continuous terminal bar between the lining cells and the branched brush cells. Small unmyelinated axons are observed to enter the gland. In contrast to Callorhynchus and Harriotta, the epidermis of Chimaera contains numerous mucous cells in addition to the epidermal glands.

About 17 000 myelinated nerve fibres supply the rostral process in Callorhynchus and most of the fibres probably innervate the ampullae besides the fibres innervating the lateral line organs and stretch receptors of the connective tissue. A

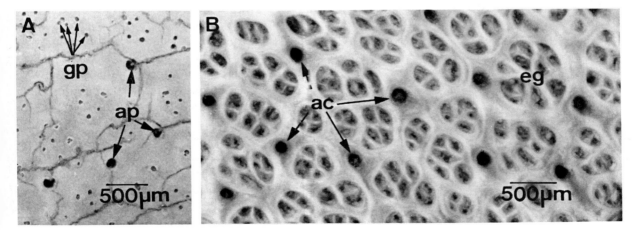

Fig. 6. Sections of area 2 of the rostral process of Callorhynchus. (A) Pores of micro-ampullae (ap) and pores of epidermal glands (gp) characterise area 2. (B) Tangential section through the basal epidermal layer of area 2; ampullary canals (ac); alveoli of the epidermal glands (eg).

122

preliminary calculation in Callorhynchus exhibits a ratio of 10 – 20 nerve fibres per ampulla.

Chimaera, Harriotta and Callorhynchus live on the sea bed where visual and olfactory orientation may not be sufficient for benthic feeding behaviour. The occurrence of macro- and micro-ampullae, the fields of micro-ampullae and their association with special epidermal glands in the rostral process of holocephali indicate that it represents a highly specialised electrosensory

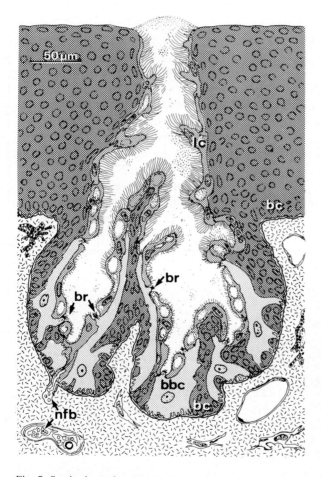

Fig. 7. Semi-schematic representation of the epidermal gland of Callorhynchus. Branched brush cells (bbc) extend from the base to the lumen of the alveolus; bundle of microvilli (br); basal epidermal cells (bc); lining cells (lc) with secretory granules and short stereocilia in the alveolus and long stereocilia in the duct and pore segment; nerve fibre bundle (nfb).

organ. The function of the epidermal glands is still obscure. Possibly they are involved in a kind of electrolyte secretion, which may be controlled by the efferent innervation. This secretion could influence the electric resistance of the epidermis and/or modulate the electric field pattern or vectors of current density.

Sensory innervation of gland duct segments in the platypus bill

Neurophysiological experiments have demonstrated that the skin of the platypus bill contains electroreceptors (Gregory et al., 1986). However, it is still an open question which of the numerous sensory structures in the bill are responsible for the electroreception.

The platypus bill is a very richly innervated sensory organ with different types of receptors (Wilson and Martin 1893; Poulton, 1894; Bohringer, 1981; Andres and von Düring, 1984). The push-rod with epidermal Merkel cell – neurite complexes, intra-epidermal vesicle chain receptors and paciniform corpuscles probably represents a specialised mechanoreceptive organ. The afferent nerve endings localised in intra-epidermal gland duct segments of specialised cutaneous glands of the bill, however, are unique in structure and occurrence as compared to all known tissue receptors in vertebrates (Andres and von Düring, 1984).

The platypus bill is characterised by three types of cutaneous glands: a mucous gland without sensory innervation (mns type), a mucous gland with sensory innervation (ms type) and a serous gland with sensory innervation (ss type) (Fig. 11). All three gland types are composed of four main segments: (1) the secretory tubules with a main and an accessory segment, (2) the subdermal segment with a coiled and an isthmic portion, (3) the dermal segment with a straight and subpapillary portion, (4) the epidermal segment with a papillary portion, a coiled sinus portion and a pore portion (Fig. 12). These segments correspond to similar segments of mammalian eccrine sweat glands. This is also true for the location and distribution of the myo-

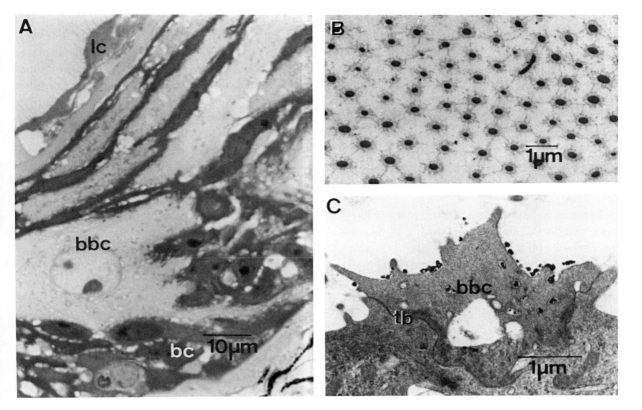

Fig. 8. Cellular composition of the epidermal glands of *Chimaera monstrosa*. (A) Semi-thin section of the secretory alveolus with basal epidermal cells (bc), branched brush cells (bbc) and lining cells with stereocilia (lc). (B) Coat of filamentous material around the stereocilia. (C) Apical cell surface of the branched brush cell bbc). Black particles characterise the surface of the brush; terminal bar (tb).

epithelial cells. In contrast to normal sweat glands, the glands of the platypus bill exhibit striking structural specialisations of the intra-epidermal gland duct segments indicating a strange function. Furthermore, the distinct mucous secretion in the mucous glands of the platypus bill never occurs in sweat glands.

The cells of the four segments differ in morphological characteristics due to a special secretory and transport function. Terminals of the autonomic nervous system are regularly observed in contact with the cells of the secretory tubules of all three types of glands.

The mucous glands without sensory duct innervation (mns type) open into a pore, which looks like a rose blossom due to the arrangement of the

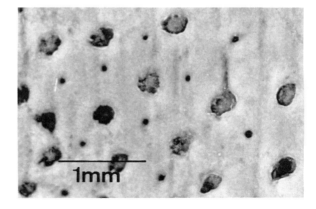

Fig. 9. Pore pattern of area 3 of the rostral process of Callorhynchus. Micro-ampullae of a simple alveolate type open into the small pores, large pores belong to the micro-ampullae of the club-shaped type. Notice the scratching stripes on the epidermal surface.

124

superficial epidermal cells (Fig. 11B). The coiled secretory tubules exhibit abundant mucous cells, cells with numerous dark granules and several mitochondria-rich cells which argue for a complex secretion varying in ionic and mucous composition. The lining cells of the duct are sealed up by a terminal bar towards the luminal surface. The subpapillary part of the dermal segment is characterised by a special enlargement of the basal cell layer due to distinct infoldings of the basal cytoplasmic membrane associated with mitochondria.

The mucous glands with sensory innervation (ms type) exhibit the largest pores with a blossom-like appearance in the scanning micrograph (Fig. 11C). The distribution pattern of the pores of the two mucous glands is mostly arranged in broad (ms glands) and smaller (mns glands) longitudinal stripes on the surface of the bill (Figs. 11A, 15A, A_1, 15B, B_1).

The secretory tubules of the ms glands contain the same types of secretory cells with an increased number of bright mucous cells. While the mns gland exhibits a 50 μm long papillary portion of the intra-epidermal duct segment the epidermal papilla of the ms gland extends about 150 μm down into

the stratum papillare of the dermis. Within this papilla a club-shaped extension with an inner and outer core is inserted between the basal cell layer and the lining cells of the duct lumen. The outer core is subdivided into an outer dark and an inner bright cell layer, both composed of flat cells. The flattened cell layer of the dark outer core presents a prominent intercellular space bridged by many desmosomes in association with its dense tonofibril system (Fig. 13). The inner core faces to the lining cells of the gland duct. It shows two or three layers of bright and polygonal epidermal cells often enlarged up to 30 μm in diameter. These cells and the bright cells of the outer core are closely attached together with interdigitations and serial desmosomes, thus forming a narrow intercellular space.

The base of the epidermal papilla is surrounded by a plexus of a few up to 30 myelinated nerve fibres forming a cuff of 50 μm around the basal part of the enlargement. This nerve fibre plexus carries the afferent innervation for the sensory endings which are located in the club-shaped enlargement. The nerve fibres penetrate 10 μm deep in the basal epidermal cell layer where they lose their myelin sheath. They terminate with very

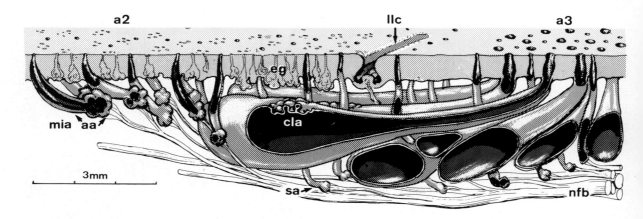

Fig. 10. Semi-schematic representation of the micro-ampulla field. The segment displays parts of area 2 and area 3 (section direction indicated in Fig. 4) of the rostral process of Callorhynchus. Micro-ampullae (mia) of the multi-alveolate type (aa) and epidermal glands (eg) with their pores characterise area 2 (a2); micro-ampullae of a simple alveolate type (sa) with straight canals and micro-ampullae of the club-shaped type (cla) with oblique canals open into area 3 (a3). Note the dense pattern of ampullary pores of area 3; nerve fibre bundle (nfb); lateral line channel (llc).

short and thin sensory nerve endings. Criteria for characterising the types of sensory endings are the structure and size of the initial nodal segment and the shape and length of the unmyelinated free intra-epidermal terminal. With regard to the diameter of the initial nodal segment two types of endings can be distinguished in the ms gland. The initial nodal segments of type 1 and type 2 have diameters of 10 μm and 6 μm, respectively. About 80 – 90% of the sensory endings are of type 1. They display enlargements of the axonal membrane due to impressive invaginations of flattened Schwann cell processes (Fig. 13). The unmyelinated parts of both types present a bulb-like swelling (5 μm) with a slender process (up to 15 μm in length, 0.8 – 1 μm in diameter). A prominent receptor matrix defined in its structural elements by Andres and von Düring (1972) lies adjacent to

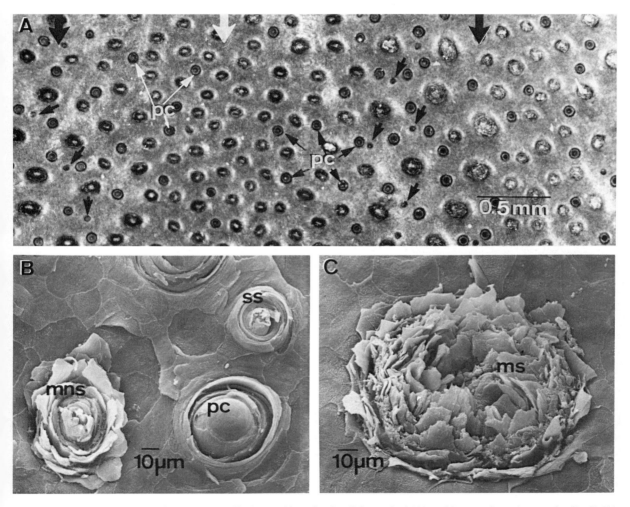

Fig. 11. Pore pattern of the Ornithorhynchus bill observed in reflecting light method (A) and in scanning micrographs (B, C) (A) Surface view of the upper bill; black arrows indicate areas with pores of large mucous glands with a sensory duct innervation; white arrow marks a field with pores of mucous glands without sensory duct innervation; pores of serous glands with sensory duct innervation (small arrows); cones of push-rod (pc). (B) Pore of the serous gland with sensory duct innervation (ss) and a mucous gland without sensory duct innervation (mns). (C) Pore of a large mucous gland with sensory duct innervation (ms). Note the blossom-like arrangement of the superficial epidermal cells.

the membrane of the bulb-like swelling. It extends with its filamentous component into the slender axonal process. The axonal bulb is located in the dark outer core, the slender axonal process terminates in invaginations of the bright outer core cells at the border to the inner core (Figs. 13, 14A,C).

The serous glands have a typical small pore (about 40 μm in diameter) surrounded by a smooth ring-like elevation of superficial epidermal cells (Fig. 11B). The gland cells in the secretory coil resemble typical sweat gland cells with dark cells bordering the lumen and clear cells more deeply situated, surrounding intercellular canaliculi. The

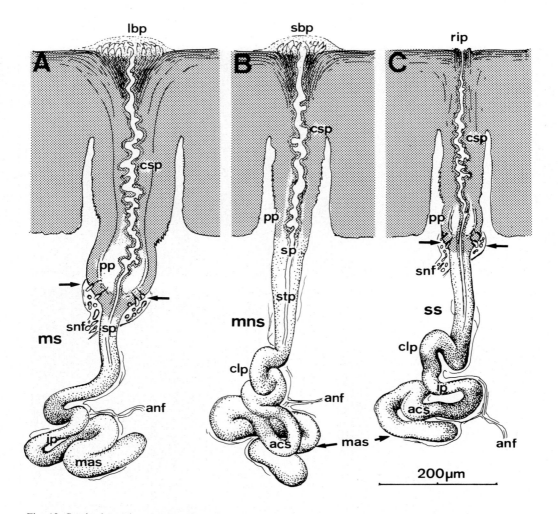

Fig. 12. Semi-schematic representation of three types of cutaneous glands of the Ornithorhynchus bill and their duct segments. (A) Mucous gland with sensory duct innervation (ms) with a large blossom-like pore (lbp). (B) Mucous gland without sensory duct innervation (mns) with a small blossom-like pore (sbp). (C) Serous gland with sensory duct innervation (ss) with a ring-like pore (rip). Secretory tubules with main segment (mas) and accessory segment (acs); subdermal segment with isthmic portion (ip) and coiled portion (clp); dermal segment with straight portion (stp) and subpapillary portion (sp); intra-epidermal segment with a papillary (pp) and a coiled sinus portion (csp) and the pore portion. Note the myelinated sensory axons (snf) and the location of the nerve terminals (arrows) in the club-like enlargement of the papillary portion of the intra-epidermal duct segment in A and C. Autonomic nerve fibres (anf) terminate at all three types of gland tubules.

epidermal papilla of the serous gland protrudes 50 µm less deep into the stratum papillare than the papilla of the ms gland. The enlargement of the papillary portion of the epidermal duct segment is smaller in size but consists of the same structural elements (Figs. 12C, 13, 14B). Its basal part is surrounded by a plexus of up to 22 afferent myelinated nerve fibres forming a cuff of 20 µm thickness. The sensory nerve fibres enter the papilla in the whole circumference to end in the enlargement.

The initial nodal segments of the myelinated axons supplying the serous gland duct also present different diameters. Four types of endings can be distinguished: type 1 with 10 µm, type 2 with 6 µm, type 3 with 2.5 – 3 µm and type 4 with 2 – 2.5 µm.

The myelinated axons of type 1 and type 2 have already been described in the ms gland. The myelinated axon of type 3 enters the basal epidermal cell layer similar to type 1 and type 2. The myelinated axon of type 4 loses its myelin sheath at the smooth epidermal border. In contrast to type 1 and type 2 the unmyelinated segments of type 3 and type 4 split up into a few unmyelinated branches (up to 15 µm and 19 µm, respectively, in length) (Fig. 13B). On average we observed in one serous gland duct the following amount of the different types of endings: four terminals of type 1, 11 terminals of type 2, five terminals of type 3 and two terminals of type 4.

The pores of the serous gland are scattered throughout the whole bill surface with higher den-

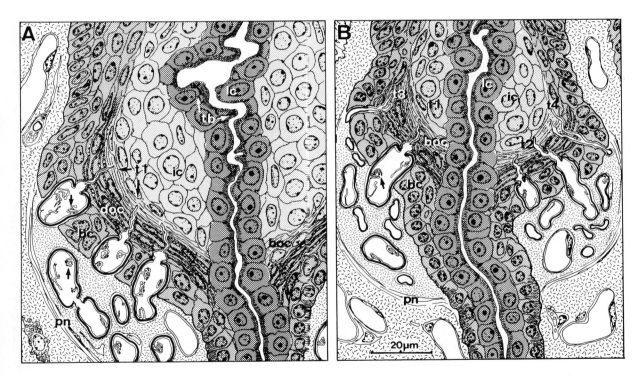

Fig. 13. Semi-schematic representation of the sensory innervated intra-epidermal duct segments of the large mucous gland (A) and the serous gland (B) of the Ornithorhynchus bill. Myelinated axons with different diameters are finally located within the basal epidermal layer or at the epidermal border. They terminate as single or branched unmyelinated axonal processes (t1; t2; t3; t4) within the bright outer core (boc); basal epidermal cell layer (bc); dark outer core (doc); inner core (ic); lining cells (lc) of the duct; terminal bar (tb). Note the distinct intercellular space of the dark outer core in contrast to the narrow intercellular space of the bright inner core. Enlargement of the axonal membrane within the initial nodal segment due to invagination of flattened Schwann cell processes (arrows); perineural sheath (pn).

sities in restricted areas such as the palatal and lip ridges (Fig. 15C, C_1, 15D, D_1). This distribution pattern is similar to the pattern of the push-rod cones but they are less numerous (Andres and von Düring, 1984).

The skin of the outer and inner bill contains altogether about 30 000 ms glands, 10 000 ss glands and 35 000 mns glands. Calculations of the total fibres of the trigeminal nerve which innervate the bill including the push-rod system and the free and encapsulated mechanoreceptors amount to 380 000 main nerve fibres of the trigeminal nerve

supplying the gland duct receptors. This is about 50% of all myelinated axons of the trigeminal nerve in platypus, emphasising the functional importance of the gland duct receptors in the bill of this monotreme.

Conclusion

Electroreceptors in fishes and amphibians present a specialised sensory cell located in the depth of a jelly-filled canal which is in synaptic contact with unmyelinated branches of a myelinated afferent

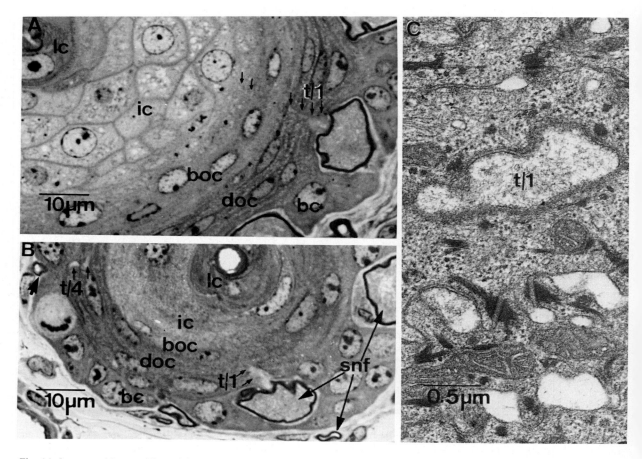

Fig. 14. Innervated intra-epidermal duct segments of a mucous (A) and a serous (B) gland of the bill of Ornithorhynchus. Myelinated sensory nerve fibres (snf). Bright axonal bulb with a thin finger-like process characterises type 1 ending (t/1); initial segment of type 4 axon (arrow) presents two filament-like endings (t/4) in the outer core of the club-shaped enlargement; lining cell of the duct (lc); inner core (ic); dark outer core (doc); bright outer core (boc). (C) Segment of the filament-like axonal process of type 1 ending (t/1) located in the bright outer core. Note the prominent filamentous material of the receptor matrix.

nerve fibre. They phylogenetically derive from the lateral line system. In contrast, electroreceptors (gland duct receptors) in monotremes are free intra-epidermal nerve fibre endings, in specialised gland duct segments, of myelinated axons from the trigeminal nerve. In spite of the striking structural differences of the elementary electroreceptors there are remarkable similarities in the distribution pattern on specialised rostral processes and in the surrounding structures of the electroreceptors involved in the sensory function.

The functional meaning of the specialised gland pores in the platypus in comparison with simple hole pores of small single salivary glands or sweat glands indicates that the blossom-like structure fixes the mucous secretion in a special location for a certain time. By this the mucous column within the gland duct is positioned to a circumscribed area of the surface. The electrolytes of the secretion are important for electric conductivity. Neuronal and hormonal stimuli may modify the electrolyte composition and concentration of the secretion in the gland duct. From this point of view it can be speculated that the micro-ampullae and the epidermal glands in holocephali build up a complex electric field with various vectors of current densities similar to the electric field of the tubular cutaneous glands in platypus bill during diving.

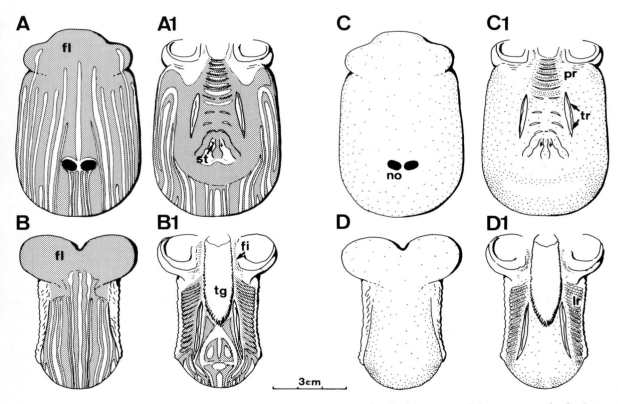

Fig. 15. Inner and outer surfaces of the Ornithorhynchus bill showing the distribution pattern of the cutaneous glands. Array of pores of the sensory mucous glands (dotted stripes) and non-sensory mucous glands (white stripes) on the outer (A, B) and the inner surfaces (A₁, B₁) of the Ornithorhynchus bill including the flap (fl). Distribution pattern of pores of the sensory serous glands on the outer faces (C, D) and the inner faces (C₁, D₁) of the Ornithorhynchus bill. The different densities of the gland pore distribution are marked by stippling. High concentrations of pores of the serous glands are present on the lip ridges (lr) and palatal ridges (pr); nostrils (no); nasopalatine duct of the vomeronasal organ (st); filiform border (fi) within the entrance to the mouth cavum; anterior segment of the tongue (tg).

In holocephali as well as platypus, sources of electricity from outside may distort the electric fields of the electrosensitive organs in specific ways. These field changes may enable the animals to detect and recognise their prey or other obstacles on the hunting grounds. Further, the impressive density of electroreceptors suggests a high resolution to detect even very small changes of the electric fields. This hypothesis is underlined by the rich innervation of the micro-ampulla field in Callorhynchus with 15 000 afferent nerve fibres and the dense innervation of the gland duct receptors of the platypus bill with about 380 000 myelinated nerve fibres, which allows a high resolution to detect even very small changes of the electric field pattern and their characteristic distortions. The scattered distribution pattern of the serous glands similar in distribution to the pushrod system argues for an electrosensory organ for short-distance detecting.

Acknowledgements

This work was supported by the Deutsche Forschungsgemeinschaft, Bionach SP 114. We wish to express our gratitude to Prof. Th.H. Bullock, Scripps Institution of Oceanography, La Jolla, CA; Dr. Peter Last, Tasmanian Fisheries Development Authority, Hobart, Tasmania; Dr. M. Stehmann, Ichthyologie Seefischerei, Zool. Institut und Museum, Hamburg; Biologische Station Espegrend, Universität Bergen, Norway, for their valuable help in getting the holocephali and elasmobranchii. We further thank Dr. W. Hayow, Dept. of Anatomy and Histology, London Hospital Medical College, London, UK; Prof. A. Iggo, Dept. of Vet. Physiology, University of Edinburgh, UK; and Dr. U. Proske, Monash University, Clayton, Australia for the platypus material. Finally we gratefully acknowledge the skillful technical assistance of Mrs. M. Löbbecke-Schumacher and Mrs. L. Augustinowski.

References

Andres, K.H. and von Düring, M. (1972) Morphology of cutaneous receptors. In: A. Iggo (Ed.), *Handbook of Sensory Physiology,* Vol. II, Springer, Berlin, pp. 3 – 28.

Andres, K.H. and von Düring, M. (1977) Interference phenomena on osmium tetroxide-fixed specimens for systematic electron microscopy. In: A. Hayat (Ed.), *Principles and Techniques of Electron Microscopy. Biol. Appl.* 8, Van Nostrand Reinhold Company, New York, pp. 246 – 261.

Andres, K.H. and von Düring, M. (1984) The platypus bill. A structural and functional model of a pattern-like arrangement of different cutaneous sensory receptors. In: W. Hamann and A. Iggo (Eds.), *Sensory Receptor Mechanisms.* World Scientific Publ. Co., Singapore, pp. 81 – 89.

Andres, K.H., von Düring, M. and Petrasch, E. (1988) The fine structure of electroreceptors in the South American blind catfish Pseudocetopsis spec. *Anat. Embryol.,* 177.

Bennett, M.V.L. and Clusin, W.T. (1978) Physiology of the ampullae of Lorenzini, the electroreceptor of elasmobranchs. In: E.S. Hodgson and R.F. Mathewson (Eds.), *Sensory Biology of Sharks, Skates and Rays.* Office of Naval Research, Arlington, VA, pp. 483 – 506.

Bodznick, D. and Smith, A.W. (1984) Somatotopy within the medullary electrosensory nucleus of the little scate, *Raja erinacea. J. Comp. Neurol.,* 225: 581 – 590.

Bodznick, D. and Boord, R.L. (1986) Electroreception in chondrichthyes. Central anatomy and physiology. In: Th.H. Bullock and W. Heiligenberg (Eds.), *Electroreception. Series in Neurobiology.* Wiley, New York, pp. 225 – 256.

Bohringer, R.C. (1981) Cutaneous receptors in the bill of the platypus *(Ornithorhynchus anatinus). Austr. Mam.,* 4: 93 – 95.

Bullock, T.H. (1982) Electroreception. *Ann. Rev. Neurosci.,* 5: 121 – 170.

Bullock, T.H. and Heiligenberg, W. (1986) *Electroreception.* Wiley, New York.

Bullock, T.H., Bodznick, D.A. and Northcutt, R.G. (1983) The phylogenetic distribution of electroreception: evidence for convergent evolution of a primitive vertebrate sense modality. *Brain Res. Rev.,* 6: 25 – 46.

Chu, Y.T. and Meng, C.W. (1979) *Monograph of Fishes of China (No. 2): A Study of the Lateral-line Canal Systems and that of Lorenzini Ampullae and Tubules of Elasmobranchiate Fishes of China.* Science and Technology Press, Shanghai.

Derbin, C. (1970) Effects de la section du nerf lateral sur les jonctions sensorineurales des ampoules de Lorenzini de la torpille, *Torpedo marmorata. J. Micros. (Paris),* 9: 119 – 126.

Derbin, C. (1974) Ultrastructure of the ampullary receptor organs in a Mormyrid fish, *Gnathonemus petersii. J. Ultrastruct. Res.,* 46: 254 – 267.

Derbin, C. and Szabo, T. (1968) Ultrastructure of an electroreceptor (knollenorgan) in the Mormyrid fish *Gnathonemus petersii. J. Ultrastruct. Res.,* 22: 469 – 484.

Derbin, C. and Denizot, J.P. (1971) Ultrastructure de l'organ ampullaire de *Gymnotus carapo* (Gymnotidae); origine et nature des mucopolysaccharides. *Z. Zellforsch.*, 113: 531 – 543.

Dijkgraaf, S. and Kalmijn, A.J. (1963) Untersuchungen über die Funktion der Lorenzinischen Ampullen an Haifischen. *Z. Vergl. Physiol.*, 47: 438 – 456.

Dotterweich, H. (1932) Bau und Funktion der Lorenzini'schen Ampullen. *Zool. Jb. Abt. Zool. Physiol.*, 50: 347 – 418.

Fields, R.D. (1982) *Electroreception in the Ratfish (Subclass Holocephali): Anatomical, Behavioral and Physiological Studies.* M.S. thesis. San Jose State University.

Fritzsch, B. and Wahnschaffe, U. (1983) The electroreceptive ampullary organs of urodeles. *Cell Tissue Res.*, 229: 483 – 503.

Gregory, J.E., Iggo, A., McIntyre, A.K. and Proske, U. (1986) Electroreceptors in the platypus. *Nature (London),* submitted.

Iggo, A. and Andres, K.H. (1982) Morphology of cutaneous receptors. *Ann. Rev. Neurosci.*, 5: 1 – 31.

Jörgensen, J.M. and Bullock, T. (1987) Organization of the ampullary organs of the African knife fish *Xenomystus nigri* (Teleostei: Notopteridae). *J. Neurocytol.*, 16: 311 – 315.

Metcalf, H.E. (1916) The innervation of the ampullae of Lorenzini in *Acanthias vulgaris. Trans. Am. Micr. Soc.*, 35: 167 – 174.

Mullinger, A.M. (1964) The fine structure of the ampullary electric receptors in *Amiurus. Proc. Roy. Soc. B.*, 160: 345 – 359.

Murray, R.W. (1960) Electrical sensitivity of the ampullae of Lorenzini. *Nature (London),* 187: 957.

Murray, R.W. (1962) The response of the ampullae of Lorenzini of elasmobranchs to electrical stimulation. *J. Exp. Biol.*, 39: 119 – 128.

Murray, R.W. (1974) The ampullae of Lorenzini. In: A. Fessard (Ed.), *Handbook of Sensory Physiology,* Vol. III/3, Springer, Berlin, pp. 125 – 144.

Poulton, E.B. (1894) The structure of the bill and hairs of *Ornithorhynchus paradoxus* with a discussion of the homologies and origin of mammalian hair. *Quart. J. Micr. Sci.,* 36: 143 – 199.

Raschi, W. (1978) Notes on the gross functional morphology of the ampullary system in two similar species of skates, *Raja erinacea* and *R. occellata. Copeia,* 1: 48 – 53.

Raschi, W. (1984) *Anatomical Observations on the Ampullae of Lorenzini from Selected Skates and Galeoid Sharks of the Western North Atlantic.* Ph.D. Thesis, College of William and Mary, Williamsburg, VA.

Retzius, G. (1898) Zur Kenntniss der Lorenzinischen Ampullen der Selachier. *Biol. Unters. N.F.,* 8: 75 – 82.

Sato, M. and Katagiri, N. (1969) Preliminary report of the fine structure of the receptor cells of the small pit-organ of the catfish *Parasilurus asotus. Jap. J. Ichthyol.,* 16: 115 – 145.

Scheich, H., Langer, G., Tidemann, C., Coles, R. and Guppy, A. (1986) Electroreception and electrolocation in platypus. *Nature (London),* 6052: 401 – 402.

Srivastava, C.B.L. and Seal, M. (1980) Electroreceptors in indian catfish teleosts. *Adv. Physiol. Sci.,* 31: 1 – 11.

Szabo, T. (1974) Anatomy of the specialized lateral line organs of electroreception. In: A. Fessard (Ed.), *Handbook of Sensory Physiology,* Vol. III/3. Springer, Berlin, pp. 13 – 58.

Szabo, T., Kalmijn, A.J., Enger, P.S. and Bullick, T.H. (1972) Microampullary organs and a submandibular sense organ in the fresh water ray, Potamotrygon. *J. Comp. Physiol.,* 79: 15 – 27.

Szamier, R.B. and Wachtel, A.W. (1970) Special cutaneous receptor organs of fish: ampullary and tuberous organs of Hypopomus. *J. Ultrastruct. Res.,* 30: 450 – 471.

Szamier, R.B. and Bennett, M.V.L. (1974) Special cutaneous receptor organs of fish. Ampullary organs of Mormyrids. *J. Morphol.,* 143: 365 – 384.

Szamier, R.B. and Bennett, M.V.L. (1980) Ampullary electroreceptors in the fresh water ray, Potamotrygon. *J. Comp. Physiol.,* 138: 225 – 230.

Wachtel, A.W. and Szamier, R.B. (1964) Special cutaneous receptor organs of fish: the tuberous organs of Eigenmannia. *J. Morph.,* 119: 51 – 80.

Wachtel, A.W. and Szamier, R.B. (1969) Special cutaneous receptor organs of fish: ampullary organs of the nonelectric catfish, Kryptopterus. *J. Morph,* 128: 291 – 308.

Waltman, B. (1966) Electrical properties and fine structure of the ampullary canals of Lorenzini. *Acta Physiol. Scand.,* Suppl. 264, 66: 3 – 60.

Wilson, J.T. and Martin, C.J. (1893) On the peculiar rod-like tactile organs in the integument and mucous membrane of the muzzle of Ornithorhynchus. *Linn. Soc. NSW MacLean Mem.,* 190 – 200.

Zakon, H. (1986) The electroreceptive periphery. In: T.H. Bullock and W. Heiligenberg (Eds.), *Electroreception.* Wiley, New York, pp. 103 – 156.

W. Hamann and A. Iggo (Eds.)
Progress in Brain Research, Vol. 74
© 1988 Elsevier Science Publishers B.V. (Biomedical Division)

CHAPTER 15

Cutaneous electroreceptors in the platypus: a new mammalian receptor

A. Iggo[a], U. Proske[b], A.K. McIntyre[b] and J.E. Gregory[b]

[a]*Department of Preclinical Veterinary Sciences, University of Edinburgh, UK and* [b]*Department of Physiology, Monash University, Clayton, Vic., Australia*

Electroreceptors are present in the skin of many species of fish and some amphibians (Andres and von Düring, 1988). They are part of the lateral line-eighth nerve system, and comprise two major types, the ampullary variety (e.g., the ampullae of Lorenzini), and tuberous organs. As Wissing et al. (1988) reported elsewhere in this volume, these receptors display both electrical and thermal sensitivity, and there is now abundant evidence for a role in electrolocation and, in the case of fish with electric organs (the Mormyrids of Africa and Gymnotids of South America), of electrocommunication (Bullock and Heiligenberg, 1986).

Electroreceptors were not known to exist in mammals but in 1986 Scheich et al. provided behavioural and neurophysiological evidence that the duck-billed platypus *(Ornithorhynchus anctinus)* is capable of electrolocation. This report has been followed up by experiments in which the characteristics of afferent fibres supplying sensory receptors in the bill of the platypus were examined by recording from dissected strands of the infraorbital nerve (Gregory et al., 1987). This nerve is a branch of the trigeminal nerve, and not part of the acoustico-lateralis system as is the case with electroreceptors in fish and amphibians.

The infraorbital nerve in the platypus is extremely large, and one estimate (Andres and von During, 1984) gives a total count of about 850 000 axons for the nerve supply of the bill, an indication of the

importance of the bill as a sensory organ. Our electrophysiological results are clear cut. Many of the afferent fibres in the infraorbital nerve carried a continuous background discharge, at frequencies in the range 20 – 50 Hz, and with interspike inter-

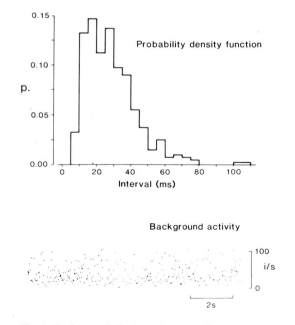

Fig. 1. Background discharge in an unstimulated electroreceptor afferent fibre dissected from the infraorbital nerve of an anaesthetised platypus. The afferent discharge is represented as an instantaneous frequency in the lower panel and as a probability density function in the graph. The mean discharge rate was 37 s⁻¹ and the coefficient of variation was 0.49.

vals which for the longer intervals were distributed approximately exponentially. Fig. 1A shows an example in which the mean firing rate was 37 s^{-1}, with a coefficient of variation of 0.49 indicating a highly irregular discharge. On some occasions the discharge was in clearly marked bursts that were not synchronous with either the cardiac or respiratory rhythms of the animal, or with stray electrical fields in the laboratory. There is, however, insufficient information to decide if there are two categories of continuously discharging electroreceptors or whether the receptors which fired in bursts were responding to some unknown source of interference.

The discharge rate could be altered by varying the temperature of the bill, and in this respect the electroreceptors were similar to other kinds of mammalian slowly adapting receptors, such as

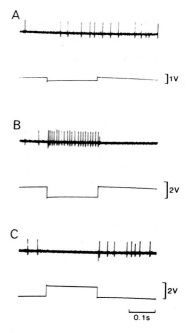

Fig. 2. The effect of applying voltage pulses to the bill of an anaesthetised platypus on the discharge of an electroreceptor. The stimulating cathode was placed on the centre of the receptive field of the unit. An anodal pulse (C) silenced the unit, whereas cathodal pulses (A and B) caused a sustained increase in the firing, that was dead beat with the more intense stimulus.

cutaneous SA1 and 2 receptors and muscle spindles. They were, however, insensitive to mechanical stimuli. The most effective stimulus was electrical. Fig. 2 shows the result of application of square wave voltage pulses to the surface of the bill. When the bill surface was explored with a roving electrode, excitation occurred when the stimulating cathode was at the most sensitive spot in the receptive field. The thresholds, under these conditions, were as low as 20 mV. Typically, in response to voltage steps maintained for several seconds, the discharge of the receptors had an early dynamic and a later static phase.

A systematic analysis of the stimulus – response relationship established clear-cut effects of stimulus intensity and polarity. For example, a receptor which had a resting discharge of 27 impulses s^{-1}, was completely silenced by a 20 mV anodal pulse applied to the centre of the receptive field whereas graded cathodal pulses of 20 mV or more progressively raised mean firing rates to a maximum of about 280 s^{-1} at 350 mV.

The platypus bill, therefore, contains many tens of thousands of electroreceptors, together with many mechanoreceptors (Gregory et al., 1987). As Andres and von Düring (1988) report in this volume, the sensory innervation of the bill is highly organised and the surface of the bill presents the appearance seen in their Fig. 11, which is a low-power view through the transmission electron microscope of the surface of fixed skin, showing several push rod (mechanoreceptors) and gland duct orifices. In order to identify the electroreceptors for morphological examination we systematically explored the receptive fields of single afferent units, using a fine wire electrode as the cathode, and in this way established that on each occasion the most sensitive spot for a receptor was the cabbage-like surface feature identified in Andres and von Düring's morphological analysis as the duct pore of a mucous secretory gland (ms gland) and not at the orifice of a push rod.

Two electroreceptors were marked by us by inserting fine entomological pins, one on each side of the sensitive spot. The animals were subsequently perfused with a glutaraldehyde – paraformalde-hyde mixture, according to the method developed by Andres and von Düring (1978). Histological processing gave the results illustrated in Fig. 3. At low power the tracks of the pins are clearly visible in semi-thin sections and outlined by the marker tracks is a structure that corresponds to an inner-vated mucous secretory gland. More detailed ex-amination of the structure (Fig. 4) reveals a pro-fuse myelinated nerve supply at the base of the ms gland, and it appears that an individual gland is supplied by several myelinated axons although serial sections have not been examined to establish

this point. The myelinated nerve fibres penetrate deeply into the basal body of the gland before ter-minating. The terminals contain an extraordinary expansion of nerve plasma membrane that is seen to be enfolded in the core of the still myelinated nerve terminal (Figs. 4B, 5). There is also a high density of mitochondria in the axoplasm. Cells ad-jacent to these terminals contain numerous small dense osmiophilic granules (melanin granules) that

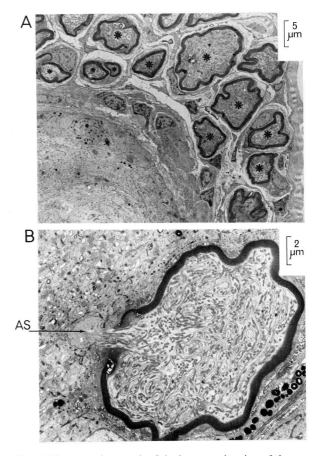

Fig. 4. Electron micrograph of the innervated region of the ms gland of Fig. 3. In the lower power illustration (A) the nerve fibres concentrated at the base of the epidermis are marked (*) and in the higher power illustration (B) the details of the myelinated sensory nerve terminal are visible. Notable features are the highly internally convoluted plasma membrane of the axon and the small papilla or spine (AS) that emerges from the myelin-ensheathed axon. This small protrusion is presumably the primary transduction site.

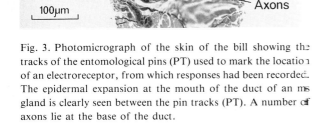

Fig. 3. Photomicrograph of the skin of the bill showing the tracks of the entomological pins (PT) used to mark the location of an electroreceptor, from which responses had been recorded. The epidermal expansion at the mouth of the duct of an ms gland is clearly seen between the pin tracks (PT). A number of axons lie at the base of the duct.

136

are absent from the deeper lying nerve plexus (Fig. 4B). The presence of the granules serves to mark the cells containing them as epidermal so that the terminals of the electroreceptors have an epidermal location.

The results thus establish that the platypus electroreceptor operates on a different principle from those already known for fish and amphibia. It seems probable that the highly modified nerve ending functions as the transducer. In fish, the transducer is a modified hair cell (neuromast) and

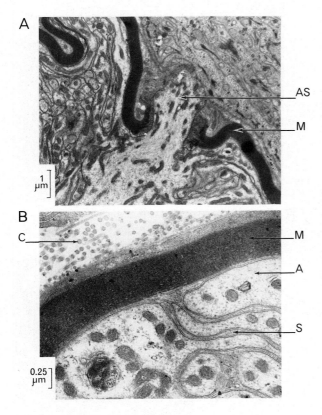

Fig. 5. (A) Electron micrograph of the axonal spine (AS) protruding into a loosely packed cellular layer adjacent to the lumen of the gland. Notice the loops of myelin and associated tongues of Schwann cytoplasm at the point of emergence, reminiscent of the paranodal region of myelinated axons. M: myelin lamellae. (B) Close up of nerve terminal. Folds of myelin leaving the innermost layer of the sheath are associated with a large area of axonal membrane. The infoldings or tongues are present only in the terminal region of the axon. C: collagen; M: myelin lamellae; S: Schwann cell cytoplasm; A: axoplasm.

activity is generated by synaptic transmission between receptor cell and afferent axon. Presumably the structure of the platypus receptor (fuller details of which are available in Andres and von Düring's (1988) paper) provides a low resistance path from the orifice of the gland duct to the nerve terminals at the epidermal base of the receptor. The final details of the transduction mechanism must await further study, but it seems likely that there is some form of local generator potential, based on activation of appropriate ionic channels. The striking and unique expansion of the area of plasma membrane (Figs. 4, 5) in the myelinated nerve terminal will undoubtedly both increase membrane capacitance and decrease overall membrane resistance. Perhaps the folds act to increase membrane surface area to aid electrogenic pumping of ions. This region is unlikely to be the site of impulse initiation and activity probably arises at the first node of Ranvier. The region of folded membrane is continuous with a membrane protrusion through the myelin lamellae at only one place (Figs. 4B, 5A). At the site where this small papilla or spine emerges, the myelin lamellae form characteristic looping connections in a manner typical of the paranodal region of a node of Ranvier (Figs. 5A, 6). The electrical resistance to longitudinal current flow at this place is no doubt high and would thus tend to cause any current to flow across the membrane of the exposed papillary process. Outward or return current would be expected to flow across the nodes of Ranvier more proximally along the myelinated axon where propagated activity is likely to be generated. The membrane of the papilla is freely exposed to the cellular matrix of a diverticulum of the gland duct, that from its histological appearance would be expected to have a low resistance. The outer wall of the gland duct, in contrast, is rich in tight intercellular junctions and, combined with the layer of collagen fibres immediately external to the myelin lamellae of the sensory nerve terminal, would be expected to offer a high resistance to current flow. There is therefore a path of low electrical resistance from the mouth of the pore down the lumen of the mucous-filled

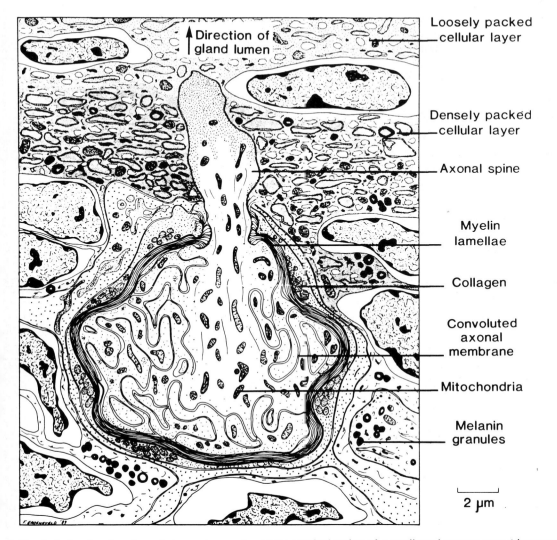

Fig. 6. A drawing, based on electron micrographs, of the terminal region of a myelinated sensory axon (electroreceptor) lying at the base of an ms gland.

gland duct to the tongue of axoplasm protruding from each myelinated axon. The path from the surface further down the duct into the depths of the gland and across the secretory surface is likely to be of high resistance as it is known that secretory cells are linked by tight junctions (Petersen, 1980). Other features of the bill skin may contribute to a channelling of current along the low-resistance path to the receptors, such as the dense tight junction boundary of the epidermal cells in the base and walls of the gland duct, the tightly packed basal epidermal cells elsewhere in the skin and the thick stratum corneum across most of the bill surface.

The most effective excitatory condition for the receptors in our experiments was to have the cathodal pole of the stimulating dipole at the orifice of the ms gland. The physiological state of the receptor terminal can probably be regarded as an unstable equilibrium, since many of the afferent fibres discharge continuously in the absence of an external stimulus. The great abundance of mitochondria in the nerve terminal is an indication of a high level of metabolic activity. They are presumably required to provide energy for the continuous ionic pumping across the heavily convoluted membrane to maintain the ongoing discharge of action potentials and stabilise the underlying depolarised state of the nerve terminal membrane. Modulation of ongoing activity in the nerve terminal would presumably facilitate the detection of small changes in the potential field surrounding the animal, and enable the receptor to signal both increases and decreases of field strength.

Acknowledgement

We would like to thank T.O. Neild for helpful discussion of the manuscript.

References

Andres, K.H. and von Düring, M. (1978) Principles and techniques of electron microscopy. *Biol. Appl. Hayat H.A.*, 8: 246 – 261.

Andres, K.H. and von Düring, M. (1984) The platypus bill. A structural and functional model of a pattern-like arrangement of different cutaneous sensory receptors. In: W. Hamann and A. Iggo (Eds.), *Sensory Receptor Mechanisms*. World Scientific Publ. Co., Singapore, pp. 81 – 89.

Andres, K.H. and von Düring, M. (1988) Comparative anatomy of vertebrate electroreceptors. In: W. Hamann and A. Iggo (Eds.), *Progress in Brain Research,* Vol. 74. Elsevier, Amsterdam, pp. 113 – 131.

Bullock, T.H. and Heiligenberg, W. (Eds.) (1986) *Electroreception.* John Wiley and Sons, New York.

Gregory, J.E., Iggo, A., McIntyre, A.K. and Proske, U. (1987) Electroreceptors in the platypus. *Nature (London),* 326: 386 – 387.

Petersen, O.H. (1980) *The Electrophysiology of Gland Cells.* Academic Press, London.

Scheich, H., Langner, G., Tidemann, C., Coles, R.B. and Guppy, A. (1986) Electroreception and electrolocation in platypus. *Nature (London),* 319: 401 – 402.

Wissing, H., Braun, H.A. and Schäfer, K. (1988) Dynamic response characteristics of the ampullae of Lorenzini to thermal and electrical stimuli. In: W. Hamann and A. Iggo (Eds.), *Progress in Brain Research,* Vol. 74. Elsevier, Amsterdam. pp. 99 – 107.

W. Hamann and A. Iggo (Eds.)
Progress in Brain Research, Vol. 74
© 1988 Elsevier Science Publishers B.V. (Biomedical Division)

CHAPTER 16

Structure and functional anatomy of visceroreceptors in the mammalian respiratory system

Monika von Düring and Karl Hermann Andres

Anatomisches Institut, Abteilung Neuroanatomie, Ruhr-Universität Bochum, 4630 Bochum, FRG

Introduction

Numerous light and electron microscopical studies have been published about the structure, localization and distribution of different visceroreceptors in the mammalian tracheobronchial tree and the lungs (Larsell, 1921; Larsell and Dow, 1933; Elftmann, 1943; Spencer and Leof, 1964; Hirsch et al. 1968; Lauweryns et al., 1969, 1972; von Düring et al., 1974; Das et al., 1978, 1979; Fox et al., 1980 Krauhs, 1984; Andres and von Düring, 1985) Physiological data and experiments concerning the afferent innervation of the tracheobronchial tree including the lung in mammals were recently reviewed (Sant'Ambrogio, 1982; Coleridge and Coleridge, 1984; Widdicombe, 1986).

The majority of afferent fibers to the tracheobronchial tree and to the lungs is of vagal origin. Recently it has been discovered in the guinea pig that there are also afferents from thoracal spinal ganglia cells (Saria et al., 1985). A systematic analysis of the vagal afferents only exists for the cat. Jammes et al. (1982) stated that 90% of the vagal afferents are unmyelinated fibers (C fibers). We confirmed their results for the vagal input in dogs, where we found a comparable relation between myelinated and unmyelinated nerve fibers. In non-human primates, however, such as rhesus monkey and grass monkey, the ratio between myelinated axons and C fibers is reduced to 1 : 3 (Fig. 1).

There are further differences in the airway morphology of mammals, such as the marked structure of the glassy membrane in primates or the lack of intraepithelial nerve endings in the trachea and extrapulmonary bronchi of the mouse (Pack et al., 1984).

It may be suspected that the quality of the afferent nerve fiber (diameter, myelination, arborization), the terminations of the fiber and its special topography within the tracheobronchial tree and the structural and cellular composition of the tissue compartments associated with the receptive complex are adjusted to the specific sensory function and the varying mechanical parameters. Furthermore we use these morphological criteria for a receptor classification (Andres and von Düring, 1972; Andres, 1973; Andres et al., 1985, 1987).

(1) Intraepithelial nerve terminals from myelinated axons of the trachea and extrapulmonary bronchi (irritant receptor)

Nerve terminals in the epithelium of the tracheobronchial tree of different mammals are known from light microscopical studies (Larsell, 1921). Electron microscopical investigations document the precise location of their terminations in close association with the terminal bar of the epithelium (Jeffery and Reid, 1973; Das et al., 1978, 1979; Laitinen, 1985). Physiological experiments (for review, see Sant'Ambrogio, 1982) indicate that these nerve terminals are rapidly adapting receptors and respond to a variety of stimuli, such as inflation and deflation of the lung, irritation of the epithelium of trachea and larger bronchi with dust or mechanical probing, and a variety of inhaled or injected chemical substances. The most used term for this type of receptor is 'rapidly adapting irri-

tant receptor' (Fillenz and Widdicombe, 1971).

In non-human primates (rhesus monkey and grass monkey) and cats we found that small nerve fiber bundles with one thin myelinated axon of $2-3$ μm diameter and a Schwann cell with $6-8$ C fibers ($0.2-0.6$ μm in diameter) enter the epithelium of the trachea and larger bronchi to ter-

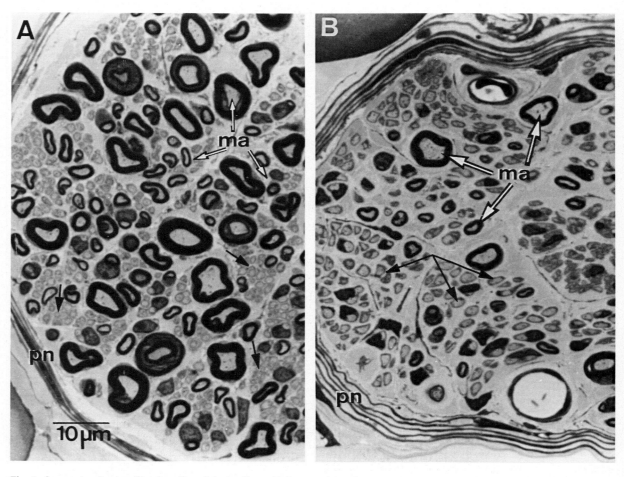

Fig. 1. Segments of nerve fiber bundles of the peribronchial nerve plexus in the main bronchus to the upper lobe in grass monkey (A) and dog (B) with myelinated (ma) and unmyelinated axons (arrows). Notice the higher number of myelinated axons in the nerve fiber bundle of grass monkey. Perineural sheath (pn).

Fig. 2. Examples of intraepithelial nerve terminals in the trachea of cat (A) and grass monkey (B, C). The course of the terminal axons (nt) parallel to the axis of the trachea is obvious in sections parallel to the surface. (A) Notice the desmosomes and attachment plaques (arrows) connecting the terminal axon (nt 1) to the surrounding epithelial cells (e); basal bodies of the cilia (bb); terminal bar (tb). (B) Nerve fiber terminal type 1 (nt 1) with varicosities (arrows) containing mitochondria and some clear vesicles; goblet cell (gc). (C) Nerve fiber terminal type 2 (nt 2) characterized by accumulations of clear and dense core vesicles.

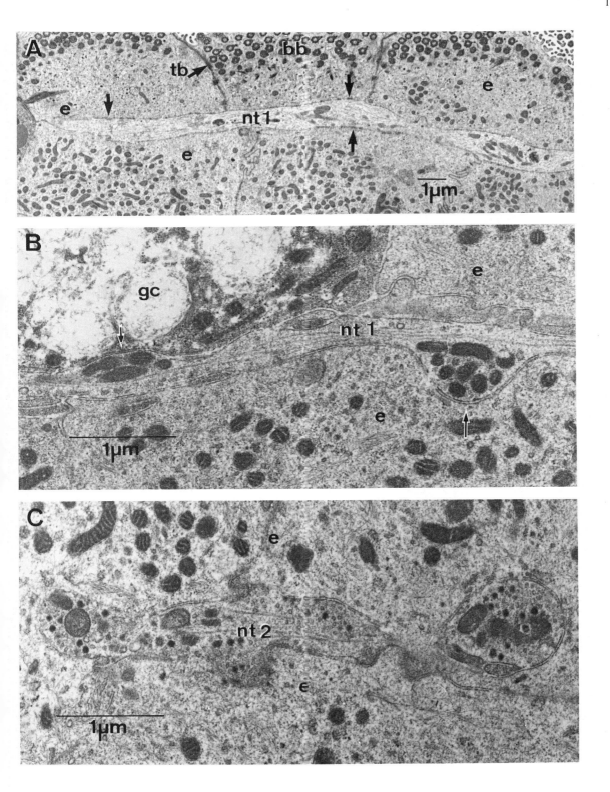

142

minate at the luminal side. We made serial semi-thin and ultrathin sections to trace the nerve fibers and to analyze the arborization of the fibers up to the termination sites. The myelinated axon loses its myelin sheath about 30 μm below the epithelial layer and splits up into 6 – 8 unmyelinated branches of 0.2 – 0.4 μm in diameter. The fine unmyelinated terminal axons of the myelinated nerve fiber and the primarily unmyelinated axons use the same Schwann cells to reach the basal epithelial cell layer. Within the epithelial cell layer the axons lie in the intercellular spaces to run straight up to the apical cell region (Fig. 3). Just below the terminal bar of the epithelial cells the axons change their course to run parallel with the long axis of the tracheobronchial tree in proximal to distal and distal to proximal directions with a length of about 300 μm. Varicosities of up to 1.2 μm in diameter occur in the course of the terminal axons, which bulge into neighboring epithelial cells. The ter-

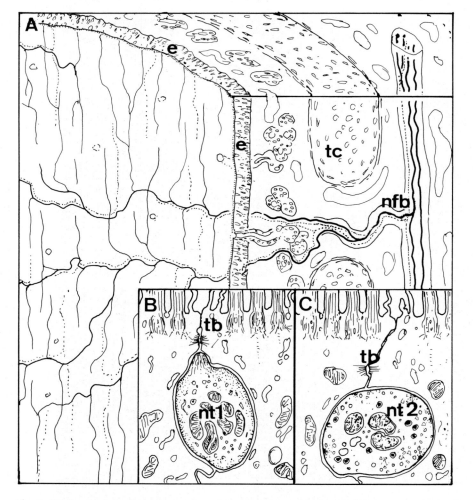

Fig. 3. (A) Semi-schematic representation of the two types of intraepithelial nerve terminals, their distribution and location in the tracheal epithelium of grass monkey. The supplying nerve fiber bundle (nfb) contains myelinated (solid lines) and unmyelinated (dotted lines) axons. Type 1 terminal (B) and type 2 terminal (C) in their characteristic topography near the terminal bar (tb) of the epithelial cells (e); tracheal cartilage (tc).

minal axons and especially the varicosities contain several mitochondria and condensations of vesicles.

With respect to the different vesicle composition we distinguish two types of nerve endings. Type 1 exhibits mainly clear vesicles. Type 2 is characterized by numerous clear and dense core vesicles (Fig. 2). The axonal segments between the varicosities show microtubules and profiles of the axoplasmic reticulum. Small attachment plaques between the axonal membrane and adjacent epithelial cells are obvious. Terminal profiles of both types of endings are observed in the entire circumference of the trachea and extrapulmonary bronchi of cat, rhesus monkey and grass monkey with a distance to the luminal surface of less than 0.9 μm (Fig. 3).

It has not been possible up to now to differentiate between the unmyelinated segments of the myelinated axon and the unmyelinated segments of the C fibers because they are very similar in size and structure. Therefore we are not able to associate our two types of nerve terminals with their related stem fibers.

Our results, however, represent a dense innervation of the epithelium of the trachea and larger bronchi with two types of nerve terminals stemming from myelinated and unmyelinated stem fibers. Immunohistochemical studies on the electron microscopical level will give additional information about these fiber types and their nerve terminals.

(2) Intraepithelial nerve terminals of myelinated fibers at the basal cell layer of the trachea (tracheal glassy membrane receptor)

In primates there is a third type of intraepithelial nerve terminal. It is located in the basal cell layer of the tracheal epithelium adjacent to the glassy membrane and restricted to the middle part of the epithelium of the posterior tracheal wall covering the paries membranaceus. The myelinated axon of 6 – 8 μm diameter can be traced to the glassy membrane where it loses its myelin sheath about 2 – 4 μm before entering the basal cell layer (Fig. 4). The nerve fiber splits up into 3 – 4 unmyelinated axonal branches and in the epithelium the terminal axons follow the circumference of the trachea for about 20 – 30 μm and terminate as free nerve endings. Therefore, a lanceolate appearance of this nerve terminal is obvious in cross sections of the trachea. Numerous mitochondria and vesicles scattered in a filamentous receptor matrix are characteristic in the afferent nerve terminal. Finger-like processes containing the receptor matrix perforate the basement lamella to come in contact with the microfilaments of the glassy membrane (Fig. 5). This is the reason why we term this nerve ending 'tracheal glassy membrane receptor'.

The function of this receptor type is not known. The distinct location of the nerve terminals between the glassy membrane and the basal epithelial cells of the posterior wall of the trachea, however, may indicate that the tracheal glassy membrane receptor measures the tension of the posterior epithelial segment during inspiration and expiration. Just this segment of the tracheal wall moves in and out during the breathing cycle and exhibits a smooth epithelial surface during inspiration and a folded surface during expiration (Fig. 5). The occurrence of the glassy membrane receptor only in primates argues for a possible function in phonation.

(3) Neuroepithelial bodies

Neuroepithelial bodies occur as single cells or in clusters. They are characterized by accumulations of dense core vesicles in the basal part of the cell body and by a close association of the cells to nerve terminals of myelinated axons. Unmyelinated axons always accompany the myelinated axons but they terminate in the connective tissue compartment below the neuroepithelial cells. Some of the neuroepithelial cells go up to the epithelial surface and bear few microvilli (Lauweryns and Peuskens, 1969; Lauweryns et al., 1972, 1977; Hung and Loosli, 1974; Wasano, 1977). The capillaries of the lamina propria adjacent to the neuroepithelial

144

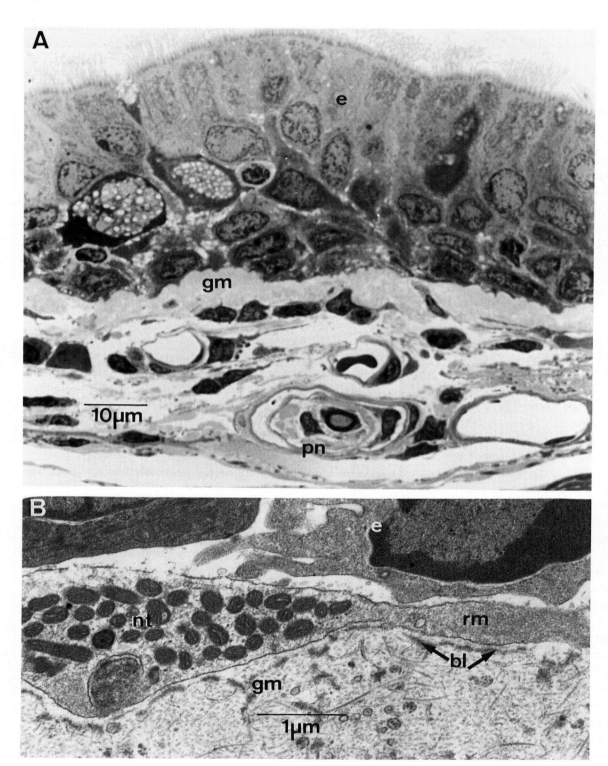

bodies exhibit endothelial fenestrations (Fig. 6) indicating that molecules up to 15 nm may pass the endothelial cells (Simionescu and Simionescu, 1983) to leave or to enter the circulatory system. The cells of the neuroepithelial bodies are considered to belong to the amine precursor uptake

and decarboxylation (APUD) system and occur in the respiratory epithelium of distal segments of the bronchial tree of mammals, including man. Due to histochemical and immunocytochemical data the dense core vesicles or the cell cytoplasm contain serotonin and a variety of regulatory peptides (for

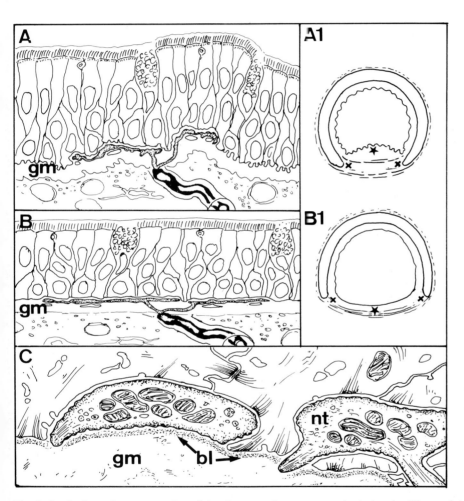

Fig. 5. Semi-schematic representation of the glassy membrane receptor in the basal cell layer of the respiratory epithelium (e) of the paries membranaceus in the posterior wall of the trachea (asterisk) of a rhesus monkey. Movements of the paries membranaceus and the covering epithelium during expiration (A, A₁) and inspiration (B, B₁) may act on the receptor membrane by stretching or relaxing the tissue. (C) Detail of the nerve terminal (nt) with its close association to the glassy membrane (gm); basement lamella (bl).

Fig. 4. Myelinated nerve fiber in the lamina propria of the trachea (A) and the related nerve terminals in the basal epithelial layer of rhesus monkey (B). (A) The myelinated axon surrounded by a perineural sheath (pn); glassy membrane (gm). (B) Nerve terminal of the glassy membrane receptor (nt) exhibiting the prominent filamentous receptor matrix (rm) in a finger-like process which contacts the glassy membrane (gm); basement lamella (bl).

146

review, see Polak and Bloom, 1984; Dayer et al., 1985). Recently, immunoreactivity for calcitonin gene-related peptide was demonstrated (Scheuermann et al., 1987).

Lauweryns et al. (1977) discussed the function of

the neuroepithelial bodies as a chemoreceptor to measure the composition of the inhaled air. The function of the neuroepithelial bodies, however, remains unclear (Pack and Widdicombe, 1984).

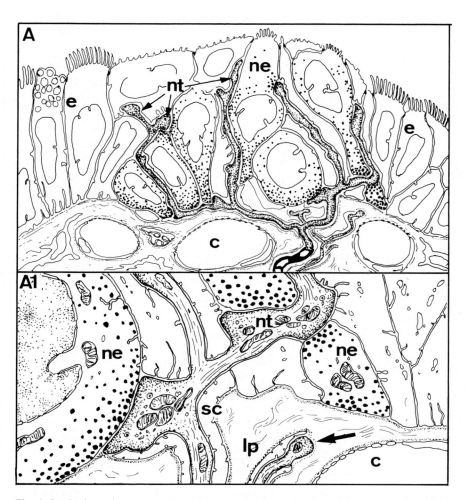

Fig. 6. Semi-schematic representation of the structural organization of the neuroepithelial body. Neuroepithelial cell (ne) in contact with nerve terminals (nt) of a myelinated axon; Schwann cell (sc); respiratory epithelium (e); lamina propria (lp) with terminating C fibers (arrow); capillary (c) with endothelial fenestrations.

Fig. 7. Myelinated nerve fiber of the smooth muscle stretch receptor (A) and the related nerve terminals (B) in the trachealis muscle of grass monkey. (A) The receptor complex with the nerve terminals (arrows) lies in series with the long axis ofthe smooth muscle cells of the trachealis muscle (tm). (B) Part of a nerve terminal of the smooth muscle stretch receptor (nt) with receptor matrix (rm). Note the close contact of the axonal membrane with the collagen fibrils (cf) of the receptor complex; elastic fibril (ef).

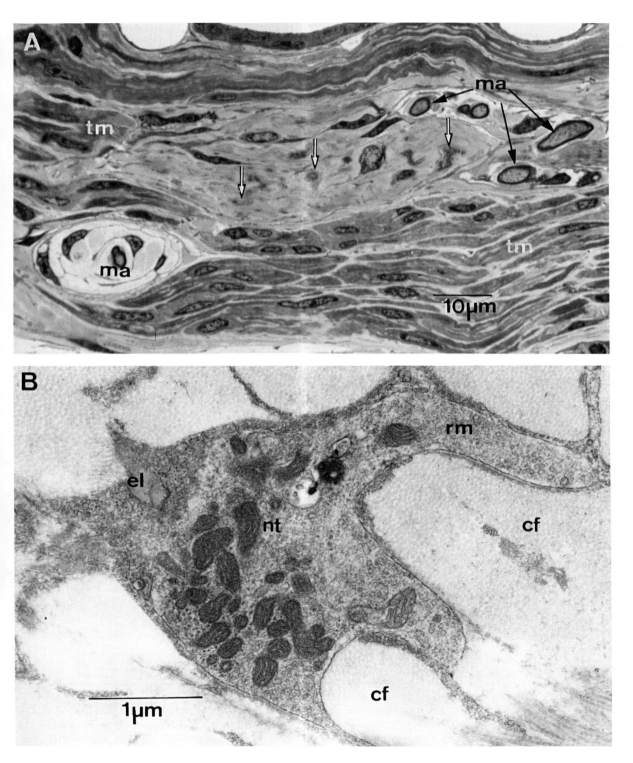

148

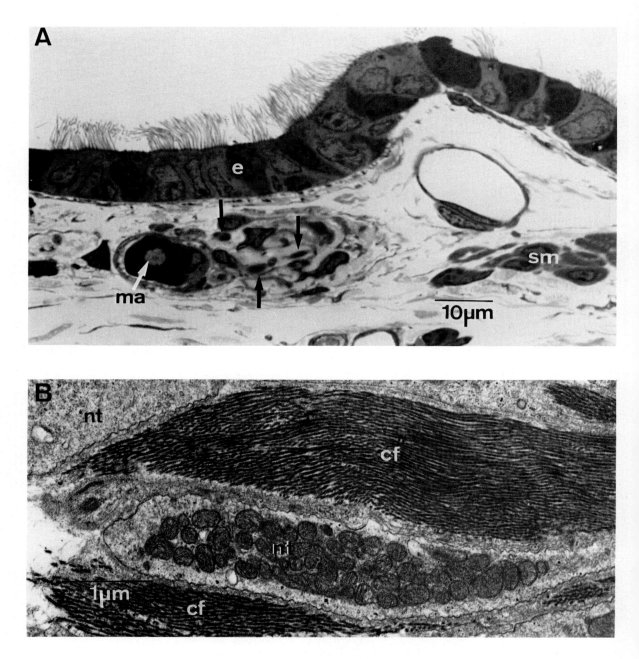

Fig. 8. Smooth muscle stretch receptor in the wall of a bronchus of the tree shrew. (A) The receptor complex lies in series with the long axis of the smooth muscle cells (sm). Note the dense microtexture of the receptor complex and the unmyelinated axonal branches (arrows) of the myelinated axon (ma); respiratory epithelium (e). (B) Profiles of the nerve terminals (nt) with characteristic features of a stretch receptor terminal as the receptor matrix, mitochondria and the contact of the terminal to collagen fibrils (cf).

(4) Nerve terminals of myelinated nerve fibers in the trachealis muscle and the smooth muscle cell layer of the bronchi (smooth muscle stretch receptor)

Physiological experiments indicate that slowly adapting receptors occur in the tracheal muscle and in the bronchial wall (for review, see Sant'Ambrogio, 1982; Ravi, 1986) and that the receptor activity varies with the bronchomotor tone, increas-ing with constriction and decreasing with dilata-tion of this tissue compartment. Two types of stretch receptors were described morphologically in the smooth muscle cell layer. Von Düring et al. (1974) showed a pulmonary stretch receptor in the bronchus wall of the rat lying in the lamina pro-pria, parallel to the smooth muscle cell layer (Fig. 13A), while Krauhs (1984) described a stretch receptor in the trachealis muscle of the dog lying in series to the long axis of the trachealis muscle.

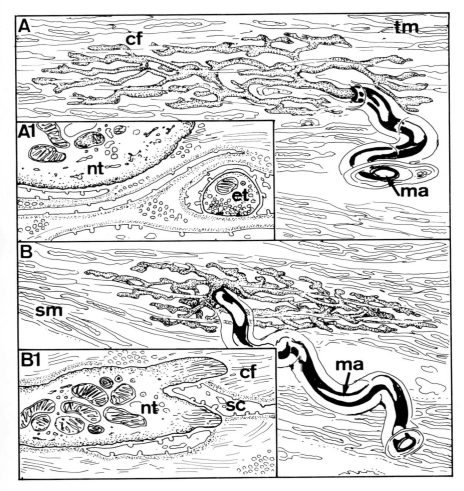

Fig. 9. Semi-schematic representation of the smooth muscle stretch receptor in the trachealis muscle of rhesus monkey (A) and in the smooth muscle cell layer of a bronchus of tree shrew (B). (A) The unmyelinated segment of the myelinated nerve fiber (ma) splits up into several branches and terminates in the dense connective tissue compartment of the receptor complex. (A1) Detail of a nerve terminal (nt) with contact to collagen fibrils (cf). Efferent nerve terminal (et) terminating at the tracheal smooth muscle cell (tm). (B) The terminal axons of the tree shrew smooth muscle stretch receptor show an intense arborization. (B1) Detail of a nerve ter-minal (nt) with association to collagen fibrils (cf); myelinated stem fiber (ma); smooth muscle cells (sm); Schwann cell (sc).

We find in our material from dog, tree shrew, grass monkey and rhesus monkey a comparable smooth muscle stretch receptor. The myelinated nerve fiber of 7 – 10 μm in diameter terminates in a conspicuous and dense connective tissue com-

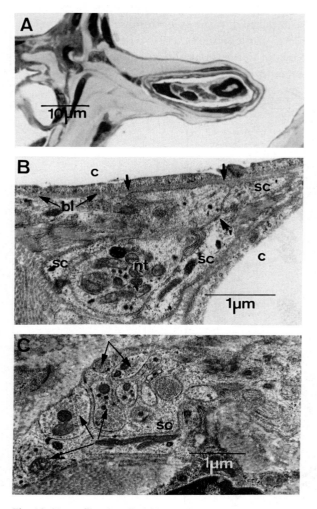

Fig. 10. Nerve fiber bundle with myelinated and unmyelinated axons in the wall of a respiratory bronchiole (A) of grass monkey and the related nerve terminals in close contact with pulmonary capillaries in the alveolar septum (B) and in the connective tissue of the alveolar septum (C). (B) Segment of a nerve terminal of the myelinated axon. Arrows indicate the close association of the nerve terminal (nt) with the basement lamella of the capillary endothelium; pulmonary capillary (c); Schwann cell (sc). (C) Terminals of a C fiber bundle (arrows) terminating in the connective tissue of an alveolar septum; Schwann cell (sc).

partment lying in series with the long axis of the trachealis muscle or with the circular smooth muscle cell layer of larger bronchi. The receptor complex is spindle-shaped with a length of about 100 μm and a diameter of about 30 – 50 μm. The nerve terminals with a diameter of 1.2 – 1.8 μm contain a large number of mitochondria, some vesicles and a prominent receptor matrix. Several areas of the axonal membrane and finger-like processes of the nerve terminals lack a Schwann cell covering. Just these areas of the axon terminals exhibit the receptor matrix and come in contact with the collagen or elastic fibers (Figs. 7, 9A). This arrangement is similar to the ultrastructural relation between nerve terminals and collagen tissue in Golgi tendon organs (Schoultz and Swett, 1972). Ruffini corpuscles (Chambers et al., 1972) and the pulmonary stretch receptor in rats (von Düring et al., 1974). The characteristic arrangement of elastic and collagen fibrils in association with the receptor complex is much more complicated in the smooth muscle stretch receptor in comparison to the above mentioned Golgi tendon organ or Ruffini corpuscle. Depending on the location of the smooth muscle stretch receptor in the tracheobronchial tree the microtexture of the connective tissue differs in the composition of collagen and elastic fibers. Collagen fiber bundles in a more rectangular course to the axis of the smooth muscle cells are associated with the nerve terminals and characterize the bronchial smooth muscle stretch receptor complex of the tree shrew (Figs. 8, 9B).

Generally speaking, any polarized arrangement of receptive structures may indicate that, depending on its configuration, either stretch or pressure may be transmitted to the transductive areas.

(5) Nerve terminals of myelinated axons at the capillary bed of the respiratory bronchioles and alveolar sacs

Unmyelinated nerve fibers within the alveolar wall of rat (Meyrick and Reid, 1971), mouse (Hung et al., 1972) and man (Fox et al., 1980) were observed with the electron microscope and confirmed a possible structural correlate to the 'J receptors from Paintal's physiological experiments (Paintal 1955, 1969, 1970).

We traced myelinated axons of $3-5$ μm in diameter up to the end of the respiratory bronchioles in rhesus monkey and grass monkey. At the end of the myelination four to six terminal axons emerge to run to the capillary wall of the respiratory bronchioles and alveolar sacs where they terminate at the capillary basement lamella. The distance between the receptor terminal and the capillary lumen was even less than 1 μm. Dense core vesicles and the receptor matrix are observed in the nerve terminals (Figs. 10B, 11A).

The position of the nerve endings argues for a function in measuring the stretching of the vascular wall. However, it cannot be excluded, considering their prominent position to the endothelial cells of the capillaries, that they are used to monitor the chemical composition of the blood.

The myelinated axons are regularly accompanied by C fiber bundles (Fig. 10A). They,

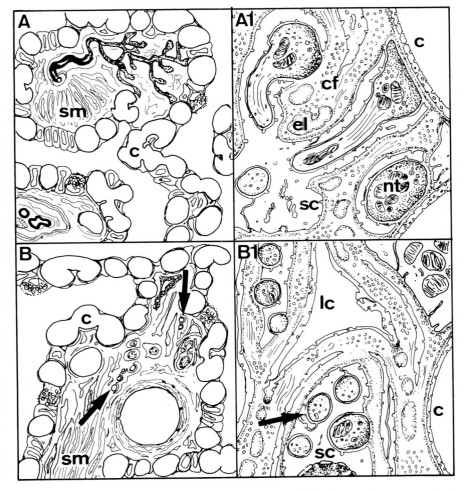

Fig. 11. Semi-schematic representation of afferent nerve terminals from myelinated axons in the alveolar ducts in close association with the pulmonary capillary bed (A/A₁) and of C fibers (arrows) in the connective tissue of the alveolar septa in the vicinity of the origin of lymphatic capillaries (B/B₁); smooth muscle cells (sm), pulmonary capillary (c); collagen (cf) and elastic (el) fibrils; nerve terminal (nt); Schwann cell (sc); lymphatic capillary (lc).

however, terminate in the connective tissue compartment of the alveolar septa (Figs. 10C, 11B). This connective tissue compartment contains the origin of the pulmonary lymphatic network (Gil and McNiff, 1981). It may be speculated that the nerve terminals of the C fibers may be involved in controlling the composition of interstitial fluid in health and disease.

(6) Nerve fiber terminals of myelinated axons in the pleura visceralis

Nerve terminations of myelinated fibers were observed in the pleura visceralis of rabbit, dog and

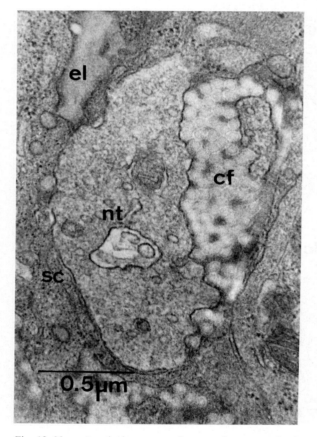

Fig. 12. Nerve terminal segment of a stretch receptor in the visceral pleura of the rat. Notice the close association of the nerve terminal (nt) to the collagen (cf) and elastic (el) fibrils; receptor matrix (rm); Schwann cell (sc).

man in methylene blue stainings (Larsell, 1922, 1935). In cats they were documented with the Bielschowsky method (McLaughlin, 1933).

Myelinated axons of $2-4$ μm diameter are observed innervating the pleura visceralis where they terminate as free Ruffini-like receptors. The arrangement of the nerve terminals with the collagen and elastic fibers of the surrounding connective tissue is very similar to the ultrastructural appearance of stretch receptors (Figs. 12, 13B).

Conclusion

Comparative studies of the structure and distribution of afferent nerve terminals in the mammalian tracheobronchial tree and the lungs show that some types of nerve endings occur in all investigated mammals. Comparative studies, in addition, elucidate that there are also striking differences such as the ratio of myelinated and unmyelinated axons of the vagal input, the prominent glassy membrane receptor in primates or the lack of intraepithelial irritant receptors in the trachea of the mouse (Pack et al., 1984). These facts must be taken into consideration if physiological results from animal experiments are compared to the respiratory system of humans.

Acknowledgements

We thank Luzie Augustinowski and Marlen Löbbecke-Schumacher for excellent technical assistance.

References

Andres, K.H. (1973) Morphological criteria for the differentiation of mechanoreceptors in vertebrates. In: J. Schwartzkopff (Ed.), *Symposium Mechanorezeption,* Abhdlg. Rhein. Westf. Akad. Wiss., Bd. 53. Westdeutscher Verlag, Wiesbaden, pp. 135 – 152.

Andres, K.H. and von Düring, M. (1972) Morphology of cutaneous receptors. In: A. Iggo (Ed.), *Handbook of Sensory Physiology,* Vol. II. Springer, Berlin, pp. 3 – 28.

Andres, K.H. and von Düring, M. (1985) Rezeptoren und nervöse Versorgung des bronchopulmonalen Systems. *Bochumer Treff,* pp. 31 – 49.

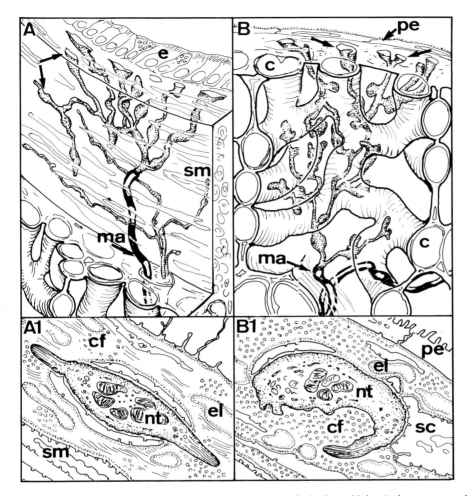

Fig. 13. Semi-schematic representation of stretch receptors in the bronchiolus (pulmonary stretch receptor) (A) and in the visceral pleura (B) of the rat. (A/A₁). The location and close association of the nerve terminals (nt) to elastic and collagen fibrils of the lamina propria are obvious; smooth muscle cells (sm) lie in parallel to the stretch receptor complex; myelinated axon (ma); respiratory epithelium (e); collagen (cf) and elastic (el) fibrils. (B/B₁) The location of the stretch receptor with its terminal branches (nt) arborizing in the lamina propria of the visceral pleura. A similar structural association between nerve terminals (nt) and collagen (cf) and elastic (el) fibrils is striking; Schwann cell (sc).

Andres, K.H., von Düring, M. and Schmidt, R.F. (1985) Sensory innervation of the Achilles tendon by group III and IV afferent fibers. *Anat. Embryol.,* 172: 145 – 156.

Andres, K.H., von Düring, M., Muszynski, K. and Schmidt, R.F. (1987) Nerve fibres and their terminals of the dura mater encephali of the rat. *Anat. Embryol.,* 175: 289 – 301.

Chambers, M.R., Andres, K.H., von Düring, M. and Iggo, A. (1972) Structure and function of the slowly adapting type II mechanoreceptor in hairy skin. *Quart. J. Exp. Physiol.,* 57: 417 – 445.

Coleridge, J.C.G. and Coleridge, H.M. (1984) Afferent vagal C fibre innervation of the lungs and airways and its functional significance. *Rev. Physiol. Biochem. Pharmacol.,* 99: 2 – 110.

Das, R.M., Jeffery, P.K. and Widdicombe, J.G. (1978) The epithelial innervation of the lower respiratory tract of the cat. *J. Anat.,* 126: 123 – 131.

Das, R.M., Jeffery, P.K. and Widdicombe, J.G. (1979) Experimental degeneration of intra-epithelial nerve fibres in the cat airways. *J. Anat.,* 128: 259 – 263.

Dayer, A.M., De Mey, J. and Will, J.A. (1985) Localization of somatostatin-, bombesin- and serotonin-like immunoreactivity in the lung of the fetal Rhesus monkey. *Cell Tissue Res.*, 239: 621–625.

von Düring, M., Andres, K.H. and Iravani, J. (1974) The fine structure of the pulmonary stretch receptor in the rat. *Z. Anat. Entwickl.-Gesch.*, 143: 215–222.

Elftman, G. (1943) The afferent and parasympathetic innervation of the lungs and trachea of the dog. *Am. J. Anat.*, 72: 1–27.

Fillenz, M. and Widdicombe, J.G. (1971) Receptors of the lungs and airways. In: E. Neil (Ed.), *Handbook of Sensory Physiology*, Vol. 3. Springer, Berlin, pp. 81–112.

Fox, B., Bull, T.B. and Guz, A. (1980) Innervation of alveolar walls in the human lung: an electron microscopic study. *J. Anat.*, 131: 683–692.

Gil, J. and McNiff, J.M. (1981) Interstitial cells at the boundary between alveolar and extraalveolar connective tissue in the lung. *J. Ultrastruct. Res.*, 76: 149–157.

Hirsch, E.F., Kaiser, G.C., Barner, H.B., Nigro, S.F., Hamouda, F., Cooper, T. and Adams, W.E. (1968) The innervation of the mammalian lung. III. Regression of the intrinsic nerves and of their afferent receptors following thoracic sympathectomy, cervical vagotomy or thoracic stripping of the vagus. *Arch. Sur.*, 96: 149–155.

Hung, K.S. and Loosli, C.G. (1974) Bronchiolar neuroepithelial bodies in the neonatal mouse lungs. *Am. J. Anat.*, 140: 191–200.

Hung, K.S., Hertwech, M.S., Hardy, J.D. and Coosli, J.D. (1972) Innervation of pulmonary alveoli of the mouse lung. An electron microscopic study. *Am. J. Anat.*, 135: 477–496.

Jammes, Y., Fornaris, E., Mei, N. and Barrat, E. (1982) Afferent and efferent components of the bronchial vagal branches in cats. *J. Auton. Nerv. Syst.*, 5: 165–176.

Krauhs, J.M. (1984) Morphology of presumptive slowly adapting receptors in dog trachea. *Anat. Rec.*, 210: 73–85.

Laitinen, A. (1985) Ultrastructural organisation of intraepithelial nerves in the human airway tract. *Thorax*, 40: 488–492.

Larsell, G. (1921) Nerve terminations in the lung of the rabbit. *J. Comp. Neurol.*, 33: 105–131.

Larsell, G. (1922) The ganglia, plexuses and nerve terminations of the mammalian lung and pleura pulmonalis. *J. Comp. Neurol.*, 35: 97–132.

Larsell, G. (1935) Nerve endings in the human pleura pulmonalis. *J. Comp. Neurol.*, 61: 407–411.

Larsell, G. and Dow, R.S. (1933) Innervation of the human lung. *Am. J. Anat.*, 52: 125–146.

Lauweryns, J., Peuskens, J., Cokelaere, M. and Theunyuck, P. (1972) Neuroepithelial bodies in the respiratory mucosa of various mammals. *Z. Zellforsch.*, 135: 569–592.

Lauweryns, J.M., Cokelaere, M., Deleersnyder, M. and Liebens, M. (1977) Intrapulmonary neuro-epithelial bodies in newborn rabbits. *Cell Tissue Res.*, 182: 425–440.

McLaughlin, A.I.G. (1933) Nerves and nerve endings in the visceral pleura of the cat. *J. Physiol. (London)*, 80: 101–104.

Meyrick, B. and Reid, L. (1971) Nerves in rat intra-acinar alveoli: an electron microscopic study. *Respir. Physiol.*, 11: 367–377.

Pack, R.J. and Widdicombe, J.G. (1984) Amine-containing cells of the lung. *Eur. J. Respir. Dis.*, 65: 559–578.

Pack, R.J., Al-Ugaily, L.H. and Widdicombe, J.G. (1984) The innervation of the trachea and extrapulmonary bronchi of the mouse. *Cell Tissue Res.*, 238: 61–68.

Paintal, A.S. (1955) Impulses in vagal afferent fibres from specific pulmonary deflation receptors. The response of these receptors to phenyl diguanide, potato starch, 5-hydroxytryptamine and nicotine, and their role in respiratory and cardiovascular reflexes. *Quart. J. Exp. Physiol.*, 40: 89–111.

Paintal, A.S. (1969) Mechanism of stimulation of type J pulmonary receptors. *J. Physiol. (London)*, 203: 511–532.

Paintal, A.S. (1970) The mechanism of excitation of type J receptors, and the J reflex. In: R. Porter (Ed.), *Breathing: Hering–Breuer centenary symposium*. Churchill, London, pp. 59–71.

Polak, J.M. and Bloom, S.R. (1984) Regulatory peptides: localization and measurement. In: K.L. Becker and A.F. Gazdar (Eds.), *The Endocrine Lung in Health and Disease*. W.B. Saunders, Philadelphia, PA, pp. 300–327.

Ravi, K. (1986) Distribution and location of slowly adapting pulmonary stretch receptors in the airways of cats. *J. Auton. Nerv. Syst.*, 15: 205–216.

Sant'Ambrogio, G. (1982) Information arising from the tracheobronchial tree in mammals. *Physiol. Rev.*, 62: 531–569.

Saria, A., Martlings, C.-R., Dalsgaard, C.-J. and Lundberg, J.M. (1985) Evidence for substance P-immunoreactive spinal afferents that mediate bronchoconstriction. *Acta Physiol. Scand.*, 125: 405–414.

Scheuermann, D.W., Timmermans, J.-P., Adriaensen, D. and De Groodt-Lasseel, M.H.A. (1987) Immunoreactivity for calcitonin gene-related peptide in neuroepithelial bodies of the newborn cat. *Cell Tissue Res.*, 249: 337–340.

Schoultz, T.W. and Swett, J.E. (1972) The fine structure of the Golgi-tendon organ. *J. Neurocytol.*, 1: 1–26.

Simionescu, N. and Simionescu, M. (1983) The cardiovascular system. In: L. Weiss (Ed.), *Histology, Cell and Tissue Biology*, 5th edn. Elsevier, Amsterdam, pp. 371–433.

Spencer, H. and Leof, D. (1964) The innervation of the human lung. *J. Anat. (London)*, 98: 599–609.

Wasano, K. (1977) Neuro-epithelial bodies in the lung of the rat and the mouse. *Arch. Histol. Japon.*, 40: 207–219.

Widdicombe, J.G. (1986) Sensory innervation of the lungs and airways. In: F. Cervero and J.F.B. Morrison (Eds.), *Progress in Brain Research*, Vol. 67, Elsevier, Amsterdam, pp. 49–64.

W. Hamann and A. Iggo (Eds.)
Progress in Brain Research, Vol. 74
© 1988 Elsevier Science Publishers B.V. (Biomedical Division)

CHAPTER 17

The effect of gastro-entero-pancreatic hormones on the activity of vagal hepatic afferent fibres

Akira Niijima

Department of Physiology, Niigata University School of Medicine, Niigata 951, Japan

Summary

The effect of intra-portal administration of gastro-entero-pancreatic hormones on the afferent activity of the hepatic branch of the vagus nerve was investigated in the rat. The experiments were conducted in vivo and in isolated and perfused liver preparations. A dose-dependent decrease in afferent discharge rate was observed after intraportal administration of glucagon and cholecystokinin; however, a dose-responsive increase in afferent activity was shown by intra-portal administration of insulin.

These results suggest the existence of vagal sensors for gastro-entero-pancreatic hormones such as insulin, glucagon and cholecystokinin in the hepato-portal system. The sensors for these substances may play a role in the regulation of food intake behaviour and nervous control of blood glucose metabolism.

Introduction

The existence of glucoreceptors in the liver was first postulated by Russek (1963) in his behavioural studies. He suggested that receptors in the liver send signals on the glucose content of portal venous blood to the central nervous system via the vagi. Electrophysiological observations of activities of vagal afferents, made in in vitro perfused guinea pig liver preparations, indicated that the mean rate of firing of afferent fibres in the hepatic branch of the vagus nerve was decreased following intra-portal administration of glucose but not of mannose or fructose (Niijima, 1969). In in vivo experiments, it was observed that a gradual increase in glucose content in the portal venous blood induced by intra-duodenal infusion of isotonic (5%) glucose solution was accompanied by a gradual decrease in afferent discharge rate in the hepatic branch of the vagus nerve, and that the mean discharge rate of glucose-sensitive fibres was inversely related to the concentration of glucose in the portal blood (Niijima, 1982). These observations demonstrate that an increase in glucose concentration in portal venous blood results in a decrease in the rate of signals from the liver to the central nervous system, perhaps to the hypothalamus via the vagus nerve and the nucleus tractus solitarius in the medulla oblongata.

On the other hand, gastro-intestinal-pancreatic hormones such as insulin, glucagon and cholecystokinin (CCK) are released into the portal venous blood, then circulate in the liver through the portal vein and exit through the hepatic vein to the systemic circulation. As insulin and glucagon are the hormones to control glucose metabolism, and CCK acts as a satiety hormone (Antin et al., 1975), it can be assumed that the vagal hepatic afferents play a role as a monitor of these hormones.

This paper is concerned with the effect of insulin, glucagon and CCK on the rate of afferent discharges in the hepatic branch of the vagus nerve in the rat.

Methods

Adult Wistar rats were used for experiments. Animals were anaesthetised with a mixture of urethane (0.7 g/kg) and chloralose (50 mg/kg). Two different types of experiments were conducted: perfusion experiments on isolated liver preparations, and experiments in vivo. In the perfusion experiments Ringer solution saturated with 95% oxygen and 5% carbon dioxide was delivered by a peristaltic pump with a flow rate of approximately 10 ml/min from a temperature-controlled (ca. 30°C) reservoir into the portal vein. The perfusion system was devised to be switched from Ringer solution to test solution and vice versa by a three-way cock placed in between the peristaltic pump and the reservoir. In the in vivo experiments a small catheter was inserted into the portal vein for the administration of insulin (regular insulin, Novo), glucagon (Novo), CCK (Squibb) and glucose (Wako).

The afferent discharge was picked up by a pair of silver wire electrodes and amplified by means of a condenser-coupled amplifier, monitored by an oscilloscope and stored on magnetic tape. All analyses of nervous activity were performed after conversion of raw data to standard pulses by a window discriminator, which separated discharge from background noise. The standard pulses were then fed to a rate meter with a reset time of 10 s for studying the time course of discharge rate. The discharge rate was displayed on an oscilloscope. The mean discharge rate was obtained during each successive 10 s for 200 s or during each successive s for 20 s and values were expressed as mean ± SE. The differences were evaluated by Student's *t* test.

Results

Effect of insulin on afferent discharge rate

Perfusion experiments. Multi-unit discharges were recorded from small nerve filaments dissected from the peripheral cut end of the hepatic branch of the vagus nerve, and multi-unit spontaneous discharges were usually observed in the isolated and perfused liver preparation. Switching from Ringer solution to insulin – Ringer solution in a concentration of 40 μU/ml to perfuse 50 ml for about 5 min caused a slow increase in afferent discharge rate. The peak value was reached about 10 min after switching back to Ringer solution. Then the discharge rate decreased slowly until it returned to control level about 30 min after switching back to Ringer solution (Fig. 1, upper trace). Perfusion by insulin – Ringer solution of a higher concentration (400 μU/ml, 50 ml) caused a larger and longer increase in discharge rate (Fig. 1, lower trace). In this particular experiment the mean discharge rate before insulin administration was 18.6 ± 1.0 impulses/s. The peak values after perfusion with insulin – Ringer solution 40 μU/ml and 400 μU/ml were 24.0 ± 0.8 impulses/s and 28.5 ± 1.2 impulses/s, respectively (Fig. 1, graph). These values showed a significant difference from each other ($P < 0.001$).

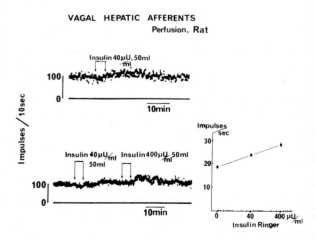

Fig. 1. Effect of insulin on the firing rate of vagal hepatic afferents. Perfusion experiment. Each pair of arrows indicates the time of perfusion with insulin – Ringer solution. The graph on the right shows the relation between the concentration of insulin and afferent discharge rate. Each point illustrates the mean ± SEM (*n* = 20).

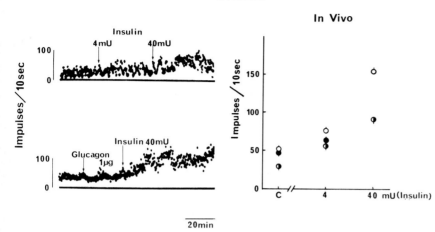

EFFECT OF INSULIN

Fig. 2. Effect of insulin on the firing rate of vagal hepatic afferents. In vivo experiment. Each arrow shows the time of injection. The figure on the right shows the relation between the dose of insulin injected into the portal vein and the afferent discharge rate (impulses/10 s). C, control values. Each point illustrates the mean ± SEM ($n = 20$).

In vivo experiments. The injection of insulin 4 mU (0.1 ml) and 40 mU (0.1 ml) caused an increase in afferent discharge rate which reached its peak value about 10–20 min after injection (Fig. 2, upper and lower traces). However, an injection of glucagon (1 μg, 0.1 ml) caused a decrease in discharge frequency. As shown in the graph in Fig. 2, the control value of discharge was 28.6 ± 3.4 impulses/10 s, and the peak values after administration of insulin 4 mU and 40 mU were 55.9 ± 4.8 impulses/10 s and 90.0 ± 5.2 impulses/10 s. The differences were significant ($P < 0.001$). Two other observations also showed a dose-dependent increase in discharge rate.

Effect of glucagon on afferent discharge rate

Perfusion experiments. Observations were made in four preparations. The upper trace in Fig. 3 shows the time course of discharge rate following successive administrations of glucagon at concentrations of 1 ng/ml, 10 ng/ml and 100 ng/ml for 10 ml. The duration of administration was approximately 1 min. The successive administrations caused a stepwise decrease in discharge rate following each administration. Closely similar results

were obtained on three other preparations. In Fig. 4, the left graph presents the relationship between glucagon concentration and afferent discharge frequency in four different preparations. It shows that the higher concentration of glucagon results in a lower frequency. In one example, afferent activities at control recording, after administration of glucagon 1 ng/ml, 10 ng/ml and

EFFECT OF GLUCAGON

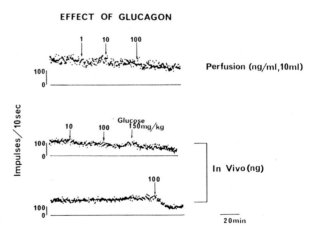

Fig. 3. Effect of injections of glucagon and glucose into the portal vein on the time course of the afferent discharge rate. Upper trace, perfusion experiment. Middle and lower traces, in vivo experiment. Each arrow shows the time of administration.

158

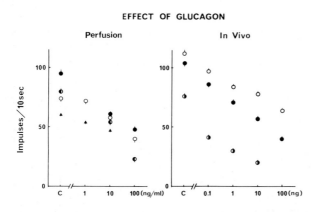

EFFECT OF GLUCAGON

Fig. 4. Relation between the dose of glucagon administered into the portal vein and the afferent discharge rate. Left, perfusion experiment. Right, in vivo experiment. Each point illustrates the mean ± SEM ($n = 20$).

100 ng/ml were 73.8 ± 2.4 impulses/10 s, 72.3 ± 2.4 impulses/10 s, 57.7 ± 2.6 impulses 10 s and 40.4 ± 2.2 impulses/10 s, respectively. The administration of glucagon 1 ng/ml gave no significant difference from the control value; however, administration of 10 ng/ml and 100 ng/ml caused a significant suppression in discharge rate ($P < 0.001$). Similar results were obtained on three other preparations.

In vivo experiments. Observations were made in six preparations. The middle trace in Fig. 3 shows the time course of discharge rate following successive injections of glucagon into the portal vein at doses of 10 ng and 100 ng, then glucose 150 mg/kg. All of these substances were dissolved with 0.1 ml saline. These successive injections caused a stepwise decrease in discharge rate following each injection. The lower trace in Fig. 3 indicates a suppression in discharge rate after an injection of glucagon 100 ng (0.1 ml). The inhibitory effect of glucagon on afferent discharge rate was also observed in four other preparations. The graphic representation in Fig. 4 shows the relationship between dose of glucagon injected into the portal vein and afferent discharge rate following each injection. In one example, discharge rate at control,

and those following injections of glucagon 100 pg, 1 ng, 10 ng and 100 ng were 103.9 ± 2.4 impulses/10 s, 85.8 ± 1.9 impulses/10 s, 70.9 ± 2.3 impulses/10 s, 57.3 ± 2.0 impulses/10 s and 39.9 ± 1.4 impulses/10 s, respectively. Each value shows a significant difference ($P < 0.001$). The other two observations in this graph represent a similar suppression by glucagon.

Effect of CCK on afferent discharge rate

The effects of CCK-8 on the discharge rate of hepatic vagal afferent fibres were observed in four preparations in perfusion experiments and in two preparations in in vivo experiments. The perfusion of CCK – Ringer solution 10 ml in concentrations of 1 ng/ml and 10 ng/ml caused a decrease in discharge rate; no change resulted from administration of Ringer solution or 0.1 ng/ml CCK – Ringer solution in perfusion experiments (Fig. 5, upper trace). The lower trace in Fig. 5 shows the time course of discharge rate following successive administrations of CCK into the portal vein at doses of 0.1 ng, 1 ng and 10 ng dissolved in 0.1 ml Ringer solution in in vivo experiments. A stepwise suppression in discharge frequency fol-

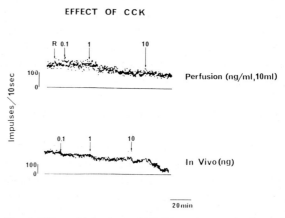

EFFECT OF CCK

Fig. 5. Effect of injections of CCK into the portal vein on the time course of the afferent discharge rate. Upper trace, perfusion experiment. R, administration of Ringer solution. Lower trace, in vivo experiment. Each arrow indicates the time of administration.

lowing each injection was observed. Fig. 6 shows the relationship between doses of CCK administered into the portal vein and afferent discharge rates in perfusion experiments (left) as well as in in vivo experiments (right). In one example in perfusion experiments the discharge rate at control and those following administration of CCK 100 pg/ml, 1 ng/ml, and 10 ng/ml were 101.0 ± 3.7 impulses/10 s, 83.1 ± 2.7 impulses/10 s, 70.6 ± 2.0 impulses/10 s and 62.9 ± 2.0 impulses/10 s, respectively. In one example of in vivo experiments the discharge rate at control and those following injection of CCK 1 ng, 10 ng and 100 ng were 100.8 ± 2.2 impulses/10 s, 78.4 ± 2.3 impulses/10 s, 68.4 ± 2.0 impulses/10 s and 44.2 ± 1.4 impulses/10 s, respectively. Another study in vivo and two other studies in perfusion experiments indicated a similar inverse relationship between CCK dose and afferent discharge rate.

Discussion

The results of the present study show that the administration of insulin into the portal vein enhances afferent activity and administration of glucagon and CCK suppresses afferent activity in the hepatic branch of the vagus nerve in vivo and in isolated and perfused liver preparations in the

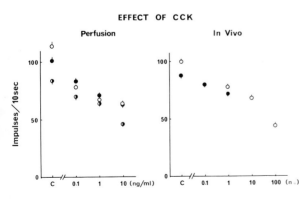

Fig. 6. Relation between the dose of CCK administered into the portal vein and the afferent discharge rate. Left, perfusion experiment. Right, in vivo experiment. Each point illustrates the mean ± SEM (n = 20).

rat. In relation to this, it has been reported that the topical application of insulin to the glucose-sensitive neurone in the lateral hypothalamic area increases its activity (Oomura, 1973) and that of glucagon causes a suppression in activity in the same type of neurone (Oomura, 1983). He explained that the dose – response relationship and low threshold for the insulin effect on the glucose-sensitive neurone imply the insulin receptor sites on the neuronal membrane, and that the inhibitory effect of glucagon on the glucose-sensitive neurone is due to the acceleration of the Na pump in the neuronal membrane because a prior application of ouabain blocks the inhibitory effect of glucagon. This explanation might be applicable for the effect of insulin and glucagon on the afferent discharge rate of vagal afferent fibres in the hepato-portal system. In addition, this type of afferent fibre possesses a similar coding mechanism from blood glucose concentration to nerve activity through Na pump activity in the neuronal membrane (Niijima, 1984) as that of glucose-sensitive neurones in the hypothalamus (Oomura et al., 1974).

It can be speculated that the glucose-sensitive afferent fibres in the hepato-portal area may have insulin receptors as glucose-sensitive neurones in the hypothalamus, and that glucagon causes an inhibition of afferent activity through Na pump activation in the membrane of glucose-sensitive afferent nerve terminals. To prove the latter mechanism, a blocking effect of ouabain on the inhibitory effect of glucagon must be observed. It might be possible to suggest that the glucose-sensitive afferent fibres in the hepato-portal area possess multimodality for sensing insulin, glucagon and CCK. However, it will be technically difficult to prove it with the recording of nerve signals from the non-myelinated single afferent fibres.

In relation to the amount of administration of insulin, glucagon and CCK, it has been reported that the concentrations of plasma insulin and glucagon are about 20 μU/ml (Steffens, 1976) and 150 pg/ml (De Jong et al., 1977) in fasting rats, and the basal level of CCK in the plasma in men was about 200 pg/ml (Rayford et al., 1978). The concentrations of these substances in the portal venous blood might be higher than these values and seem to be comparable to the doses of these substances used in the experiments.

As described before, Russek (1963) reported that the increase in glucose content in the portal venous blood suppresses food intake, and the reduction in nerve signals of the vagal hepatic afferents accompanies the increase in glucose content of the portal venous blood (Niijima, 1982); the anorexic effect of CCK and glucagon might be explained by a similar mechanism. Satiation after feeding might be due to the release of CCK, glucagon and other gastro-intestinal-pancreatic hormones into the portal venous blood which may modulate the frequency of the afferent discharges in the hepatic branch of the vagus nerve.

References

Antin, J., Gibbs, J., Holt, J., Young, R.C. and Smith, G.P. (1975) Cholecystokinin elicits the complete behavioral sequence of satiety in rats. *J. Comp. Physiol. Psychol.,* 89: 784 – 900.

De Jong, A., Strubbe, J.H. and Steffens, A.B. (1977) Hypothalamic influence on insulin and glucagon release in the rat. *Am. J. Physiol.,* 233: E380 – E388.

Niijima, A. (1969) Afferent impulse discharges from glucoreceptors in the liver of guinea-pig. *Ann. N.Y. Acad. Sci.,* 157: 690 – 700.

Niijima, A. (1982) Glucose-sensitive afferent nerve fibres in the hepatic branch of the vagus nerve in the guinea-pig. *J. Physiol. (London),* 322: 315 – 323.

Niijima, A. (1984) Afferent discharges from glucose sensors in the liver. In: W. Hamann and A. Iggo (Eds.), *Sensory Receptor Mechanisms.* World Scientific, Singapore, pp. 203 – 206.

Oomura, Y. (1973) Central mechanism of feeding. In: M. Kotani (Ed.), *Advances in Biophysics.* Tokyo University Press, Tokyo, pp. 65 – 142.

Oomura, Y. (1983) Glucose as a regulator of neural activity. In: A.J. Szabo (Ed.), *Advances in Metabolic Disorders,* Vol. 10. Academic Press, New York, pp. 31 – 65.

Oomura, Y., Ooyama, H., Sugimori, M., Nakamura, T. and Yamada, Y. (1974) Glucose inhibition of glucose sensitive neurone in the rat lateral hypothalamus. *Nature (London),* 247: 284 – 286.

Rayford, P.L., Schafmyer, A., Teichmann, R.K. and Thompson, J.C. (1978) Cholecystokinin radioimmunoassay. In: S.R. Bloom (Ed.), *Gut Hormones.* Churchill Livingstone, Edinburgh, pp. 208 – 212.

Russek, M. (1963) An hypothesis on the participation of hepatic glucoreceptors in the control of food intake. *Nature (London),* 197: 79 – 80.

Steffens, A.B. (1976) Influence of oral cavity on insulin release in the rat. *Am. J. Physiol.,* 230: 1411 – 1415.

W. Hamann and A. Iggo (Eds.)
Progress in Brain Research, Vol. 74
© 1988 Elsevier Science Publishers B.V. (Biomedical Division)

CHAPTER 18

The responses of chemoreceptors with medullated and non-medullated fibres to chemical substances and the mechanical hypothesis

A.S Paintal

DST Centre for Visceral Mechanisms, V.P. Chest Institute, University of Delhi, Delhi 110 007, India

Introduction

The hypothesis that all sensory receptors are stimulated by mechanical deformation of the generator region of the sensory receptor complex and not by an action of a chemical transmitter on the generator region (Fig. 1) has been advanced from time to time (Paintal, 1967, 1971a, 1972 1973, 1976, 1977). This hypothesis arose from experiments, on aortic chemoreceptors, designed to test the earlier suggestion that certain chemical substances sensitize, stimulate or depress sensory receptors by an action on the regenerative region of the sensory receptor complex and not on the generator region. From information gathered a that time (Paintal, 1964) it followed that the greater responsiveness of the endings of non-medullated fibres to chemical substances must be due to the regenerative region of these fibres being more susceptible to the effects of such substances than the regenerative region of the endings with medullated fibres. The aortic chemoreceptors were chosen as the test object because this group of sensory receptors not only had both medullated and non-medullated fibres but the receptors of both types of fibres responded in an identical manner to the same natural stimulus, i.e., hypoxia (Paintal and Riley, 1966; Paintal, 1967). The results showed clearly that for a given dose of

acetylcholine (ACh) or phenyldiguanide the aortic chemoreceptors with medullated fibres were either unaffected or if they were stimulated the resulting responses were much smaller than those yielded by endings with non-medullated fibres. These unequivocal observations which are reproduced in Fig. 2 supported the hypothesis that chemical substances produce their effects by an action on the regenerative region of the sensory receptors, i.e., the region where the propagated impulses were initiated (see Paintal, 1964) (Fig. 1).

These results, which were presented at the Wates symposium in July 1966 at Oxford, were published subsequently (Paintal, 1967, 1968). Soon after Fidone and Sato (1969) repeated the observations on carotid chemoreceptors and reported results which were quite the opposite of those reported by Paintal (1967). They reported that carotid chemoreceptors with A fibres had a lower threshold to ACh than carotic chemoreceptors with C fibres. This conclusion by Fidone and Sato resulted from a new technique for measuring conduction velocities of nerve fibres — the so-called 'monotopic' technique. Using this technique they found that the conduction velocities of the A fibres of chemoreceptors ranged from 4 to 53 m/s with a median at 16 m/s.

Thus there is a striking difference between the conduction velocities of the medullated fibres of

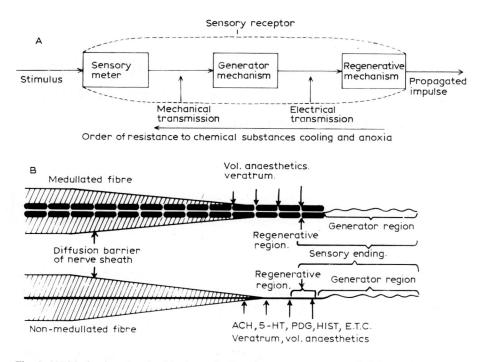

Fig. 1. (A) Mechanisms involved in the excitation of sensory receptors and their relative resistance to chemical substances, cooling and anoxia (Paintal, 1971a). Note the scheme envisages that the generator region is stimulated by mechanical deformation and not by any chemical transmitter. (B) Schematic diagram of sensory endings consisting of the generator region and the regenerative region which is the first node in the case of medullated fibres showing the probable site of action of injected drugs at the regenerative region where there is no diffusion barrier. A greater variety of drugs affect the endings of non-medullated fibres because the fibres themselves are susceptible to these drugs (Paintal, 1964).

aortic (Paintal and Riley, 1966) and carotid (Fidone and Sato, 1969) chemoreceptors. This difference could be, as suggested by Fidone and Sato (1969), due to a dissimilarity between the aortic and carotid chemoreceptors or it could be due to a difference in the method of measuring conduction velocities of nerve fibres. Since the latter possibility was more likely, the conduction velocity values obtained by using the conventional and 'monotopic' techniques were compared on the same fibres. As shown below it is clear that the conduction velocity values obtained using the 'monotopic' technique are far greater than those obtained using the conventional technique.

Methods

The experiments were carried out in 1970 on cats anaesthetised with chloralose (75 mg/kg) after induction with trichlorethylene. The electrophysiological set-up consisted of two Tektronix type 122 preamplifiers, one Devices stimulator and two Tektronix 422 oscilloscopes placed one above the other, for recording two sweeps, at slow and fast speeds simultaneously, with a 70 mm recording camera.

Two methods of measuring conduction velocities of individual fibres in filaments dissected off the vagus nerve were used (Fig. 3). In the conven-

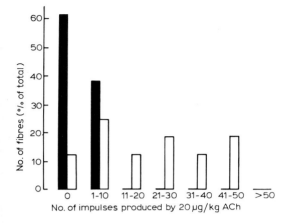

Fig. 2. Responses of chemoreceptors with medullated fibres (black columns) and non-medullated fibres (open columns) to 20 μg/kg ACh injected into the ascending aorta. The abscissa indicates the total number of impulses generated by ACh and the ordinate the number of fibres (% of total) that yielded the responses with different intensities. The data were obtained from dose–response curves (Paintal, 1967). The total number of medullated fibres was 13, the number of non-medullated fibres 16.

measured. The distance between these electrodes which was about 4 mm was measured with a measuring micrometer. When using this technique channel 1 of both oscilloscopes was connected to the output of the preamplifier of the proximal electrode and channel 2 of both oscilloscopes was connected to the output of the preamplifier of the distal electrode. The sweep of the second 422 oscilloscope was set at much higher sweep speed than the first. In both oscilloscopes the two channels, 1 and 2, were set in the chopped mode (chopping frequency, 100 kHz) thereby ensuring that there was no error in the temporal events displayed on the two channels. This was further facilitated by the fact that the sweeps were recorded either as frames (photographic paper still) or with the photographic paper moving horizontally (i.e., same direction as the sweeps). This ensured that there was no error in the alignment of the two traces on the fast sweep oscilloscope. The measurements of the intervals between two impulses were made using a measuring micrometer.

tional method (Fig. 3A), a pair of stimulating electrodes were placed under the vagosympathetic trunk low in the neck and square pulses of 0.1–0.2 ms duration were delivered through a Devices Isolator stimulator (Mk IV). A pair of silver–silver chloride recording electrodes were placed under filaments dissected off the vagus nerve near the nodose ganglion. These were connected to one preamplifier with a band pass of 0.2 Hz to 10 kHz. The conduction distance between the stimulating and recording electrodes which was usually about 60 mm was measured with a pair of dividers.

The second method for measuring conduction velocities of the same fibres consisted of a set of three electrodes on which the filaments were placed. They were connected to two preamplifiers in the manner shown in Fig. 3B. This is the 'monotopic' technique used by Fidone and Sato (1969). In this method the time for conduction of an impulse between the two proximal electrodes (the distal electrode is common to both) is

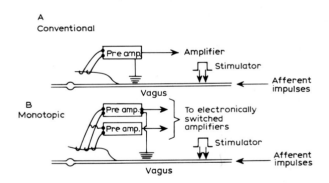

Fig. 3. Methods used for measuring the conduction velocities of individual fibres of the vagus nerve. (A) The conventional arrangement with the stimulating electrodes on the vagus nerve low in the neck and a pair of recording electrodes with a filament near the nodose ganglion. (B) The 'monotopic' technique for measuring the conduction velocity of individual fibres. Here the aim is to measure the time taken for an impulse to travel from the proximal recording electrode, connected to one differential amplifier, to the distal recording electrode connected to another differential amplifier (as shown in Figs. 4 and 5); note the common most distal (third) electrode connected to both preamplifiers (see Fidone and Sato, 1969).

The temperature of the paraffin pool in which the recording end of the vagus lay was measured with a thermistor set-up. This was about 1°C less than the rectal temperature, i.e., the temperature of the main length of the vagus. Corrections for temperature differences in conduction velocities were made using a Q_{10} of 1.6 (Paintal, 1965).

Results

The conduction velocities of ten medullated and non-medullated fibres were measured carefully using both methods. The values yielded by the 'monotopic' technique were absurdly high in all of them. For example, as shown in Fig. 4, whether one uses the foot or the peak of the impulse, the conduction velocity values (conduction distance 4 mm) amount to 200–700 m/s whereas the actual conduction velocity of this fibre was 36 m/s. Similarly in the case of non-medullated fibres the values obtained were also very high. For example, Fig. 5A shows an impulse in a non-medullated fibre, at the arrow, that was conducted over a distance of 65 mm from the stimulating to the recording electrode. The conduction velocity estimated from Fig. 5A amounts to 2.2 m/s. However, in Fig. 5B, which is a sweep that is ten times faster than in Fig. 5A, the conduction velocity measured monotopically amounts to about 27 m/s. The actual value obtained depended on

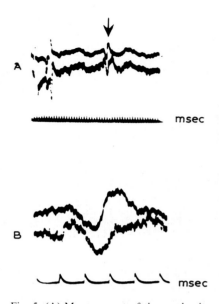

Fig. 5. (A) Measurement of the conduction velocity of a non-medullated fibre (impulse shown by arrow) using the conventional method. The conduction distance was 65 mm. Estimated conduction velocity 2.2 m/s. (B) The same impulses on an expanded sweep on another oscilloscope as recorded by the 'monotopic' method (see Fig. 3B); the distance between the two electrodes was 4 mm. Estimated conduction velocity 26.7 m/s. In three other sweeps the conduction velocities by this method were 13.3, 5.7 and 57.0 m/s.

the shapes of the individual impulses. For example in the case of this fibre the conduction velocity values were 13.3, 5.7 and 57 m/s in three other consecutive sweeps.

Discussion

From the results (e.g., Figs. 4 and 5) it is certain that the 'monotopic' technique yields a gross overestimate of the actual conduction velocity of nerve fibres, be they medullated or non-medullated. This conclusion is specially relevant in the case of the non-medullated fibres because if the fibres that Fidone and Sato (1969) thought were medullated (from their 'monotopic' measurements) were in fact non-medullated then this would explain (keeping in mind the observations on aortic chemoreceptors (Paintal, 1967)) why they concluded that their so-called A fibre chemorecep-

"Monotopic" recording

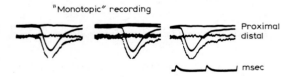

Proximal
distal

msec

Fig. 4. Records of individual impulses with the 'monotopic' method. The impulses were from a pulmonary stretch fibre with a conduction velocity of 36 m/s as measured by the conventional method shown in Fig. 3A. Note the interval between any pair of impulses (arriving at the proximal and distal electrode) in any of the three pairs of sweeps is hard to measure. However whether one uses the start or the peak of the impulse the estimated conduction velocity over a conduction distance (i.e., distance between the two electrodes) of 4 mm ranges from 222 to 710 m/s.

tors were more sensitive to ACh than their C fibre chemoreceptors. From a variety of data given below it is almost certain that the vast majority of chemoreceptors thought by them to have A fibres were probably chemoreceptors with non-medullated fibres. Not only is this conclusion tenable on the basis of the present results but it is also consistent with the information already available on the subject. For example De Castro (1951) showed that in the carotid nerve 17.5% of the medullated fibres had a diameter of $1.5 - 2.8$ μm, 79% a diameter of $3 - 5$ μm; only 3.5% had a diameter of $6 - 8$ μm, i.e., far less than that expected from the results of Fidone and Sato (1969). Ten years later Eyzaguirre and Uchizono (1961) obtained results that were in general agreement with the observations of De Castro (1951). Eyzaguirre and Uchizono (1961) further observed that the relative number of medullated fibres was far less in the portion of the carotid nerve close to the carotid body than in the middle part of the carotid nerve. They determined the relative numbers of medullated and non-medullated fibres in three sections of the carotid nerve by counting all the fibres in a sample of 15 electron micrographs. In Table 1 are shown the counts of fibres in the carotid nerve close to the

TABLE 1

Ratio of non-medullated fibres to medullated fibres in the carotid nerve at two levels. The first two lines show the number of fibres counted in sections made at the origin (near glomus) and in the middle of the nerve, respectively (Eyzaguirre and Uchizono, 1961). The last line gives the number of medullated fibres that would have been counted in the middle of the nerve had the number of non-medullated fibres counted been 603.

Section level	Number of non-medullated fibres	Number of medullated fibres	Ratio
Origin (i.e., near glomus)	603	122	4.94
Middle	404	191	2.11
Middle	603 (assumed)	285 (expected)	2.11

glomus and in the nerve near the middle of its length, i.e., before the branch to the carotid sinus was given off so that this part contains the fibres to both the glomus and the sinus. From the counts Eyzaguirre and Uchizono obtained the ratio of non-medullated to medullated fibres which is given in the last column. Had they counted the same number of non-medullated fibres in the middle of the nerve (i.e., 603), then, as shown in the last line of Table 1, the corresponding number of medullated fibres that would have been counted would have been about 285. This figure (285) would have included the 122 medullated fibres destined to reach the carotid body (first line of Table 1), leaving 163 fibres destined for the carotid sinus, i.e., carotid baroreceptors. Assuming that the medullated fibres at the glomeral end were all from chemoreceptors (which is unlikely: see below) then the maximum possible ratio of medullated chemoreceptor fibres to medullated baroreceptor fibres can be 122:163, i.e., 1:1.3. This ratio is in the opposite direction of that derived by Fidone and Sato (1969) which was 2:1 (2/3 chemoreceptors, 1/3 baroreceptors). The actual ratio of carotid chemoreceptor fibres (medullated) to baroreceptor fibres will be even less than 1:1.3 for two reasons. First the count (603) of non-medullated fibres in the middle of the carotid nerve would include non-medullated fibres destined for carotid baroreceptors. Second, as shown by De Castro (1951), medullated fibres also innervate the arteries and arterioles of the glomus in addition to the cells of the glomus.

From the above it is clear that the correlation of the electrophysiological observations of Fidone and Sato (1969) with the histological observations of Eyzaguirre and Uchizono (1961) as done in Fig. 6 of their paper (Fidone and Sato, 1969) is hard to justify.

The relative conduction velocities of the baroreceptors and chemoreceptors shown by them in their Fig. 6 (Fidone and Sato, 1969) is also quite inconsistent with the relative spike heights of carotid chemoreceptors and baroreceptors. Ever since the classical work of Erlanger and Gasser

(1937) it is known that the spike heights of medullated nerve fibres are inversely related to their conduction velocities (or fibre diameters). Thus since in records of impulses from the whole intact carotid nerve (thereby avoiding injury to nerve fibres) the spike heights of carotid baroreceptors have invariably been found to be much larger than those of carotid chemoreceptor fibres by several investigators (e.g., see Euler et al., 1939; Duke et al., 1952; Landgren et al., 1954) it must follow that the conduction velocities (and fibre diameter) of baroreceptors are much larger than those of chemoreceptors. It needs to be pointed out that sometimes in dissected filaments from the carotid nerve, or aortic nerve, one can obtain spikes from chemoreceptor fibres that are larger than those from baroreceptors but this is due to relative injury to the nerve fibres and variable recording conditions. In any case this is an exception and not the rule.

Finally there are two sources of direct evidence obtained by Gallego and Belmonte (1984) and Kirkwood et al. (1985) which are quite contrary to the observations of Fidone and Sato (1969). Gallego and Belmonte (1984) carried out their experiments on an in vitro preparation of the petrosal ganglion connected to the carotid body. They recorded impulses intracellularly from the ganglion cells and identified 101 cells as belonging to chemoreceptor fibres on the basis of their excitation by stimuli known to stimulate chemoreceptors. An additional 60 cells were assumed to belong to chemoreceptor fibres on the basis of certain properties of the soma. In spite of some uncertainty caused by the inclusion of the latter group it is nevertheless clear from their Fig. 3 (Gallego and Belmonte, 1984) that 94% of the actual and assumed chemoreceptor fibres had conduction velocities less than 18 m/s. However, even this value (which is far lower than the values of $25 - 53$ m/s in 17% of the fibres of Fidone and Sato (see their Fig. 6)) is much higher than the maximum of 9 m/s obtained by Kirkwood et al. (1985) in 36 chemoreceptor units using a different technique; in only one unit the conduction velocity was 15 m/s. It should be

noted that Kirkwood et al. (1985) made their observations in vivo and they used spike triggered averaging of either the extracellular field potential recorded through a microelectrode in the petrosal ganglion or the impulses recorded from the cut peripheral end of the IXth nerve. The conduction velocity values of $19 - 44$ m/s in baroreceptor fibres and $1 - 9$ m/s in chemoreceptor fibres obtained by them are in close agreement with the corresponding values of conduction velocities of aortic baroreceptor and chemoreceptor fibres (Paintal, 1953; Paintal and Riley, 1966). As pointed out by Gallego and Belmonte (1984), the conduction velocities obtained by them also correspond to the values in the aortic nerve (Paintal, 1953; Paintal and Riley, 1966) on the one hand and differ from those obtained by Fidone and Sato (1969) on the other.

From the above it follows that, if, as seems likely the so-called A fibres of chemoreceptors of Fidone and Sato (1969) were in fact non-medullated fibres, the earlier conclusion that the endings of non-medullated fibres are far more sensitive to the effects of ACh (Paintal, 1967) stands uncontradicted. It was essentially because of the contradictory conclusion of Fidone and Sato (1969) that the observations showing the greater sensitivity of endings of non-medullated fibres to chemical substances (Paintal, 1967) fell into the background. This also resulted in the mechanical hypothesis of stimulation of chemoreceptors (Fig. 6) (Paintal, 1967) also falling into the background in spite of the fact that evidence had been provided subsequently showing that the aortic chemoreceptors have certain properties that are like mechanoreceptors, e.g., their Q_{10} was about 2.5, i.e., similar to that of mechanoreceptors (Paintal, 1971b) (Fig. 6). On the other hand, the search for transmitters at chemoreceptors has continued with much interest and several candidate transmitters have been tested and discarded from time to time (see Eyzaguirre et al, 1983). It would seem that a simple method of testing a candidate transmitter substance would be to see whether it stimulates endings with medullated fibres as intensely as the

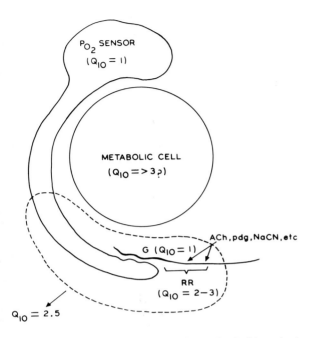

Fig. 6. Schematic diagram outlining the mechanical hypothesis of mechanism of initiation of impulses at arterial chemoreceptors. G, generator region; RR, regenerative region of the sensory receptor complex. Lowering of local pO_2 owing to a fall in oxygen availability is sensed by the pO_2 sensor, which by producing a suitable physical change at the generator region leads to the production of a generator potential (note no role of a chemical transmitter is envisaged in this hypothesis). The generator current initiates a propagated impulse at the regenerative region. Chemical substances such as ACh phenyldiguanide (pdg) and NaCN produce their excitatory effect by acting on the regenerative region. The temperature coefficient (Q_{10}) of the whole sensory receptor complex (enclosed by dashed line) is 2.5. Likely Q_{10}s of the other components are also shown (Paintal, 1973).

endings with non-medullated fibres. This is quite easy to do in the case of aortic chemoreceptors. If it does then one could justifiably entertain the idea that it might be acting on the generator mechanism of the sensory receptor complex (see Fig. 1). So far no such substance has been found, hence the need to consider seriously the hypothesis of mechanical transmission at chemoreceptors (Fig. 6) and other receptors (Paintal, 1976).

Summary and conclusions

The importance of earlier observations (Paintal, 1967) showing that chemoreceptors with non-medullated fibres are far more sensitive to chemical substances than chemoreceptors with medullated fibres has been re-established through recent measurements of conduction velocities of nerve fibres. The existence of such a difference in sensitivity in the case of any particular chemical substance makes that substance an unlikely candidate transmitter for initiation of impulses at chemoreceptors.

Until a candidate transmitter that excites endings with both types of fibres is found it might be worth while considering seriously the mechanical hypothesis of stimulation of chemoreceptors and other sensory receptors (Paintal, 1971a).

Acknowledgement

I am grateful to Dr. Ashima Anand for invaluable discussions.

References

De Castro, F. (1951) Sur la structure de la synapse dans les chémorecepteurs: leur mécanisme d'excitation et rôle dans la circulation sanguine locale. *Acta Physiol. Scand.* 22: 14 – 43.

Duke, H.N., Green, J.H. and Neil, E. (1952) Carotid chemoreceptor impulse activity during inhalation of carbon monoxide mixtures. *J. Physiol. (London),* 118: 520 – 527.

Erlanger, J. and Gasser, H.S. (1937) *Electrical Signs of Nervous Activity.* University of Pennsylvania Press, Philadelphia, PA, pp. 172 – 173.

Euler, U.S.v., Liljestrand, G. and Zotterman, Y. (1939) The excitation mechanism of chemoreceptors of the carotid body. *Skand. Arch. Physiol.,* 83: 132 – 152.

Eyzaguirre, C. and Uchizono, K. (1961) Observations on the fibre content of nerves reaching the carotid body of the cat. *J. Physiol. (London),* 159: 268 – 281.

Eyzaguirre, C., Fitzgerald, R.S., Lahiri, S. and Zapata, P. (1983) Arterial chemoreceptors. In: J.T. Shepherd and F.M. Aboud (Eds.), *Handbook of Physiology. The Cardiovascular System III.* Williams and Wilkins, Baltimore, MD, pp. 557 – 621.

Fidone, S.J. and Sato, A. (1969) A study of chemoreceptor and baroreceptor A- and C-fibres in the cat carotid nerve. *J. Physiol. (London)*, 205: 527 – 548.

Gallego, R. and Belmonte, C. (1984) Chemoreceptor and baroreceptor neurones in the petrosal ganglion. In: D.J. Pallot (Ed.), *The Peripheral Arterial Chemoreceptors.* Croom Helm, London, pp. 1 – 7.

Kirkwood, P.A., Nisimaru, N. and Sears, T.A. (1985) Carotid sinus nerve afferent discharges in the anaesthetised cat. *J. Physiol. (London)*, 360: 44P.

Landgren, S., Liljestrand, G. and Zotterman, Y. (1954) Impulse activity in the carotid sinus nerve following intracarotid injections of sodium-iodo-acetate, histamine hydrochloride, lergitin, and some purine and barbituric acid derivatives. *Acta Physiol. Scand.*, 30: 149 – 160.

Paintal, A.S. (1953) The conduction velocities of respiratory and cardiovascular afferent fibres in the vagues nerve. *J. Physiol. (London)*, 121: 341 – 359.

Paintal, A.S. (1964) Effects of drugs on vertebrate mechanoreceptors. *Pharmacol. Rev.*, 16: 341 – 380.

Paintal, A.S. (1965) Block of conduction in mammalian myelinated nerve fibres by low temperatures. *J. Physiol. (London)*, 180: 1 – 19.

Paintal, A.S. (1967) Mechanism of stimulation of aortic chemoreceptors by natural stimuli and chemical substances. *J. Physiol. (London)*, 189: 63 – 84.

Paintal, A.S. (1968) Some considerations relating to studies on chemoreceptor responses. In: R.W. Torrance (Ed.), *Arterial Chemoreceptors.* Blackwell, Oxford, pp. 253 – 260.

Paintal, A.S. (1971a) Action of drugs on sensory nerve endings. *Ann. Rev. Pharmacol.*, 11: 231 – 240.

Paintal, A.S. (1971b) The responses of chemoreceptors at reduced temperatures. *J. Physiol. (London)*, 217: 1 – 18.

Paintal, A.S. (1972) Cardiovascular receptors. In: E. Neil (Ed.), *Handbook of Sensory Physiology,* Vol. III/I. Springer-Verlag, Berlin, pp. 1 – 45.

Paintal, A.S. (1973) Vagal sensory receptors and their reflex effects. *Physiol. Rev.*, 53: 159 – 227.

Paintal, A.S. (1976) Natural and paranatural stimulation of sensory receptors. In: Y. Zotterman (Ed.), *Sensory Functions of the Skin.* Pergamon Press, Oxford, pp. 3 – 12.

Paintal, A.S. (1977) Effects of drugs on chemoreceptors, pulmonary and cardiovascular receptors. *Pharmacol. Ther.*, B, 3: 41 – 63.

Paintal, A.S. and Riley, R.L. (1969) Responses of aortic chemoreceptors. *J. Appl. Physiol.*, 21: 543 – 548.

W. Hamann and A. Iggo (Eds.)
Progress in Brain Research, Vol. 74
© 1988 Elsevier Science Publishers B.V. (Biomedical Division)

CHAPTER 19

Mechanisms of chemotransmission in the mammalian carotid body

S.J. Fidone, C. Gonzalez[*], B.G. Dinger and G.R. Hanson

Departments of Physiology, and Pharmacology and Toxicology, University of Utah School of Medicine, 410 Chipeta Way, Research Park, Salt Lake City, Utah 84108, USA

Introduction

The carotid bodies are small (< 1.0 mg) paired organs located near the bifurcations of the common carotid arteries; they lie in variable anatomical relationship with these vessels in different animal species. The organ is usually spherical, ovoid, or discoid and is innervated both by the carotid sinus nerve (CSN), a branch of the glossopharyngeal nerve (9th cranial nerve), and by the ganglioglomerular (sympathetic) nerve of the nearby superior cervical ganglion. Fig. 1 schematically illustrates the prominent microscopic features of the mammalian carotid body. The organ contains two types of parenchymal cells, one of which (type I or glomus cell) contains numerous dense-cored vesicles and receives synaptic-like contacts from sensory fibers of the carotid sinus nerve (CSN; see Fidone and Gonzalez, 1986). The other cell type (type II or sustentacular cell) lacks any distinguishing cytoplasmic organelles or innervation, and occurs in capsule-like arrays surrounding one or more type I cells. The morphological differences between these two cell types have provided the hypothetical basis for ascribing a more direct role in chemoreception for the type I cells and a supporting, or glial-like, function for the

type II cells. However, in spite of recent advances in carotid body chemoreception, the precise roles of the type I and type II cell still remain to be elucidated. Morphologically, the axon terminals of the CSN can be postsynaptic, presynaptic or reciprocally synaptic to the type I cells (McDonald and Mitchell, 1975). In addition, these cells in some species may also receive limited synaptic inputs from both preganglionic and postganglionic sympathetic fibers (not shown in the figure).

It is now well established that several transmitter candidates are contained within the type I

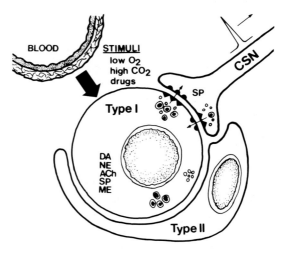

Fig. 1. Schematic representation of mammalian carotid body. See text for explanation.

[*] *Present address: Departamento de Fisiología y Bioquímica, Facultad de Medicina, Valladolid, Spain.*

cell/nerve ending complex, including biogenic amines (dopamine, DA; norepinephrine, NE; acetylcholine, ACh; and perhaps serotonin, 5-HT) and neuropeptides (substance P, SP; met-enkephalin, ME). Two perennial issues pertaining to arterial chemoreception concern, first, whether type I cells are the sole transducer elements in this sensory receptor, and second, what are the functions of the several putative neurotransmitters contained in these cells. In the following sections we discuss some findings from our recent studies of glomus cells and their contents of multiple neuroactive agents. In addition to examining the hypothesis that glomus cells are the locus of chemotransduction, our experiments have, in particular, focused attention on the effects of natural stimuli (hypoxia, hypercapnia and decreased pH) on the synthesis, storage and release of putative neurotransmitters, and their specific receptor sites within the chemosensory tissue.

The transduction of chemosensory stimuli in the carotid body

Several important observations have been made that probably relate to the transductive processes which occur in the carotid body. For example, the carotid body has been shown to have the highest blood flow per unit weight of any organ in the body, and the tissue exhibits a correspondingly high O_2 consumption (see Fidone and Gonzalez, 1986, for review). Particularly noteworthy is the finding from spectrometric and fluorometric studies (Mills, 1975) that the type I cells may contain a cytochrome oxidase with a very low affinity for oxygen, such that at a pO_2 of 140 torr it is already reduced by $10-40\%$, and is completely reduced at a pO_2 of $7-9$ torr. These observations, and the fact that metabolic poisons (e.g., NaCN, dinitrophenol, etc.) are powerful chemostimulants, have led to the suggestion that the transduction mechanisms in this tissue, at least for hypoxia, are linked to the energetic metabolism of the organ (Mulligan and Lahiri, 1981). We have examined this hypothesis by studying the effects of natural

and pharmacological stimulation on the metabolism of glucose and ATP in the carotid body.

Glucose consumption in the carotid body was determined by measuring the accumulation of 2-deoxy-^{3}H-glucose-6-phosphate from tracer amounts of labelled 2-deoxy-^{3}H-glucose (^{3}H-2DG). In addition, we studied the accumulation of ^{3}H-2DG in the non-chemosensory tissue of the nodose sensory ganglion for comparison. The rate of ^{3}H-2DG phosphorylation in carotid body (64

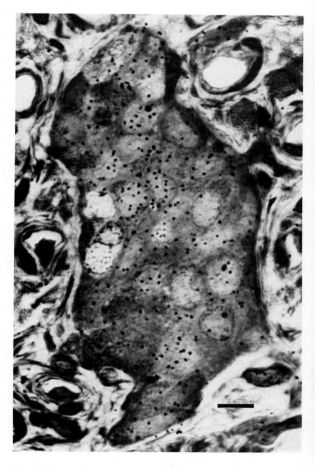

Fig. 2. Autoradiograph localizing ^{3}H-2DG uptake to lobule of type I/type II cells in normal rabbit carotid body. Following incubation, carotid bodies were washed for 30 min in 100% O_2-Tyrode to eliminate non-phosphorylated ^{3}H-2DG. The tissue was processed for autoradiography of water-diffusible substances according to the method of Fidone et al. (1977). Scale = 10 μm.

nmol/g/min) and nodose ganglion (42 nmol/g/min) was linear for more than 30 min during incubation in 100% O_2-equilibrated (control) media, indicating that tracer amounts of ^{3}H-2DG (2 μM) do not interfere with glucose metabolism. The results from autoradiography (Fig. 2) show that ^{3}H-2DG uptake is localized to lobules of type I and type II cells in the carotid body. The incidence of silver grains is low over nearby connective tissue and blood vessels. Following chronic (14 days) CSN denervation, the amount of ^{3}H-2DG uptake and its pattern of distribution within the carotid body is identical to normal, unoperated tissue. These data suggest that the basal metabolism of the carotid body is not altered in the absence of CSN axons and terminals, and that lobules of type I/type II cells account for nearly all of the glucose consumption in the carotid body.

Carotid bodies incubated for 5 or 10 min in media equilibrated with 20% O_2 in N_2 (a chemosensory stimulus in vitro) exhibited increases in ^{3}H-2DG phosphorylation of 34% ($P < 0.001$) and 45% ($P < 0.02$), respectively; nodose ganglia similarly treated yielded values ($+11\%$ and -3%, respectively) which were not significantly different from those obtained with control media. The inability of hypoxia to alter glucose consumption in the nodose ganglia agrees with the results of Ksiezak and Gibson (1981) who showed that glucose utilization in rat brain slices and synaptosomes was unaffected by similar levels of hypoxia. These findings emphasize the unique sensitivity of the carotid body to reduced ambient oxygen.

In closely related studies, the concentration of adenosine triphosphate (ATP) was measured in cat carotid bodies which were exposed for 5 min to either 100% O_2 equilibrated media or 20% O_2 in N_2 equilibrated media (Obeso et al., 1985). The results showed that hypoxia reduced the concentration of ATP in the carotid body by 21%. Experiments in which the carotid body was stimulated by CN^- (10^{-4} M) or 2-deoxyglucose (2 mM 2DG; 5 mM sodium pyruvate; zero glucose) reduced ATP levels by similar amounts and also showed that changes in ATP were correlated with increases in ^{3}H-DA release (synthesized from ^{3}H-tyrosine) and CSN activity.

The findings that natural physiological stimuli of the carotid body increase glucose metabolism and deplete ATP stores, while similar stimulation of other nervous tissue is ineffective, suggest that the intermediary metabolism of the carotid body is uniquely sensitive to chemostimulation, and moreover, that chemotransduction in the organ involves fundamental metabolic processes. Furthermore, the demonstration that ^{3}H-2DG uptake in the carotid body occurs primarily in parenchymal cell lobules in both normal and CSN-denervated organs indicates that type I cells are centrally important to the transduction of chemosensory stimuli.

The function of catecholamines in the carotid body

Numerous studies have established the existence of catecholamines (CA) in type I cells of the carotid body. In recent years, particular attention has focused on the role of the CAs, most notably DA, in the chemoreception process (for review of these studies, see Fidone and Gonzalez, 1986). Because it is well recognized that the actions of a given putative neurotransmitter are reflected in its metabolic response to natural stimulation (Orrego, 1979), we have undertaken studies to characterize the effects of hypoxic stimulation on the synthesis of CAs by the carotid body and to monitor directly the release of CAs from this organ as a function of the intensity of hypoxic stimulation and electrical activity of the CSN.

Catecholamine synthesis

Cat and rabbit carotid body incubated in media equilibrated with 100% O_2 and containing ^{3}H-tyrosine (5 – 40 μM) synthesize ^{3}H-DA and ^{3}H-NE (Fidone and Gonzalez, 1982; Rigual et al., 1986). Under these resting conditions, the rates of ^{3}H-DA and ^{3}H-NE synthesis (^{3}H-tyrosine = 40 μM) were approximately 10 and 0.5 nmol/g tissue/h, respectively, in the cat, while in the rabbit the rates were 12.10 (^{3}H-DA) and 0.85 (^{3}H-NE) nmol/g tissue/h, which yielded ^{3}H-DA:^{3}H-NE ratios of 20 and 14.24 for these species. These data suggest a low turnover of NE in the carotid body which is consistent with the findings of Belmonte et al. (1977), who found low levels of dopamine-β-hydroxylase (the synthetic enzyme for conversion of DA to NE) in the cat carotid body. Moreover, it has been demonstrated that exposure of cats to hypoxia resulted in decreased carotid body DA without any change in NE content (Fitzgerald et al., 1983), suggesting a slow rate of NE utilization during hypoxia.

In other experiments, we studied the synthesis of ^{3}H-DA and ^{3}H-NE 12 – 15 days following transection of the CSN or removal of the superior cervical ganglion (sympathectomy). After either procedure the rate of ^{3}H-DA synthesis was unaffected, which supports the idea that carotid body type I cells are the site of DA synthesis and storage. Chronic CSN denervation, however, resulted in an increase in the synthesis of ^{3}H-NE, a finding which may be due to sprouting of sympathetic fibers, which has been reported to occur following degeneration of CSN axons and terminals (Vazquez-Nin et al., 1978). Sympathectomy reduced ^{3}H-NE synthesis by 40% in the cat and 80% in the rabbit, owing to the degeneration of noradrenergic axons, which primarily innervate the carotid body vasculature, but also a few type I cells. The ^{3}H-NE synthesis which remains following sympathectomy probably occurs in type I cells, although it is unclear whether DA and NE synthesis are segregated between subgroups of type I cells (see Stensaas et al., 1981).

The effects of natural stimulation on CA synthesis were studied by exposing unanesthetized, unrestrained animals in a chamber to hypoxic gas mixtures (10% or 14% O_2 in N_2) for 3 h prior to removal and incubation of carotid bodies in ^{3}H-tyrosine. The hypoxic carotid bodies (10% O_2 in N_2 breathing) exhibited increases in ^{3}H-DA synthesis of 100% in the cat and 72% in the rabbit, but no change in ^{3}H-NE synthesis. Less severe

hypoxia (14% O_2 in N_2 breathing) resulted in a 53% increase in ^{3}H-DA synthesis (rabbit), again with unaltered ^{3}H-NE synthesis. No alterations in synthesis were observed when ^{3}H-dopa was used as a precursor, and this finding is in agreement with that found for other catecholaminergic systems (see Fidone et al., 1982a). The ability of the carotid body to increase the synthesis of ^{3}H-DA (from ^{3}H-tyrosine) in response to hypoxia appears to be a unique feature of this organ, since in our parallel experiments, the rate of ^{3}H-CA synthesis in superior cervical ganglia was unaffected by hypoxia, and the studies of others have shown that catecholaminergic tissues exhibit either unaltered or decreased synthesis of CA with hypoxia (Davis and Carlsson, 1973). The elevated ^{3}H-DA synthesis induced in the carotid body by hypoxia was unaffected 12 – 15 days following CSN transection or sympathectomy, and carotid bodies exposed in vitro to alternating hypoxic and normoxic media similarly displayed an increased rate of ^{3}H-DA synthesis, thereby demonstrating the intrinsic response properties of the organ, independent of humoral factors in vivo.

The specific increase in ^{3}H-DA synthesis which occurs shortly after a hypoxic episode probably results from increased release of endogenous DA, and subsequent removal of feedback inhibition exerted by DA at the level of tyrosine hydroxylase (TH), the rate limiting step in catecholamine synthesis. In related experiments, it was shown that the activity of TH in the carotid body is increased 48 h following a hypoxic episode, which suggests that additional long-term adjustments in CA metabolism in the carotid body may also occur in particular situations, such as residence at high altitude (Gonzalez et al., 1979a, b, 1981). These latter experiments also demonstrated that the basal levels of TH are elevated and the ability of a hypoxic episode to increase TH activity is enhanced 12 – 15 days following CSN denervation while, in contrast, TH induction by hypoxia is blocked after removal of the superior cervical ganglion (Gonzalez et al., 1979b). Thus, the CSN and the sympathetic innervation appear to exert a reciprocal control over long-term changes in TH activity.

Catecholamine release

Fig. 3A illustrates the data obtained from a typical experiment designed to measure the basal and stimulus evoked release of ^{3}H-DA from the rabbit carotid body in vitro (Fidone et al., 1982b). Organs were incubated for 2 h in 100% O_2-equilibrated Tyrode's solution containing ^{3}H-tyrosine prior to the experiment. The release of DA is measured as the sum of ^{3}H-DA plus ^{3}H-DOPAC (3,4-dihydroxyphenyl acetid acid, the principal DA catabolite in the carotid body). Chemoreceptor discharge was simultaneously recorded with a suction electrode. The amount of ^{3}H-DA released in excess of the basal release is proportional to the strength of the stimulus for each of three 5-min stimulus periods consisting of superfusion media equilibrated with 100% N_2, 30% O_2 in N_2, and 10% O_2 in N_2, respectively. Likewise, comparison of the summated nerve discharge for each stimulus period (see Fig. 3A, insets) reveals responses which parallel the stimulus strength. In Fig. 3B, data compiled from multiple experiments show that release of ^{3}H-DA from rabbit carotid body increased with decreasing dissolved O_2 and that a linear relationship exists between DA release and CSN activity. Comparative experiments with cat carotid body also demonstrated that ^{3}H-DA release and CSN discharge increased in parallel, with the exception that during severe hypoxia ($[O_2] \leq 10\%$), the release of ^{3}H-DA increased markedly without any further increase in CSN discharge (Rigual et al., 1986). Finally, the release of ^{3}H-DA evoked by hypoxia was similar following chronic CSN denervation or sympathectomy, except that ^{3}H-DA release was somewhat reduced during high intensity stimulation. Nonetheless, these data for denervated preparations demonstrate the ability of type I cells to respond to hypoxia independent of neural activity.

The relationship between the intensity of the low O_2 stimulus, on the one hand, and ^{3}H-DA release and chemosensory activity on the other, suggest a

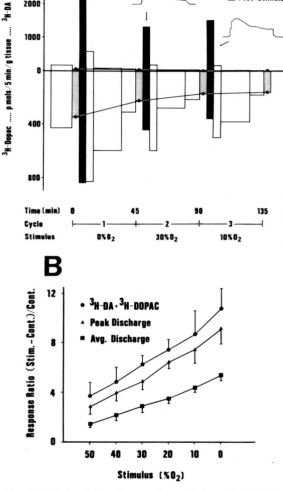

Fig. 3. Effects of low O_2 on release of dopamine (DA) and chemoreceptor discharge recorded from rabbit carotid body during superfusion of organ in vitro. (A) Release of ^{3}H-DA and efflux of ^{3}H-DOPAC during 3 stimulus cycles of 0% O_2, 30% O_2, and 10% O_2. Each stimulus cycle consisted of a 5-min control period (superfusion with 100% O_2-equilibrated media), 5 min stimulus, and post-stimulus periods of 5, 10 and 20 min. Chemoreceptor discharge during each 5-min stimulus period is shown by insets. (B) Relationships between total ^{3}H-DA release (^{3}H-DA + ^{3}H-DOPAC), peak (max) chemoreceptor discharge, and mean chemoreceptor discharge during stimulus periods are indicated. Response ratio is net stimulus-induced change in release or discharge (i.e., stimulus – control/control). From Fidone et al. (1982b).

role for DA in the mechanisms of chemoreception. Although our data do not provide incontrovertible evidence for a *causal* relationship between DA release and chemosensory activity, the correspondence between these two phenomena in normal Tyrode media suggests that DA participates in an important way in the overall genesis of the chemoresponse. Furthermore, DA receptors (D-2) are known to be located on the sensory neural elements in the carotid body (as well as the type I cells; see Fidone and Gonzalez, 1986). However, it must also be considered that some agent in addition to DA, perhaps one of the neuropeptides present in this organ, may be released to excite the sensory nerve endings. Other possible roles of DA in the mammalian carotid body should also be considered. DA may act as a 'modulator' of the chemoresponse, its presence in the carotid body being required for optimal chemosensitivity. This might be achieved through modifications of ionic permeabilities in the sensory nerve membrane, which could change the threshold to natural stimuli.

Acetylcholine and chemoreception

It is well established that small quantities of cholinergic agonists and antagonists profoundly alter chemoreceptor discharge. In addition, neurochemical investigations indicate that the metabolic machinery necessary for ACh synthesis, storage and inactivation are associated with type I cells and that afferent fibers of the CSN are nearly devoid of cholinergic activity (see Fidone and Gonzalez, 1986, for review). Furthermore, it has been demonstrated that an ACh-like substance is released upon stimulation of the organ in vitro (Eyzaguirre and Zapata, 1968).

While ACh may play a role in carotid body chemoreception, the precise actions of this substance in the sensory process has been elusive, particularly with respect to the locus of its specific effects on type I cells vs. afferent nerve terminals. Previous attempts to demonstrate pharmacologically the chemosensory involvement of ACh have

not been convincing, since neither the sites of action of the applied drugs, nor the nicotinic vs. muscarinic nature of the cholinergic receptors were clearly differentiated (see Fidone and Gonzalez, 1986). An additional problem is that exogenous ACh enhances chemosensory discharge in the cat (Fidone et al., 1968), while similar doses in the rabbit produce inhibition of discharge (Monti-Bloch and Eyzaguirre, 1980; Docherty and McQueen, 1979). Because of these uncertainties, we have undertaken ligand binding studies in an effort to clarify the localization and characteristics of nicotinic and muscarinic ACh receptors in the carotid body.

In earlier studies, we characterized and localized putative nicotinic receptors in the cat carotid body with ^{125}I-α-bungarotoxin (^{125}I-α-BGT; $K_D = 5.56$ nM, $B_{max} = 9.21$ pmol/g tissue) and muscarinic receptors in the rabbit carotid body with ^{3}H-quinuclydinylbenzilate (^{3}H-QNB; $K_D = 71.46$ pM, $B_{max} = 9.23$ pmol/g tissue). These biochemical and autoradiographic studies showed that nicotinic sites in the cat and muscarinic sites in the rabbit are localized within lobules of type I and type II parenchymal cells (Dinger et al., 1985, 1986). We found that chronic CSN denervation did not change the number of ^{125}I-α-BGT binding sites in the cat or ^{3}H-QNB binding sites in the rabbit, but degeneration of the sympathetic fibers from the superior cervical ganglion reduced the specific ^{125}I-α-BGT binding in the cat and ^{3}H-QNB binding in the rabbit by approximately 50%. These latter results may reflect the presence of presynaptic cholinergic receptors associated with sympathetic terminals, because in other sympathetically innervated tissues, muscarinic and nicotinic drugs can modulate the evoked release of catecholamines (Westfall, 1977).

More recently, we have examined muscarinic binding sites in the cat and nicotinic binding sites in the rabbit, in an effort to test the correspondence between the pharmacological effects of cholinergic drugs in each of these species and the number of nicotinic versus muscarinic receptors and their location within the carotid body cell lobules. Binding was assayed at a single concentration of radioligand (either 11.00 nM ^{125}I-α-BGT or 350 pM ^{3}H-QNB), chosen in accordance with our earlier studies to provide near saturation of the nicotinic or muscarinic sites, with minimal non-specific binding. Non-specific binding of ^{125}I-α-BGT is identical in cat and rabbit chemosensory tissue, suggesting that the toxin is equally accessible to the carotid bodies in both species. The portion of the total binding displaceable by 10^{-3} M ACh (specific binding) is 6.25 pmol/g of tissue in the cat carotid body, which is similar to that found in our earlier studies (Dinger et al., 1985). In contrast, specific ^{125}I-α-BGT binding in the rabbit carotid body amounts to only 0.54 pmol/g, or 8.6% of cat specific binding.

Comparisons of the binding of ^{3}H-QNB (350 pM) in normal rabbit and cat carotid body also showed that non-specific binding in the presence of 10^{-6} M atropine was comparable in the two species, indicating equal access of the ligand. The specific binding of ^{3}H-QNB in rabbit carotid body amounted to 6.78 $\pm$ 0.72 pmol/g of tissue, while under identical binding conditions, 3.77 $\pm$ 0.47 pmol/g was specifically bound in cat carotid body. Thus, assuming identical dissociation constants (K_D) for ^{3}H-QNB in the cat and rabbit, the data indicate a 55.6% relative abundance of specific binding sites in the cat as compared to the rabbit chemosensory tissue. In the rabbit, muscarinic sites account for over 90% of the total cholinergic receptor population. Conversely, nicotinic receptors dominate cat carotid bodies by approximately 2 to 1 over muscarinic sites.

Cholinergic receptor coupling to catecholamine release and chemoreceptor discharge

Because specific α-BGT and QNB binding sites are localized primarily within glomerular lobules in the carotid body, but are absent from the sensory terminals of the CSN, it follows that the type I cells are the most likely site for these receptors. We have therefore investigated whether the dominant receptor subtype in each animal, that is, nicotinic receptors in the cat and muscarinic receptors in the rabbit, are able to modulate both the release of DA from the type I cells and CSN chemoreceptor discharge. We found that in cat carotid body, α-BGT (50 nM) depressed the increase in chemosensory discharge (30 – 50% reduction) and the release of DA ($\sim$50% decrease) elicited by nicotine (10^{-5} M) as well as low O$_2$ (Dinger et al., 1985). In contrast to this dominant excitatory effect of nicotinic agents on discharge and release in the cat, our preliminary data with muscarinic agents in the rabbit carotid body suggest a very different effect on chemoreceptor discharge and ^{3}H-DA release. In 100% O$_2$-equilibrated superfusion media, basal release was unaffected by the muscarinic agonist, bethanechol (100 μM), but during normal hypoxia, bethanechol severely reduced the evoked release and CSN discharge, and this effect could be reversed by atropine (0.5 μM; Fidone et al., in press). These data suggest that muscarinic receptors in this species primarily inhibit DA release.

In sum, rabbit carotid bodies are dominated by inhibitory muscarinic receptors to an extent which correlates with the ability of ACh to depress the CSN discharge. Cat carotid bodies in contrast contain mostly nicotinic cholinergic sites which mediate a large excitatory response to nicotinic drugs. A substantial population of ^{3}H-QNB binding sites in cat chemosensory tissue is not associated with the sympathetic or sensory innervation, and the function and localization of these muscarinic sites remain obscure. Nonetheless, it is noteworthy that the increase in ^{3}H-DA release produced in the cat by nicotinic receptors, and the antagonistic effects of muscarinic agents on release in the rabbit, correspond to the actions of nicotinic and muscarinic agents on CSN impulse activity in these two species. A similar antagonistic effect on catecholamine release by nicotinic and muscarinic receptors has been described for isolated bovine adrenal chromaffin cells (Derome et al., 1981), while in other species it has been found that adrenal chromaffin cell secretion is stimulated by both nicotinic and muscarinic agents (Role and Perlman, 1983).

The response of neuropeptides to chemoreceptor stimulation

The neuropeptides met- and leu-enkephalin (ME, LE) have been localized to the type I cells with immunohistochemical techniques, while substance P (SP)-like immunoreactivity (SPLI) has been reportedly found in both nerve fibers and 20% of the type I cells (see Hanson et al., 1986, for references). Little is known regarding the role of these substances in carotid body function, but recent pharmacological studies suggest that administration of exogenous neuropeptides is able to modify chemoreceptor activity of both in vivo and in vitro carotid body preparations (see Hanson et al., 1986), and consequently these substances are thought to play a role in the genesis of the normal chemoresponse. In studying the role of SP and enkephalin in the carotid body, an important step is to determine the response of the endogenous neuropeptides to natural stimuli which are known to alter the physiological activities of this organ. We recently investigated whether the levels of SP and ME in the carotid body are responsive to a physiological stimulus (Hanson et al., 1986). In these experiments, unanesthetized rabbits were exposed in a flow chamber to either air or 5% O_2 in N_2 for two 30-min periods, with a 20-min interval. The rabbits were then anesthetized and respired with the given gas mixture during surgical removal of the carotid body and nearby nodose ganglia, which served as control. The levels of SP and ME were assayed using standard RIA techniques.

As shown in Fig. 4, animals exposed to hypoxia had significantly reduced levels of both SPLI and MELI in their carotid bodies, compared to animals exposed only to room air in the chamber. These results suggest that SP and ME may be involved in the regulation and/or mediation of carotid body chemoreception. The implicit assumption is that decreases in neuropeptide levels during the relatively short period of exposure to hypoxia are indicative of increased release and subsequent rapid proteolysis. Such an assumption may not be unreasonable, since the relatively rapid changes in

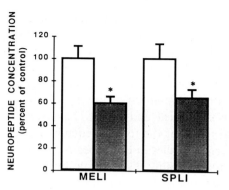

Fig. 4. Effects of hypoxia on neuropeptide concentrations in the carotid body. Rabbits were exposed to two 30-min periods of either 5% O_2 (hypoxia) or air. Immediately following this treatment, carotid bodies were surgically removed and assayed for MELI and SPLI. Each mean represents 7–9 samples. The control values for MELI and SPLI concentrations were 63.2 and 2.97 ng/mg protein, respectively. $P < 0.025$. Open column: room air; dark column: hypoxia (from Hanson et al., 1986).

peptide concentrations which we observed in this study are unlikely to be due to alterations in protein synthesis; Harmer and Keen (1981) have shown that 8 h after complete blockade of protein synthesis, the SP levels in dorsal root ganglia remain unchanged.

Preliminary experiments have also been initiated to investigate the effects of chronic section of the carotid sinus nerve (CSN) and chronic sympathectomy on neuropeptide levels in the carotid body. Our initial results suggest that 12–15 days following section of the CSN, the basal (unstimulated) level of SPLI in the carotid body is significantly increased, in spite of the loss of CSN SPLI. On the other hand, it appears that the level of MELI in the carotid body is reduced following CSN section. Following chronic sympathectomy (12–15 days), the basal peptide levels in the carotid body were likewise increased in the case of SPLI, and decreased for MELI. These preliminary results on changes in carotid body peptide following chronic denervations of the organ suggest long-term trophic effects of these nerves on transmitter regulation, and are reminiscent of similar actions we earlier reported for the trophic effects of these nerves on carotid body biogenic amines (Gonzalez et al., 1979b).

Neuropeptide levels (SPLI and MELI) in nodose ganglia were unchanged after exposure of the animal to the hypoxic episode. Although our experiments do not rule out possible non-specific effects of hypoxia on the carotid body, such as those unrelated to direct changes in chemoreception (e.g., local tissue hypoxia, blood pressure changes, hormonal and temperature effects, etc.), the lack of effect of hypoxia on neuropeptides in nodose ganglia suggests that tissue peptide stores may be resistant to such sequelae, and that changes observed in carotid body peptide levels reflect a true physiological response dependent on altered chemoreceptor drive.

Concluding remarks

The results of our studies of chemotransduction and chemotransmission in the carotid body are summarized schematically in Fig. 5. Our findings

are illustrated to show the cellular contents of neurotransmitters, the locations of specific receptors, the actions of chemoreceptor stimuli on putative neurotransmitter metabolism, as well as the trophic effects following chronic CSN denervation and sympathectomy. Since the inception of our research more than a decade ago, the problem of chemical transmission in the carotid body has gradually evolved from what we perceived then to be the study of an elegantly simple receptor system (with a single sensory transmitter), to what we now recognize is a complex synaptic apparatus in which the concerted actions of multiple neuroactive agents determine the net sensory activity on the CSN. What remains to be demonstrated, however, is the precise role of each of these agents, and their interactions, in the process of chemosensation.

References

Belmonte, C., Gonzalez, C. and Garcia, A. (1977) Dopamine beta hydroxylase activity in cat carotid body. In: H. Acker,

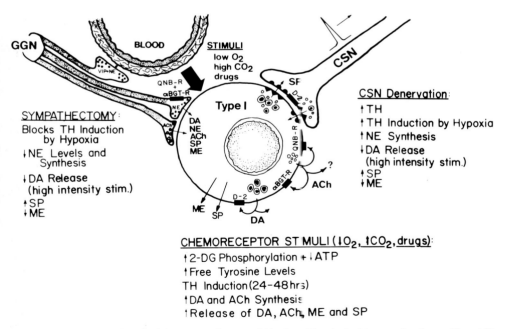

Fig. 5. Schematized type I cell of the mammalian carotid body, with principal innervation from afferent fibers of the CSN and limited synaptic contacts from sympathetic fibers of the ganglioglomeruler nerve (GGN). See text for explanation.

178

S. Fidone, D. Pallot, C. Eyzaguirre, D.W. Lubbers and R.W. Torrance (Eds.), *Chemoreception in the Carotid Body*. Springer, Berlin, pp. 99 – 105.

Davis, J.N. and Carlsson, A. (1973) Effect of hypoxia on tyrosine and tryptophan hydroxylation in unanesthetized rat brain. *J. Neurochem.*, 20: 913 – 915.

Derome, G., Tseng, R., Mercier, P., Lemarre, I. and Lemarre, S. (1981) Possible muscarinic regulation of catecholamine secretion mediated by cyclic GMP in isolated bovine adrenal chromaffin cells. *Biochem. Pharmacol.*, 30: 855 – 860.

Dinger, B., Gonzalez, C., Yoshizaki, K. and Fidone, S. (1985) Localization and function of cat carotid body nicotinic receptors. *Brain Res.*, 339: 295 – 304.

Dinger, B.G., Hirano, T. and Fidone, S.J. (1986) Autoradiographic localization of muscarinic receptors in rabbit carotid body. *Brain Res.*, 367: 328 – 331.

Docherty, R.J. and McQueen, D.S. (1979) The effects of acetylcholine and dopamine on carotid chemosensory activity in the rabbit. *J. Physiol. (London)*, 288: 411 – 423.

Eyzaguirre, C. and Zapata, P. (1968) The release of acetylcholine from carotid body tissues. Further study on the effects of acetylcholine and cholinergic blocking agents on the chemosensory discharge. *J. Physiol. (London)*, 195: 589 – 607.

Fidone, S.J. and Gonzalez, C. (1982) Catecholamine synthesis in rabbit carotid body in vitro. *J. Physiol (London)*, 333: 69 – 79

Fidone, S.J. and Gonzalez C. (1986) Initiation and control of chemoreceptor activity in the carotid body. In: N. Cherniack and J.G. Widdicombe (Eds.), *Handbook of Physiology, Respiration*, vol. I. American Physiological Society, Washington, DC.

Fidone, S.J., Sato, A. and Eyzaguirre, C. (1968) Acetylcholine activation of carotid body chemoreceptor A fibers. *Brain Res.*, 9: 374 – 376.

Fidone, S.J., Weintraub, S., Stavinoha, W.B., Sterling, C. and Jones, L. (1977) Endogenous acetylcholine levels in the cat carotid body and the autoradiographic localization of a high affinity component of choline uptake. In: H. Acker, S. Fidone, D. Pallot, C. Eyzaguirre, D.W. Lubbers and R.W. Torrance (Eds.), *Chemoreception in the Carotid Body*. Springer, Berlin, pp. 106 – 113.

Fidone, S.J., Gonzalez, C. and Yoshizaki, K. (1982a) Effects of hypoxia on catecholamine synthesis in rabbit carotid body in vitro. *J. Physiol. (London)*, 333: 79 – 93.

Fidone, S.J., Gonzalez, C. and Yoshizaki, K. (1982b) Effects of low oxygen on the release of dopamine from the rabbit carotid body in vitro. *J. Physiol. (London)*, 333: 93 – 110.

Fidone, S., Gonzalez, C., Dinger, B., Almaraz, L., Rigual, R. and Hanson, G. (in press) Transmitter interactions in peripheral arterial chemoreceptors. In: S. Lahiri (Ed.), *Chemoreceptors and Reflexes in Breathing, Comroe Memorial Symposium*. Oxford University Press, London.

Fitzgerald, R.S., Garger, P., Haner, M.C., Raff, M. and Fet-

cher, L. (1983) Effect of hypoxia and hypercapnia on catecholamine content in cat carotid body. *J. Physiol. Respirat. Environ. Exercise Physiol.*, 54: 1408 – 1413.

Gonzalez, C., Kwok, Y., Gibb, J.W. and Fidone, S. (1979a) Effects of hypoxia on tyrosine hydroxylase activity in rat carotid body. *J. Neurochem.*, 33: 713 – 719.

Gonzalez, C., Kwok, Y., Gibb, J.W. and Fidone, S.J. (1979b) Reciprocal modulation of tyrosine hydroxylase activity in rat carotid body. *Brain Res.* 172: 572 – 576.

Gonzalez, C., Kwok, Y., Gibb, J. and Fidone, S. (1981) Physiological and pharmacologic effects on TH activity in rabbit and cat carotid body. *Am. J. Physiol.* 240: R38 – R43.

Hanson, G.R., Jones, L.F. and Fidone, S. (1986) Physiological chemoreceptor stimulation decreases enkephalin and substance P in the carotid body. *Peptides*, 7: 767 – 769.

Harmer, A. and Keen, P. (1981) Chemical characterization of substance P-like immunoreactivity in primary afferent neurons. *Brain Res.* 220: 203 – 207.

Ksiezak, H.J. and Gibson, G.E. (1981) Oxygen dependence of glucose and acetylcholine metabolism in slices and synaptosomes from rat brain. *J. Neurochem.* 37: 305 – 314.

McDonald, D.M. and Mitchell, R.A. (1975) The innervation of glomus cells, ganglion cells and blood vessels in the rat carotid body: a quantitative ultrastructural analysis. *J. Neurocytol.* 4: 177 – 230.

Mills, E. (1975) Metabolic aspects of chemoreceptor function. In: M.J. Purves (Ed.), *The Peripheral Arterial Chemoreceptors*. Cambridge University Press, London, pp. 373 – 386.

Monti-Bloch, L. and Eyzaguirre, C. (1980) A comparative physiological and pharmacological study of cat and rabbit carotid body chemoreceptors. *Brain Res.*, 193: 449 – 470.

Mulligan, E. and Lahiri, S. (1981) Mitochondrial oxidative metabolism and chemoreception in the carotid body. In: C. Belmonte, D. Pallot, H. Acker and S. Fidone (Eds.), *Arterial Chemoreceptors, Proc. 6th Int. Meeting*. Leicester University Press, Leicester, pp. 316 – 326.

Obeso, A., Almaraz, L. and Gonzalez, C. (1985) Correlation between adenosine triphosphate levels, dopamine release and electrical activity in the carotid body: support for the metabolic hypothesis of chemoreception. *Brain Res.*, 348: 64 – 68.

Orrego, F. (1979) Criteria for the identification of central neurotransmitters and their application to studies with some nerve tissue preparations in vitro. *Neuroscience*, 4: 1037 – 1057.

Rigual, R., Gonzalez, E., Gonzalez, C. and Fidone, S. (1986) Synthesis and release of catecholamines by the cat carotid body in vitro. Effects of hypoxic stimulation. *Brain Res.*, 374: 101 – 109.

Role, L.W. and Perlman, R.L. (1983) Both nicotinic and muscarinic receptors mediate catecholamine secretion by isolated guinea-pig chromaffin cells. *Neuroscience*, 10: 979 – 985.

Stensaas, L.J., Stensaas, S.S., Gonzalez, C. and Fidone, S.J.

(1981) Analytical electronmicroscopy of granular vesicles in the carotid body of the normal and reserpinized cat. In: C Belmonte, D. Pallot, H. Acker and S. Fidone (Eds.), *Arteria Chemoreceptors, Proc. 6th Int. Meeting*. Leicester University Press, Leicester, pp. 176 – 186.

Vazquez-Nin, G.H., Costero, I., Echevarria, O.M., Aguilar, R

and Barroso-Moguel, R. (1978) Innervation of the carotid body. An experimental quantitative study. *Acta Anat.*, 102: 12 – 28.

Westfall, T.C. (1977) Local regulation of adrenergic neurotransmission. *Physiol. Rev.*, 57: 659 – 728.

W. Hamann and A. Iggo (Eds.)
Progress in Brain Research, Vol. 74
© 1988 Elsevier Science Publishers B.V. (Biomedical Division)

CHAPTER 20

Multiple messenger candidates and marker substances in the mammalian Merkel cell – axon complex: a light and electron microscopic immunohistochemical study

W. Hartschuh[a] and E. Weihe[b]

[a]*Dermatological Clinic, University of Heidelberg, FRG and* [b]*Department of Anatomy, Johannes Gutenberg-Universität, Mainz, FRG*

Introduction

According to the APUD theory (Pearse, 1986), cells of the diffuse neuroendocrine system (DNES) are essentially characterized by containing amines, peptides and marker substances like neuron-specific enolase (NSE) and chromogranin A (CGA). While the search for amines in Merkel cells of mammalian skin has been unsuccessful in mammals (Hartschuh and Grube, 1979; Hartschuh et al., 1986), there is evidence for the presence of serotonin in Merkel cells in the marine eel (Zaccone, 1984). The demonstration of opioid (enkephalin) and non-opioid (VIP) peptides (Hartschuh et al., 1986) and of NSE (Gu et al., 1981) in Merkel cells of mammalian skin supports the concept of Pearse (1986) to classify the Merkel cell as a member of the DNES. On the other hand, immunohistochemistry failed to visualize CGA in Merkel cells (Pearse, 1986) although by immunoblotting considerable quantities of CGA were measured in extracts of bovine skin (Nolan et al., 1985).

To resolve this controversy as regards CGA and in order to evaluate our previous assumptions that the Merkel cell may contain a multiplicity of peptide messenger candidates, most likely in the secretory granules (Hartschuh et al., 1986), we used a highly sensitive light microscopic (LM) and

electron microscopic (EM) immunohistochemical approach. A parallel purpose of this study was to determine the differential distribution of a variety of more or less selective neuroendocrine markers like neurofilament, synaptophysin, cytokeratin 18, protein S-100 and neuron-specific enolase either in the Merkel cell or in the associated axon or in both. By the comparison of the histotopography of immunostained peptides, CGA and neuroendocrine markers, we expected to find out the most appropriate immunohistochemical marker of the Merkel cell and to get further insight into the complex chemoanatomy and possible functional spectrum of the Merkel cell – axon complex at various developmental stages.

Material and methods

For LM immunohistochemistry, adult and fetal skin of pig snout ($n = 10$) and adult human finger ($n = 4$) as well as finger from different developmental stages ($n = 2$ for each stage investigated) were fixed by immersion in Bouin's solution, dehydrated in propan-2-ol and embedded in paraplast. Cytokeratin 18 immunostaining was performed on cryostat sections of unfixed, frozen tissue. Sequential sections were incubated in a humid chamber with primary antisera at room temperature and for periods ranging from 1 to

24 h. For visualizing immunoreactions, species-specific biotinylated secondary antisera and streptavidin – biotinylated horseradish peroxidase (HRP) complexes (Amersham) were used. For EM immunocytochemistry, the pre-embedding technique on vibratome sections (40 μm thick) of tissues fixed in Bouin with the addition of 2% glutaraldehyde was employed. Sections were immunoreacted with the streptavidin – biotin-HRP method and postfixed in osmium tetroxide, dehydrated in ethanol and embedded in EPON 812. Ultrathin sections were obtained from selected areas containing immunopositive Merkel cells as assessed by LM evaluation of semi-thin sections.

Primary antisera

(a) Neuroendocrine marker substances

Polyclonal antisera against porcine and bovine CGA (Immunonuclear, INC), NSE (INC), protein S-100 (Dakopatts) and against neurofilament (NF, Dakopatts) were used. Monoclonal antibodies against synaptophysin (Boehringer, Mannheim) and cytokeratin 18 (Progen, Heidelberg) were also employed.

(b) Peptides

Antisera/antibodies against a variety of opioid peptide sequences derived from the opioid precursors proenkephalin (PRO-ENK) and prodynorphin (PRO-DYN) were used as described in detail elsewhere (Weihe et al., 1985, in press). Polyclonal antisera against the following non-opioid peptides were employed: vasoactive intestinal polypeptide (VIP, Hartschuh et al., 1983) peptide histidine isoleucine (PHI, Itoh et al., 1983) rat and human calcitonin-gene-related peptide (CGRP, Amersham, Peninsula). A monoclonal antibody against substance P (SP, Serotec) was also employed.

Polyclonal antisera were applied in working dilutions ranging from 1:6000 to 1:40 000. Working dilutions of monoclonal antibodies (ascites) ranged from 1:50 to 1:200.

Routine specificity tests were carried out by preabsorbing antisera against peptides and markers with homologous and a variety of heterologous antigens (Weihe et al., 1985, in press). The immunoreactions obtained were only abolished by the respective antigens. Poly-L-lysine (Sigma) added to the diluted antisera (a mandatory novel control procedure suggested by Scopsi et al., 1986) did not affect the immunostaining indicating absence of non-specific immunoreactions as regards the basic peptides immunoreacted in our study.

Results

Peptides

Opioid and non-opioid peptide immunoreactivities were regularly absent from the axonal component of the Merkel cell – axon complex. There was no clear evidence for the presence of opioid immunoreactive (ir) material in Merkel cells of pig and man (Table 1).

TABLE 1

Distribution of (ir) peptides and neuroendocrine marker substances in the Merkel cell – axon complex of pig skin

	Merkel cell		Axon	
	Fetal	Adult	Fetal	Adult
Peptides				
VIP	–	+	–	
PHI	–	+	–	
CGRP	+	+	–	
SP	+	+	–	
PRO-ENK	–	–	–	
PRO-DYN				
Marker				
CGA	+	+	–	
Cytokeratin 18	+	+	–	
NSE	+	+	+	
S-100	+	+	+	
Neurofilament	–	–	+	
Synaptophysin	?	?	? (*)	

+ immunopositive; – immunonegative; ? immunostaining questionable; * immunopositive in adult guinea-pig.

In contrast, Merkel cells were stained with antisera against non-opioid peptides whereby the immunostaining depended on the developmental stage and varied between man and pig. Thus, (ir) VIP and PHI were only present in Merkel cells of adult pig whereas (ir) SP and CGRP were present in adult and fetal Merkel cells. Staining with SP and CGRP antisera was less intense than that obtained with VIP/PHI antisera. In adult and fetal (week 9–21) human skin, the staining for SP and CGRP was questionable.

Adjacent sections alternately stained for the different peptides revealed codistribution of (ir) VIP, PHI, SP, and CGRP in a similar number of Merkel cells. The immunostaining of peptides predominated in the basal cytoplasm (Fig. 1) facing the axon terminal but was also present in the opposite part of the cell. This pattern corresponded well with the fact that on the ultrastructural level, (ir) peptides prevailed in Merkel granules which are well known to be preferentially accumulated in the juxta-axonal cytoplasm.

Neuroendocrine marker substances

Unlike peptides, neuroendocrine marker substances were heterogeneously distributed to the Merkel cell and/or to the axon (see Table 1). There were no differences in the staining pattern between adult and fetal pig skin. Results were similar in human skin with the exception of the staining for CGA which was much stronger in fetal than in adult Merkel cells. The average number of Merkel cells immunostained for markers restricted to the Merkel cell, i.e., CGA and cytokeratin 18, or present in both Merkel cell and axon, i.e., NSE and S-100 (Fig. 5), equalled that of Merkel cells stained by antisera against peptides (Table 1). The absence of neurofilament (NF) from the Merkel cell and its presence in the axon ending could be unequivocally evaluated on the LM level (Fig. 6). The presence of (ir) synaptophysin in Merkel axons could be clearly demonstrated in perfusion-fixed guinea-pig skin but not in immersion-fixed pig and human skin.

The immunostaining for CGA in Merkel cells was particularly strong in fetal and in adult pig skin which exceeded the strength of immunoproducts obtained with all other antisera used in this study. The extreme intensity of the (ir) CGA made it impossible to discern concentration differences between juxta-axonal and opposite parts of individual cells (Figs. 2, 3). Human Merkel cells were stained with the antiserum against bovine but not with that against porcine CGA whereas in pig Merkel cells both antisera produced similar patterns.

EM immunostaining for CGA clearly revealed that the immunoreactions were located in the Merkel cell granules (Fig. 4). Staining intensity varied between individual secretory granules. There was no evidence for the presence of CGA in the associated axon. The entire population of Merkel cells was found to be CGA (ir). In fetal but not in adult pig skin CGA (ir) Merkel cells were not restricted to the basal part of epidermal cones but were also found to be disseminated in the upper epidermis, albeit in much lower numbers.

Discussion

This study has added important novel aspects to the knowledge of the chemoanatomy of the Merkel cell–axon complex at different developmental stages. Firstly, the presence in the Merkel cell of neuropeptides which have not been found before in this cell, i.e., CGRP and SP, has been documented and our preliminary findings showing (ir) PHI in Merkel cells of pig and man (Hartschuh et al., 1986) have been substantiated. Secondly, the open question about the possible occurrence of CGA in mammalian Merkel cells (Pearse, 1986) could be resolved. We provided evidence for the co-occurrence of CGA and various peptides in the entire Merkel cell population. Co-localization of CGA and peptides in the secretory granules can be anticipated but warrants electron microscopical double labeling immunocytochemistry. Thirdly, further comparative information regarding the complexity of neuroendocrine marker substances

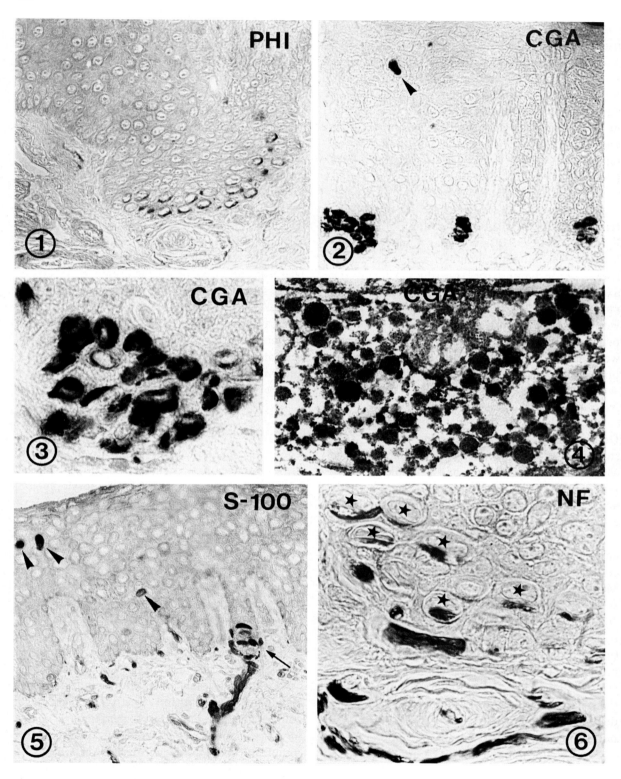

in the Merkel cell – axon complex has been contributed.

Evidence for a multiple peptide messenger system

The demonstration of PHI (see Itoh et al., 1983) was anticipated because it is contained in the same precursor as VIP, a peptide of the glucagon-secretin family which we recently detected in pig and human Merkel cells (Hartschuh et al., 1983).

More surprising was our finding concerning SP and CGRP which have wide distribution in the central and peripheral nervous system and co-exist in primary sensory neurones (Lundberg and Hökfelt, 1986) and, in guinea pig also with PRO-DYN opioid peptides (Weihe et al., 1985, in press; Weihe, 1987). In contrast to earlier findings in rodents (Hartschuh et al., 1986), we obtained no evidence in this study for the presence of opioid peptides in pig and human Merkel cells. However, we would not like to rule out this possibility because the sensitivity of our opioid antisera used

may be too low to detect opioids in pig and human Merkel cells or immersion fixation may be insufficient to preserve opioid peptides. On the other hand, there may be true interspecies variations in the peptidic phenotype of Merkel cells since we were unable to clearly visualize VIP/PHI or SP and CGRP in perfusion-fixed rodent Merkel cells. The differences in the immunostaining of VIP/PHI in fetal vs. adult pig skin may be due to true developmental differences in transcription or post-translational processing or may simply reflect methodological differences in the stainability of fetal vs. adult tissue.

In extension of our previous hypothesis, we postulate that the Merkel cell contains a very complex messenger setting of peptides (and possibly additional mediators like biogenic amines) which probably will turn out to even exceed the spectrum established here. It may act as a cocktail of transmitters or modulators to fulfil the assumed mechanoreceptive role of the Merkel cell – axon complex (see Hartschuh et al., 1986). Paracrine/autocrine (Grube, 1986) or even endocrine functions of multiple peptides in this still enigmatic cell are also conceivable.

Chromogranin A, an additional messenger candidate and optimal marker of the Merkel cell?

Our demonstration of CGA in the Merkel cell is further support of the view that it is a member of the DNES (Pearse, 1986). In analogy to the knowledge and hypothesis about the function of CGA in various other neuroendocrine cells and in conjunction with the location of CGA in secretory granules of the Merkel cell we postulate similar roles of CGA in mammalian Merkel cells. Thus, CGA may be involved in packaging of regulatory peptides into secretory granules (Rosa et al., 1985), in the sequestration and mobilization of calcium from secretory vesicles during stimulus-secretion coupling (Benedum et al., 1986) or may even act as a precursor for multiple biologically active peptides (Iacangelo et al., 1986). Such a precur-

---

Fig. 1. PHI (ir) Merkel cells at the base of an epidermal cone of glabrous snout. The strongest staining in the basal part of the cells. Adult pig (× 180).

Fig. 2. CGA (ir) Merkel cells at the base of epidermal cones, single CGA (ir) Merkel cell (arrow head) in the higher epidermis. Glabrous snout, fetal pig (× 180).

Fig. 3. CGA (ir) Merkel cells. The nuclear region is spared out from the strong overall staining of the cytoplasm. Epidermal cone from glabrous snout. Fetal pig (× 500).

Fig. 4. EM micrograph showing part of a Merkel cell with CGA (ir) secretory granules. Note variable immunostaining of individual granules. Fetal pig. Stained with lead citrate and uranyl acetate (× 47 000).

Fig. 5. Single S-100 (ir) Merkel cells in the higher epidermis (arrow heads). Merkel cells in the basal epidermis can hardly be distinguished from (ir) axon endings (arrow). Glabrous snout, fetal pig (× 180).

Fig. 6. Neurofilament (NF) (ir) dermal nerve fibers and NF (ir) axon endings contacting unstained Merkel cells (asterisks). Glabrous snout skin, pig (× 800).

sor – product relationship has been recently described between CGA and pancreastatin (Eiden, 1987). Apart from considering multiple functions of CGA in the Merkel cell we would like to stress the argument that it can be regarded as a marker substance of Merkel cells in skin and oral mucosa (Gauweiler et al., 1987). Thus, CGA immunohistochemistry offers an ideal tool to selectively stain and quantify Merkel cells at least in some mammals.

Functional implications of cytokeratin, NSE, S-100 and synaptophysin

While the wide distribution of these compounds in the nervous system and in a variety of neuroendocrine cells is well established their physiological role is not very well elucidated. For example, there are speculations that NSE facilitates interaction with positively charged cytoskeletal proteins (Forss-Petter et al., 1986). Synaptophysin may not just be regarded as a marker of synaptic and secretory vesicles in neuronal endings or neuroendocrine cells but may also have important functions in the process of vesicle formation and exocytosis (Wiedenmann et al., 1986). Their precise role in the Merkel cell – axon complex and possible functional interactions with Merkel cell peptides and CGA offers an interesting aspect of future Merkel cell research.

Acknowledgements

Preliminary aspects of this study have been presented at the Joint International Meeting of the European Society for Dermatological Research and the Society for Investigative Dermatology in Geneva (1986) and at the Second World Congress of Neuroscience in Budapest (1987). The study was supported by the Stifterverband für die Deutsche Wissenschaft and the German Research Foundation (DFG Grant We 910/2-1). For superb technical assistance we are indebted to U. Egner and A. Leibold.

References

Benedum, U.M., Baeuerle, P.A., Konecki, D.S., Frank, R., Powell, J., Mallet, J. and Huttner, W.B. (1986) The primary structure of bovine chromogranin A: a representative of a class of acidic secretory proteins common to a variety of peptidergic cells. *EMBO J.,* 5: 1495 – 1502.

Eiden, L.E. (1987) Is chromogranin a prohormone? *Nature (London),* 325: 301.

Forss-Petter, S., Danielson, P. and Sutcliff, J.G. (1986) Neuron-specific enolase: complete structure of rat mRNA, multiple transcriptional start sites, and evidence suggesting post-transcriptional control. *J. Neurosci. Res.,* 16: 141 – 156.

Gauweiler, B., Hartschuh, W., Nohr, D. and Weihe, E. (1987) Neuronal and non-neuronal histotopography of peptides and chromogranin in oral mucosa, tongue, and dental pulp of pig. *Neuroscience,* 22 (Suppl.): S814.

Grube, D. (1986) The endocrine cells of the digestive system: amines, peptides and modes of action. *Anat. Embryol.,* 175: 151 – 162.

Gu, J., Polak, J.M., Tapia, F.J., Marangos, P.J. and Pearse, A.G.E. (1981) Neuron-specific enolase in the Merkel cell of mammalian skin. *Am. J. Pathol.,* 104: 6368.

Hartschuh, W. and Grube, D. (1979) The Merkel cell – a member of the APUD cell system? *Arch. Dermatol. Res.,* 265: 115 – 122.

Hartschuh, W., Weihe, E., Yanaihara, N. and Reinecke, M. (1983) Immunohistochemical localization of vasoactive intestinal polypeptide (VIP) in Merkel cells of various mammals: evidence for a neuromodulator function of the Merkel cell. *J. Invest. Dermatol.,* 81: 361 – 364.

Hartschuh, W., Weihe, E. and Reinecke, M. (1986) The Merkel cell. In: J. Bereiter-Hahn, A.G. Matoltsy and K.S. Richards (Eds.), *Biology of the Integument,* Vol. 2, Vertebrates, Springer-Verlag, Berlin, pp. 605 – 620.

Hartschuh, W., Weihe, E., Yanaihara, N. and Yanaihara, C. (1986) PHI/PHM-like immunoreactivities in Merkel cells and nerves of pig snout: colocalization with VIP-like immunoreactivity. *J. Invest. Dermatol.,* 87: 144.

Hartschuh, W., Egner, U., Leibold, A., Nohr, D. and Weihe, E. (1987) Light and electronmicroscopic immunocytochemistry reveals localization of chromogranin A-like immunoreactivities in cutaneous Merkel cells. *Neuroscience,* 22 (suppl.): S814.

Iacangelo, A., Affolter, H.-U., Eiden, L.E., Herbert, E. and Grimes, M. (1986) Bovine chromogranin A a sequence and distribution of its messenger RNA in endocrine tissues. *Nature (London),* 323: 82 – 86.

Itoh, N., Obata, K., Yanaihara, N. and Okamoto, H. (1983) Human prepovasoactive intestinal polypeptide contains a novel PHI-27-like peptide, PHM-27. *Nature (London),* 304: 547 – 549.

Lundberg, J.M. and Hökfelt, T. (1986) Multiple co-existence of peptides and classical transmitters in peripheral autonomic and sensory neurons – functional and pharmacological implications. In: T. Hökfelt, K. Fuxe and B. Pernow (Eds.), *Progress in Brain Research,* Vol. 68. Elsevier, Amsterdam, pp. 241 – 262.

Nolan, A.J., Trojanowski, J.Q. and Hogue-Angeletti, R. (1985) Neurons and neuroendocrine cells contain chromogranin: detection of the molecule in normal bovine tissues by immunochemical and immunohistochemical methods. *J. Histochem. Cytochem.,* 33: 791 – 798.

Pearse, A.G.E. (1986) The diffuse neuroendocrine system: peptides, amines, placodes and the APUD theory. In: T. Hökfelt, K. Fuxe and B. Pernow (Eds.), *Progress in Brain Research,* Vol. 68. Elsevier, Amsterdam, pp. 25 – 31.

Rosa, P., Hille, A., Lee, R.W.H., Zanini, A., De Camilli, P. and Huttner, B. (1985) Secretogranins I and II: two tyrosine-sulfated secretory proteins common to a variety of cells secreting peptides by the regulated pathway. *J. Cell Biol.,* 101: 1999.

Scopsi, L., Wang, B.-L. and Larsson, L.-I. (1986) Nonspecific immunocytochemical reactions with certain neurohormonal peptides and basic peptide sequences. *J. Histochem. Cytochem.,* 34: 1469 – 1475.

Weihe, E. (1987) Peripheral innervation of the heart. In: Th. von Arnim and A. Maseri (Eds.), *Silent Ischemia.* Steinkopf Verlag, Darmstadt, pp. 7 – 18.

Weihe, E., Hartschuh, W. and Weber, E. (1985) Prodynorphin opioid peptides in small somatosensory primary afferents of guinea-pig. *Neurosci. Lett.,* 58: 347 – 352.

Weihe, E., Nohr, D., Hartschuh, W., Gauweiler, B. and Fink, T. (in press) Multiplicity of opioidergic pathways related to cardiovascular innervation: differential contribution of all three opioid precursors. In: K.O. Stumpe and K. Kraft (Eds.), *Proceedings of the Satellite Symposium to the 11th Scientific Meeting of ISH 1986, Opioid Peptides and Blood Pressure Control.* Springer, Berlin.

Wiedenmann, B., Franke, W.W., Kuhn, C., Moll, R. and Gould, V.E. (1986) Synaptophysin: a marker protein for neuroendocrine cells and neoplasms. *Proc. Natl. Acad. Sci. USA,* 83: 3500 – 3504.

Zaccone, G. (1984) Immunohistochemical demonstration of neuron-specific enolase in the nerve endings and skin receptors of marine eels. *Histochem. J.,* 16: 1231 – 1236.

W. Hamann and A. Iggo (Eds.)
Progress in Brain Research, Vol. 74
© 1988 Elsevier Science Publishers B.V. (Biomedical Division)

CHAPTER 21

Immunohistochemical evidence for a co-transmitter role of opioid peptides in primary sensory neurons

Eberhard Weihe, Donatus Nohr and Wolfgang Hartschuh[a]

Anatomical Institute, University of Mainz, 6500 Mainz, FRG, and [a] Dermatological Clinic, University of Heidelberg, 6900 Heidelberg, FRG

Introduction

Small-diameter primary sensory neurons not only transmit nociceptive messages to central neurons, but are also active in the periphery in mediating axon-reflex mechanisms and inflammation response (for review see Besson and Chaouch, 1987; Foreman, 1987; Zieglgänsberger, 1987). The tachykinin substance P (SP) is a strong candidate to fulfil such central and peripheral transmitter functions in mammals (Lembeck and Donnerer, 1985). Other tachykinins play a similar role, in particular neurokinin A (NKA) which is derived from the same preprotachykinin molecule as SP (Lundberg and Hökfelt, 1986). In the rat, two preprotachykinin mRNAs encoding SP and NKA and one only encoding SP have been recently sequenced (Krause et al., 1987). This situation points to the diversity of products which can be generated from one sensory precursor family alone. However, the chemical coding of sensory neurons seems to be even more complex because neuropeptides like calcitonin gene-related peptide (CGRP) and cholecystokinin (CCK) are also present in primary afferents where they apparently co-exist and co-function with tachykinins (see Lundberg and Hökfelt, 1986).

Furthermore, there is recent evidence provided by radioimmunological (Boticelli et al., 1981) and immunohistochemical investigations that opioid peptides are not only expressed in embryonic and

in cultured (Sweetnam et al., 1986) but also in adult sensory ganglia, at least of guinea-pig (Weihe et al., 1985). Opioid peptides are derived from three precursors, i.e., prodynorphin (PRO-DYN) (Goldstein, 1984), pro-enkephalin (PRO-ENK), and proopiomelanocortin (POMC) (see Millan and Herz, 1985). It appeared that primary sensory opioid peptides are derived from PRO-DYN but not from PRO-ENK or POMC and there was preliminary evidence for co-existence with SP and CGRP in spinal and trigeminal ganglionic cells (Weihe et al., 1985, 1986). Moreover, opioid peptides were detected in skin extracts and localized in cutaneous nerves (Weihe et al., 1983, 1985). However, the exact molecular forms, interspecies variations and peripheral distributions of sensory opioid peptides and their interrelationships with tachykinins and CGRP are still unclear. Therefore, the main aim of this study was to answer these open questions by using a highly sensitive light microscopic (LM) immunohistochemical approach. In addition, we introduce a novel concept of opioid involvement in peripheral and central primary sensory neurotransmission.

Material and methods

LM immunohistochemical procedure

Tissues of non-colchicine-treated adult guinea-pigs (6), rats (15), cats (2), dogs (2), pigs (2) and rabbit

(1) were fixed by perfusion or immersion with aldehyde solutions, dehydrated in propan-2-ol, and embedded in paraffin. In order to determine co-existence patterns, adjacent 4 – 6-µm thick sections were alternately incubated with the various primary antisera. Biotinylated species-specific secondary antisera, streptavidin – biotin peroxidase complexes (Amersham), and the chromogen diaminobenzidine (Dakopatts) were used for visualization of immunoreactions. For further details see Weihe et al. (1986, 1988a,b).

Primary antisera and their specificities

(1) Anti-tachykinins: anti-SP (Serotec, rat, monoclonal) and anti-NKA (Peninsula, rabbit, polyclonal); anti-SP partly cross-reacted with NKA and anti-NKA with SP, but not with opioid peptides, CGRP or various other neuropeptides.

(2) Anti-CGRP (Peninsula, Amersham; rabbit, polyclonal) did not differentiate between the different molecular forms of rat or human CGRP (Brain et al., 1986) and cross-reacted neither with opioids nor with tachykinins.

(3) Antisera against opioid peptides (OP); (a) anti-Met-enkephalyl-Arg-Gly-Leu (MRGL; rabbit, polyclonal) was specific for PRO-ENK sequences containing MRGL. (b) anti-DYN A 1 – 17, anti-DYN A 1 – 8, anti-DYN B, anti-alpha-neoendorphin (anti-NEO; rabbit, polyclonal) were all specific for PRO-DYN fractions containing the respective sequences. (c) anti-Leu-enkephalin (LE; rabbit, polyclonal) was non-selective in differentiating PRO-ENK and PRO-DYN but detected specifically and collectively the entire opioid potential contained in both precursors. Anti-LE (Seralab; mouse, monoclonal) had the advantage of staining the pentapeptides without recognizing dynorphins or NEO (Cuello et al., 1984). None of the antisera against the opioids cross-reacted with SP, NKA or CGRP. Specificities and sources of antisera against the various opioids are described in more detail elsewhere (see Weihe et al., 1985, 1986, 1988a,b).

Results

Characterization of opioid peptides in spinal and trigeminal ganglionic cells of different species

Several molecular forms of opioid peptides (OP) derived from PRO-DYN, i.e., ir-DYN A 1 – 17, ir-DYN B, and ir-NEO were found in numerous small- (< 20 µm), less numerous medium- (20 – 40 µm), and a few large- (> 40 µm) diameter ganglionic cells of cervical, thoracic and lumbosacral spinal ganglia and of trigeminal ganglia from guinea-pig, cat, dog, but not rat. The non-selective polyclonal anti-LE revealed identical patterns. This form of ir-LE and all PRO-DYN-specific ir-OP were found to co-exist with each other. As a distinct feature, ir-DYN A 1 – 8 ganglionic cells were absent. The number of PRO-DYN-specific and LE-ir cells varied between 5 and 15% per section plane of one ganglion and was higher in lumbosacral than in thoracic, cervical or trigeminal ganglia.

In rabbit, only a few OP-ir sensory ganglionic cells were seen. The PRO-DYN-specific and LE immunostaining was much stronger in guinea-pig than in the other species. The intensity of cellular staining varied among individual cells from very weak to very strong.

PRO-ENK-OP-specific (MRGL) immunostaining of sensory ganglionic cells was absent in all species investigated except the pig in which a few MRGL-ir trigeminal ganglionic cells were visualized. PRO-DYN-OP-specific immunostaining in pig sensory ganglia was equivocal.

The use of the monoclonal anti-LE (only applied in guinea-pig) revealed less numerous ir cells than the polyclonal anti-LE or the PRO-DYN-OP-specific antisera.

Interrelation of ir-PRO-DYN-OP with ir-SP/NKA and ir-CGRP in spinal and trigeminal ganglia (Table 1)

SP- and CGRP-ir cell populations appeared to be almost completely overlapped. In contrast, co-existence of ir-PRO-DYN-OP with ir-SP or ir-CGRP was restricted to a subpopulation of ganglionic cells (Fig. 2). SP/CGRP-ir and opioid-ir cell populations also occurred independently of each other. Co-existence of ir-PRO-DYN-OP with ir-SP/CGRP was more frequent in small and medium-sized than in large ganglionic cells. Staining in large cells was more granular and weaker than in small and medium-sized cells in which the immunoproduct was usually confluent. In appropriate thin (< 4 μm) consecutive sections, co-existence of ir-PRO-DYN-OP, ir-SP and ir-CGRP in identical ganglionic cells was determined. Not infrequently, the intensities of opioid and tachykinin immunostaining were reciprocal.

As a rule, OP-ir fibers were less frequent than SP/CGRP-ir fibers. They were co-distributed within the ganglia, dorsal roots and spinal nerves. Opioid fiber staining appeared to be mostly confined to non-myelinated C and a population of thinly myelinated A-δ fibers, whereas ir-SP/CGRP, in addition, was present in a population of thickly myelinated fibers within the A-δ range and in a few A-β fibers. The pattern of ir-NKA was identical to that of ir-SP. Likewise, partial co-existence of ir-OP and ir-NKA was observed. This situation was typical of the guinea-pig. Principally similar co-existence/co-distribution patterns were seen in the cat but have not yet been evaluated in rabbit, dog or pig.

TABLE 1

Relative proportions of sensory neurons characterized by either a single or a combinatory peptide phenotype[a]

SP	$-/+$
CGRP	$-/+$
PRO-DYN-OP	$+$
SP/CGRP	$+++++$
SP/PRO-DYN-OP	$+++$
CGRP/PRO-DYN-OP	$+++$
PRO-ENK-OP	$-$

[a] Spinal/trigeminal ganglia of guinea-pig.

Interrelation of ir-PRO-DYN-OP and ir-SP/CGRP in spinal dorsal horn and trigeminal complex (guinea-pig vs. rat)

In the dorsal horn (particularly in laminae I and IV/V) of all segments of spinal cord and in equivalent regions of the trigeminal complex, PRO-DYN-specific OP-ir nerve fibers were less frequent than SP/CGRP-ir nerve fibers but did not occur independent of the latter (Fig. 1). This pattern was similar in guinea-pig and rat except for one distinct difference, namely, that PRO-DYN-specific OP-ir fibers and LE-ir fibers were frequently present in the Lissauer zone of guinea-pig but almost absent in that of rat. PRO-ENK-specific MRGL-ir fibers were virtually absent from the Lissauer zone. In contrast, SP- and CGRP-ir fibers were equally frequent in the Lissauer zones of rat and guinea-pig.

Interrelation of OP-ir and SP/CGRP-ir innervation in selected peripheral regions

The peripheral pattern is exemplarily described for the guinea-pig. Almost similar results were found in other species, except in rat, where ir-PRO-DYN-OP seemed to be absent from sensory type fibers. The most powerful antiserum to reveal OP-ir fibers in the periphery was the non-selective anti-LE. The staining with the PRO-DYN-OP-specific antisera was principally similar but more variable and somewhat less frequent. Interestingly, ir-DYN A 1–8 was present in some fibers although it was absent from sensory perikarya. In contrast, PRO-ENK-specific MRGL-ir fibers were mostly absent from these regions. The OP-ir nerve fibers were very thin, apparently C, as well as small A-δ fibers and were only present in areas where SP/CGRP-ir nerve fibers also occurred (Fig. 3). As a rule SP/CGRP-ir fibers outnumbered the co-distributed OP-ir fibers and consisted of C fibers and of A-δ fibers of various diameters. The co-distributed OP-ir and SP/CGRP-ir fibers occurred in somatic and visceral tissues (1) unrelated to target structures, apparently as 'free nerve endings' and (2) in

192

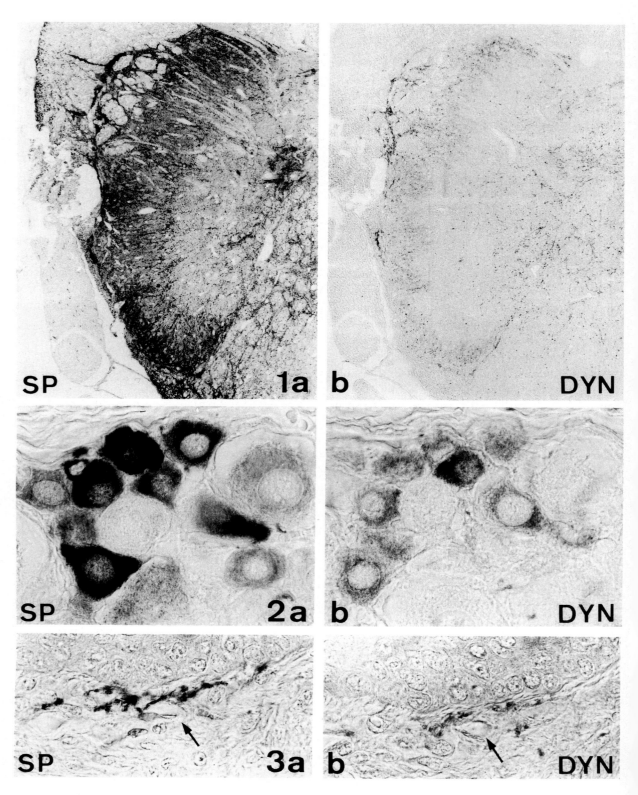

more or less close association with various target cells.

Targets

The common peripheral targets (see also Fig. 4) of OP-ir and SP/CGRP-ir nerve fibers included the endothelium and pericytes of capillaries and pericytic venules, smooth muscle of the micro-vasculature (arterioles, muscular venules), mast cells, basophils, some local immune cells and non-vascular smooth muscle (tracheobronchial, ureter, urethra, dermal smooth muscle strands). In contrast to the microvasculature, macrovascular segments and systemic blood vessels were rarely innervated by OP-ir fibers whereas the SP/CGRP innervation was very rich. Many somatic tissues (glabrous and hairy skin, cornea, eye, deep tissues like ligaments, tendons, joint capsules) and visceral tissues like urinary tract, and restricted cardiac regions (see Weihe, 1987) received innervation by SP/NKA/CGRP/OP-ir fibers. The opioid innervation was prominent in pelvic viscera. The lamina propria of the urinary tract (including renal pelvis) and of the entire respiratory tract received a particularly dense innervation with co-distributed SP/NKA/CGRP/OP-ir fibers. A similar accumulation of ir fibers was observed in papillary and subepidermal regions of guinea-pig and cat skin, where capillaries and venules received a dense supply with fibers containing these peptides.

Discussion

Multiplicity and co-existence patterns of primary sensory opioids

In extension of previous investigations (Weihe et al., 1985, 1986), the present study shows that the chemical coding of a subpopulation of small-diameter (C, A-δ) primary sensory neurons includes co-existing opioid peptides, tachykinins (SP, NKA) and CGRP at both their central and peripheral endings (Fig. 4). This chemoanatomical constellation was found to be typical of the guinea-pig which, in addition, seems to contain CCK in capsaicin-sensitive neurons exhibiting this particular combinatory peptide phenotype (Gibbins et al., 1987). We have to be aware that combinatory sets of peptides (Kawatani et al., 1986) and other possible transmitters like glutamate which is a strong candidate (cf. Zieglgänsberger, 1986; Besson and Chaouch, 1987) may be even more complex and not strictly fixed to, but interchangeable between, the respective populations including rare single peptide phenotypes.

Our findings of PRO-DYN opioid peptides in sensory ganglionic cells of cat are in good agreement with the accumulation of DYN B in sacral primary afferent fibers observed upon ligation of the dorsal roots (Basbaum et al., 1986). By the use of radioimmunoassay (RIA), the same authors measured higher levels of ir-DYN B in sacral than in other spinal ganglia, which is concordant to similar segmental variations revealed in our study and by Sweetnam et al. (1986) who used explant extracts of murine dorsal root ganglia. In spite of colchicine treatment, Basbaum et al. (1986) could not visualize DYN B containing sensory ganglionic cell bodies in the cat. Therefore, it is particularly noteworthy that in our study, colchicine was unnecessary to 'lighten up' opioid staining of sensory perikarya. On the other hand, we did not succeed in visualizing ir-OP in spinal or trigeminal ganglionic cells or in the Lissauer tract of the rat, although the use of RIA revealed DYN-ir material in extracts of rat spinal ganglia (Boticelli et al., 1981). The mouse is a further species which encodes PRO-DYN-OP in primary sensory neurons.

Figs. 1 – 3. LM micrographs of adjacent sections (a/b) showing the interrelation of immunoreactivities to substance P (SP) and dynorphin A 1 – 17 (DYN) in the guinea-pig. (1) Co-distribution in fibers of lamina I and lamina IV/V of the dorsal horn (L5). Note higher frequency of SP-ir fibers. (2) Co-existence in small-diameter dorsal root ganglionic cells (L5). (3) Co-distribution in small-diameter subepidermal nerve fibers of skin. Note close relation of ir fibers to a venule (arrow) and higher density of SP-ir fibers.

The number of such neurons expressing ir-DYN seems to increase with the duration of explants of neonatal ganglia (Sweetnam et al., 1986). Ligation experiments in explant cultures of guinea-pig spinal ganglia revealed transport of DYN in central as well as peripheral branches (Gibbins et al., 1987).

The fact that we found ir-MRGL in pig trigeminal sensory cells in conjunction with the demonstration of ir-met-enkephalin as well as of ir-DYN and ir-NEO in extracts of human spinal ganglia (Przewlocki et al., 1983) may indicate that the opioid phenotype in mammalian sensory neurons not only involves PRO-DYN but also PRO-ENK opioid peptides. However, in none of the other species we obtained evidence for the presence of any PRO-ENK-specific opioid peptides in ganglionic cells. We cannot exclude the possibility that sensory PRO-ENK processing is silent. Even co-existence of PRO-DYN and PRO-ENK is not an unlikely possibility (see Weihe et al., 1988a,b).

The question arises which molecular forms of PRO-DYN-OP are posttranslationally processed in sensory neurons. The fact that DYN A 1 – 8 appeared to be present in sensory terminals but not in cell bodies indicates that it is cleaved from DYN A 1 – 17 in transit or in the terminals. There, both forms of DYN A together with NEO and LE could be acting as sensory transmitters. In contrast, Sweetnam et al. (1986) observed ir-DYN A 9 – 17 in murine sensory perikarya which may indirectly reflect cleavage of DYN A 1 – 8 in the soma.

Our evidence for the presence of the authentic pentapeptide leu-enkephalin (LE) is supportive of the view that there may be a dynorphinergic or neoendorphinergic pathway for sensory LE (Weihe et al., 1985). The spectrum of PRO-DYN-OP detected immunohistochemically correlates well with chromatographic characterization of opioid peptides in skin and nerve extracts where LE, DYN A 1 – 8, DYN B and NEO could be bioassayed (Weihe et al., 1983, 1985, and unpublished). On the other hand, PRO-ENK opioid peptides also seemed to be present in these extracts. Puzzlingly, we found ir-MRGL in some cutaneous nerves around hairs (unpublished). This points to the necessity of using the combination of retrograde/anterograde tracing and immunohistochemistry in order to differentiate sensory from sympathetic and parasympathetic opioid pathways in the periphery (see Weihe, 1987; Weihe et al.,

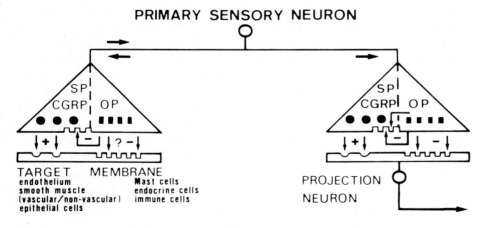

Fig. 4. Schematic diagram summarizing our hypothesis on the assumed antinociceptive co-transmitter role of primary sensory opioid peptides. Opioid peptides (OP) may act (1) on presynaptic external or internal autoreceptors to inhibit the release of their excitatory (nociceptive) co-transmitters (SP, CGRP) at both peripheral and spinal endings; (2) on postsynaptic receptors present on central (e.g., spinal) projection neurons to inhibit their excitability to the excitatory co-transmitters; (3) on postjunctional peripheral receptors where they may equally inhibit the excitability of various peripheral target cells. Further considerations see text.

1988b; Häppölä et al., 1987). Nonetheless, the presence in sensory neurons of endogenous opioid ligands known to act on different receptors, namely LE preferentially on δ and DYN/NEO preferentially on x (see Paterson et al., 1984; Goldstein 1984; Millan and Herz, 1985), points to the conclusion that both receptor types may be crucial in primary sensory nociceptive processing.

Possible opioid autoinhibition of primary sensory (nociceptive) neurotransmission (Fig. 4)

Based on the established co-existence patterns, we deduce a modulatory or co-transmitter role of sensory opioids in concert with SP, NKA and CGRP which should be operational at peripheral as well as at central endings. While these co-transmitter candidates are known to co-function and to be co-released from the antipodal endings, in the case of SP, apparently upon selective noxious stimulation (Gamse and Saria, 1985; Brain et al., 1986; Helme et al., 1986; Duggan et al., 1987; Oku et al., 1987), there is no direct experimental evidence that this is also true for the sensory opioid peptides. Nevertheless, their presence in sensory neurons tempts us to assume their release.

One target of centrally and peripherally released opioid peptides may be the releasing terminal itself. In that case, they would act on presynaptic opioid autoreceptors (Weihe et al., 1985). The presence of presynaptic opioid receptors on spinal and trigeminal terminals of primary afferents containing SP has been demonstrated (Ninkovic and Hunt, 1985). It was postulated that they are accessed by opioid peptides released by spinal interneurons and then mediate inhibition or attenuation of the release of SP resulting in antinociception (see Millan, 1986; Zieglgänsberger, 1986; Besson and Chaouch, 1987). Since CGRP promotes mechanical nociception by potentiating the spinal release of SP from afferent terminals (Oku et al., 1987) an opioid-induced attenuation of this mechanism is also conceivable. As there seems to be some selectivity of peptide transmitter candidates (SP, CCK, CGRP, somatostatin) to

mechano-, thermo- or chemonociception (Wiesenfeld-Hallin, 1986; Duggan et al., 1987; Hill et al., 1987), we may postulate differential antinociceptive potencies of sensory opioid peptides depending on these modalities of nociception. CCK has nociceptive as well as antinociceptive properties and puzzlingly, its antinociceptive action can be antagonized by naloxone (Hill et al., 1987). This is particularly interesting in the light of the co-existence of CCK and DYN in sensory neurons of guinea-pig (Gibbins et al., 1987).

Presynaptic opioid receptors were also shown to be present on peripheral terminals where they seem equally to mediate attenuation of the release of SP reflected in a decrease of antidromically induced extravasation by exogenously applied opioid agonists (Lembeck and Donnerer, 1985; Wei et al., 1986). We propose that the close interrelation of opioid and tachykinin innervation with venular and capillary endothelium may be of key significance in neurogenic mechanisms of extravasation.

Interestingly, peripheral presynaptic opioid receptors are also present on SP containing vagal afferents (Laduron, 1984). The release of SP, probably in combination with NKA and CGRP, from peripheral terminals of the vagal nerve seems to play a crucial role in vagally induced edema, inflammation and non-vascular smooth muscle constriction of tracheobronchial tissue (see Lundberg and Hökfelt, 1986).

Since we have preliminary evidence that opioid peptides are not only contained in primary sensory afferents of the somatic and visceral spinal and trigeminal system but also in the vagal sensory neurons (unpublished), we postulate the general principle of endogenous opioid autoinhibition of the release of excitatory co-transmitters like SP from various primary sensory afferents (Fig. 4). According to the pharmacological action profile of exogenous opioids on central as well as on peripheral endings of a variety of visceral and somatic primary afferents, we conclude a similar action profile of endogenous opioids. Thus, we would expect that they produce spinal and peripheral antinociception, attenuation of axon-reflex mechanisms, i.e., of protein extravasation, reflex tracheo-bronchoconstriction or reflex spasms of urinary tract. Effects on other primary sensory functions like baroreception and chemoreception are also conceivable (Weihe, 1987). In addition, we postulate interference of primary collaterals containing opioid peptides with reflex mechanisms mediated by primary sensory SP collaterals at the level of pre- and paravertebral sympathetic ganglia (Matthews et al., 1987).

The very recent demonstration by Frank and Sudha (1987) of the presence of stereospecific opioid receptors, located on the intracellular surface of sensory A and C fiber axons, opens the intriguing possibility that such internal opioid receptors are also present in sensory terminals and used by endogenous opioids.

The inhibitory action profile of opioid peptides (see Millan and Herz, 1985; Zieglgänsberger, 1986) suggests that endogenous sensory opioid peptides shorten the duration of the action potential and inhibit or attenuate by this mechanism the central and peripheral release of an excitatory co-transmitter, e.g., SP. However, in experiments in which depressant effects of exogenous opioids on mouse sensory neurons in culture were blocked by pertussis toxin an opioid-induced prolongation of the action potential has been demasked (Crain et al., 1987). This is compatible with the view that an excitatory effect of opioids is also possible. It may explain the paradox of opioid-induced peripheral hyperalgesia (Van der Kooy, 1986). Arguments against such hyperalgesic functions of peripheral opioids can be deduced from experiments of Russell et al. (1987) who provided electrophysiological evidence for inhibitory effects of peripherally applied opiates on afferent discharges from inflamed knee joint of cat. Stereospecific antinociceptive peripheral actions of opiates, apparently involving sensory fibers, are also reported in the polyarthritic rat (Stein et al., 1988). The functional significance of endogenous primary sensory opioid ligands and receptors may be more important in neurogenic inflammation than under normal conditions.

Possible postsynaptic (central) and postjunctional (peripheral) effects of primary sensory opioids

Different classes of opioid receptors are thought to be operational on the dendrites and somata of spinothalamic projection neurons in laminae I and V which are regarded as second-order nociceptive neurons (see Zieglgänsberger, 1986; Millan, 1986; Besson and Chaouch, 1987). Therefore it is plausible to assume that opioid peptides, released from primary sensory afferents containing only opioid peptides or combinatory sets with other peptides, would postsynaptically inhibit the excitability of these neurons to the co-released or parallelly released primary nociceptive transmitter candidates SP/NKA/CGRP/CCK. Effects of primary sensory OP on the complex circuitry of inhibitory and excitatory neurons in the substantia gelatinosa (see Millan, 1986; Zieglgänsberger, 1986) must be expected but details cannot be outlined here.

Interestingly, the antinociceptive effects of experimental electroacupuncture can be blocked by intrathecally applied antibodies against DYN or ENK depending on the frequencies used (Han et al., 1987). Likewise, the nociceptive effects upon noxious heat stimulation can be blocked by antibodies against SP (Duggan et al., 1987). Therefore, we speculate that the specific state of the membrane potential regulates the composition of the released sensory transmitter cocktail and vice versa. The antinociceptive effect of electroacupuncture could be mediated by a selective activation of the sensory opioid component resulting in postsynaptic inhibition of secondary nociceptive neurons or in presynaptic autoinhibition of the nociceptive primary afferent itself. On the other hand, propriospinal opioid peptides, particularly dynorphins, which respond to acute and chronic pain with an increase (see Millan, 1986; Weihe et al., 1988a), may be equally or even more important.

If opioid peptides were released from sensory terminals in the periphery, they could reach a variety of target membranes (Fig. 4). However, in contrast to the established postjunctional peripheral action profile of the co-transmitters

SP/NKA/CGRP (Foreman, 1987; Besson and Chaouch, 1987), it is not clear whether opioid peptides could evoke postjunctional effects because the knowledge about the presence of stereospecific opioid receptors on these target cells is sparse. There are reports that certain immune cells possess opioid receptors and even express opioid peptides (Morley and Kay, 1986). Thus, a neuroimmunomodulatory function of primary sensory opioids in conjunction with the other sensory peptides is conceivable (Fink et al., 1987). Interestingly, there is also evidence for a sensory – endocrine axis (Amann and Lembeck, 1986), in which endogenous opioids may also be involved (Millan and Herz, 1985). In addition, a trophic role of peptides has been reported which may be linked to axon-reflex mechanisms (see Weihe et al., 1988).

Opioid-induced release of histamine from mast cells has been known for a long time and sensory opioids may have the same effect. Thus, they could act synergistically with SP to induce histamine release (Foreman, 1987). Sensory endogenous opioid ligands and receptors may be involved in histamine and non-histamine mediated pruritus, a complicating side effect of opiate therapy. On the whole, the possibility of postjunctional effects of sensory opioid peptides in the periphery needs to be further elucidated. Nonetheless, the present study has revealed the most likely targets for such actions (Fig. 4).

General conclusions and perspectives

We introduce the concept that there is a functionally important tandem constellation of transmitters in a perhaps specific nociceptive population of primary sensory afferents consisting of (1) an inhibitory transmitter family, the opioid peptides, and (2) an excitatory transmitter family, the tachykinins. The presence of the inhibitory opioid peptides and of presynaptic opioid receptors implies the novel principle of presynaptic primary sensory autoinhibition. Other transmitter candidates (e.g., glutamate, or additional peptides) may act synergistically with either of the two op-

posite components. The balance of this 'transmitter cocktail' may be crucial in nociceptive/antinociceptive cybernetics and axon-reflex mechanisms. Its disbalance may be of principal pathophysiological significance, particularly in chronic inflammatory processes involving pain. On the other hand, therapeutical maneuvers such as acupuncture, electro-acupuncture, physiotherapy and even pharmacological therapy used for the relief of pain may, inter alia, act by rebalancing a disturbed transmitter composition of primary sensory afferents in both their peripheral and central endings. With respect to minimization of drug side effects, a selective peripheral approach in the pharmacological treatment of localized inflammatory skin diseases or arthritis could be particularly attractive.

Acknowledgements

This study was supported by the Deutsche Forschungsgemeinschaft (DFG Antrag We 910/2-1), Stifterverband für die Deutsche Wissenschaft and Schering A.G., Berlin. For generous supply of antisera we would like to thank A. Herz and coworkers R.M. Arendt, C. Gramsch, V. Höllt, B. Seizinger, D.C. Liebisch (Munich), A. Goldstein (Stanford) and E. Weber (Oregon). For excellent technical assistance we thank A. Leibold and U. Egner.

References

Amann, R. and Lembeck, F. (1986) Capsaicin sensitive afferent neurons from peripheral glucose receptors mediate the insulin-induced increase in adrenaline secretion. *Naunyn-Schmiedeberg's Arch. Pharmacol.*, 334: 71 – 76.

Basbaum, A.I., Cruz, L. and Weber, E. (1986) Immunoreactive dynorphin B in sacral primary afferent fibers of the cat. *J. Neurosci.*, 6: 127 – 133.

Besson, J.-M. and Chaouch, A. (1987) Peripheral and spinal mechanisms of nociception. *Physiol. Rev.*, 67: 67 – 186.

Boticelli, L.J., Cox, M. and Goldstein, A. (1981) Immunoreactive dynorphin in mammalian spinal cord and dorsal root ganglia. *Proc. Natl. Acad. Sci. U.S.A.*, 78: 7783 – 7786.

Brain, S.D., MacIntyre, I. and Williams, T.J. (1986) A second form of human calcitonic gene-related peptide which is a po-

198

tent vasodilator. *Eur. J. Pharmacol.,* 124: 349–352.

Crain, S.M., Shen, K.-F. and Chalazonitis, A. (1987) Enhanced excitatory effects of opioids on sensory neurons after treatment of mouse spinal cord-ganglion explants with pertussis toxin or forskolin. *Neuroscience,* 22, Suppl.: S409.

Cuello, A.C., Milstein, C., Couture, R., Wright, B., Priestley, J.V. and Jarvis, J. (1984) Characterization and immunocytochemical application of monoclonal antibodies against enkephalins. *J. Histochem. Cytochem.,* 32: 947–957.

Duggan, A.W., Morton, C.R., Zhao, Z.Q. and Hendry, I.A. (1987) Noxious heating of the skin releases immunoreactive substance P in the substantia gelatinosa of the cat: a study with antibody microprobes. *Brain Res.,* 403: 345–349.

Fink, T., Nohr, D., Leibold, A. and Weihe, E. (1987) Peptidergic innervation of guinea-pig lymph nodes: chemoanatomical link for sensory and autonomic neuroimmunomodulation? *Neuroscience,* 22, Suppl.: S814.

Foreman, J.C. (1987) Peptides and neurogenic inflammation. *Br. Med. Bull.,* 43: 386–400.

Frank, G.B. and Sudha, T.S. (1987) Effects of enkephalin applied intracellularly on action potentials in vertebrate A and C nerve fibre actions. *Neuropharmacology,* 26: 61–66.

Gamse, R. and Saria, A. (1985) Potentiation of tachykinin-induced plasma protein extravasation by calcitonin gene-related peptide. *Eur. J. Pharmacol.,* 114: 61–66.

Gibbins, I.L., Furness, J.B. and Costa, M. (1987) Pathway-specific patterns of the co-existence of substance P, cholecystokinin and dynorphin in neurons of the dorsal root ganglia of the guinea-pig. *Cell Tissue Res.,* 248: 417–437.

Goldstein, A. (1984) Biology and chemistry of the dynorphin peptides. In: S. Udenfriend and J. Meienhofer (Eds.), *The Peptides.* Academic Press, New York, pp. 96–137.

Han, J.S., Fei, H. and Sun, S.L. (1987) New evidence showing differential release from spinal cord of enkephalin and dynorphin by low and high frequency electroacupuncture stimulation. *Neuroscience,* 22, Suppl.: S315.

Häppölä, O., Soinila, S., Päivärinta, H. and Panula, P. (1987) Met-enkephalin-Arg-Phe- and met-enkephalin-Arg-Gly-Leu-immunoreactive nerve fibres and neurons in the superior cervical ganglion of the rat. *Neuroscience,* 21: 283–295.

Helme, R.D., Koschorke, G.M. and Zimmermann, M. (1986) Immunoreactive substance P release from skin nerves in the rat by noxious thermal stimulation. *Neurosci. Lett.,* 63: 295–299.

Hill, R.G., Hughes, J. and Pittaway, K.M. (1987) Antinociceptive action of cholecystokinin octapeptide (CCK 8) and related peptides in rats and mice: effects of naloxone and peptidase inhibitors. *Neuropharmacology,* 26: 289–300.

Kawatani, M., Nagel, J. and deGroat, W.C. (1986) Identification of neuropeptides in pelvic and pudendal nerve afferent pathways to the sacral spinal cord of the cat. *J. Comp. Neurol.,* 249: 117–132.

Krause, J.E., Chirgwin, J.M., Carter, M.S., Xu, Z.S. and Her-

shey, A.D. (1987) Three rat preprotachykinin mRNAs encode the neuropeptides substance P and neurokinin A. *Proc. Natl. Acad. Sci. U.S.A.,* 84: 881–885.

Laduron, P.M. (1984) Axonal transport of opiate receptors in capsaicin-sensitive neurons. *Brain Res.,* 294: 157–160.

Lai, Y.-L. and Cornett, A.F. (1987) Substance P-inducing massive postmortem bronchoconstriction in guinea-pig lungs. *J. Appl. Physiol.,* 62: 746–751.

Lembeck, F. and Donnerer, J. (1985) Opioid control of the function of primary afferent substance P fibres. *Eur. J. Pharmacol.,* 114: 241–246.

Lundberg, J.M. and Hökfelt, T. (1986) Multiple co-existence of peptides and classical transmitters in peripheral autonomic and sensory neurons – functional and pharmacological implications. In: T. Hökfelt, K. Fuxe and B. Pernow (Eds.), *Progress in Brain Research,* Vol. 68. Elsevier, Amsterdam, pp. 241–262.

Matthews, M.R., Connaughton, M. and Cuello, A.C. (1987) Ultrastructure and distribution of substance P-immunoreactive sensory collaterals in the guinea-pig prevertebral sympathetic ganglia. *J. Comp. Neurol.,* 258: 28–51.

Millan, M.J. (1986) Multiple opioid systems and pain. *Pain,* 27: 303–349.

Millan, M.J. and Herz, A. (1985) The endocrinology of the opioids. *Neurobiology,* 26: 1–83.

Morley, J.E. and Kay, N. (1986) Neuropeptides as modulators of immune function. *Psychopharmacol. Bull.,* 22: 1089–1092.

Ninkovic, M. and Hunt, S.P. (1985) Opiate and histamine H1 receptors are present on some substance P containing dorsal root ganglion cells. *Neurosci. Lett.,* 53: 133–137.

Oku, R., Satoh, M., Fujii, N., Otaka, A., Yajima, H. and Tagaki, H. (1987) Calcitonin gene-related peptide promotes mechanical nociception by potentiating release of substance P from the spinal dorsal horn in rats. *Brain Res.,* 403: 350–354.

Paterson, S.J., Robson, L.E. and Kosterlitz, H.W. (1984) Opioid receptors. In: S. Udenfriend and J. Meienhofer (Eds.), *The Peptides.* Academic Press, New York, pp. 147–184.

Przewlocki, R., Gramsch, C., Pasi, A. and Herz, A. (1983) Characterization and localization of immunoreactive dynorphin, alpha-neoendorphin, met-enkephalin and substance P in human spinal cord. *Brain Res.,* 280: 95–103.

Russell, N.J.W., Schaible, H.-G. and Schmidt, R.F. (1987) Opiates inhibit the discharges of fine afferent units from inflamed knee joint of the cat. *Neurosci. Lett.,* 76: 107–112.

Stein, C., Millan, M.J., Shippenberg, T.S. and Herz, A. (1988) Peripheral effects of fentanyl upon nociception in inflamed tissue of the rat. *Neurosci. Lett.,* 84: 225–228.

Sweetnam, P.M., Wrathall, J.R. and Neale, J.H. (1986) Localization of dynorphin gene product-immunoreactivity in neurons from spinal cord and dorsal root ganglia. *Neuroscience,* 18: 947–955.

Van der Kooy, D. (1986) Hyperalgesic functions of peripheral opiate receptors. *Ann. N.Y. Acad. Sci.,* 467: 154–168.

Wei, E.T., Kiang, J.G., Buchan, P. and Smith, T.W. (1986) Corticotropin-releasing factor inhibits neurogenic plasma extravasation in the rat paw. *J. Pharmacol. Exp. Ther.,* 238: 783–789.

Weihe, E. (1987) Peripheral innervation of the heart. In: T. v. Arnim and A. Maseri (Eds.), *Silent Ischemia.* Steinkopf Verlag, Darmstadt, pp. 7–18.

Weihe, E., McKnight, A.T., Corbett, A.D., Hartschuh, W., Reinecke, M. and Kosterlitz, H.W. (1983) Characterization of opioid peptides in guinea-pig heart and skin. *Life Sci.,* 33, Suppl. 1: 711-714.

Weihe, E., Hartschuh, W. and Weber, E. (1985) Prodynorphin opioid peptides in small somatosensory primary afferents of guinea-pig. *Neurosci. Lett.,* 58: 347–352.

Weihe, E., Leibold, A., Nohr, D., Fink, T. and Gauweiler, B. (1986) Co-existence of prodynorphin-opioid peptides and substance P in primary sensory afferents of guinea-pig. *NIDA Res. Monogr.,* 75: 295–298.

Weihe, E., Millan, M.J., Leibold, A., Nohr, D. and Herz, A. (1988a) Co-localization of proenkephalin- and prodynorphin-derived opioid peptides in laminae IV/V spinal neurons revealed in arthritic rats. *Neurosci. Lett.,* 85: 187–192.

Weihe, E., Nohr, D., Hartschuh, W., Gauweiler, B. and Fink, T. (1988b) Multiplicity of opioidergic pathways related to cardiovascular innervation: differential contribution of all three opioid precursors. In: K.O. Stumpe and K. Kraft (Eds.), *Opioid Peptides and Blood Pressure Control.* Springer, Berlin.

Wiesenfeld-Hallin, Z. (1986) Substance P and somatostatin modulate spinal cord excitability via physiologically different sensory pathways. *Brain Res.,* 372: 172–175.

Zieglgänsberger, W. (1986) Central control of nociception. In: V.B. Mountcastle, F.E. Bloom and S.R. Geiger (Eds.) *Handbook of Physiology, The Nervous System IV.* Williams and Wilkins, Baltimore, MD, pp. 581–645.

W. Hamann and A. Iggo (Eds.)
Progress in Brain Research, Vol. 74
© 1988 Elsevier Science Publishers B.V. (Biomedical Division)

CHAPTER 22

Chemical factors in the sensitization of cutaneous nociceptors

R.H. Cohen[*] and E.R. Perl

Department of Physiology, University of North Carolina, Chapel Hill, NC 27514, USA

Introduction

Nociceptors have been categorized into different types according to the receptive tissue, the conduction velocity of their afferent fibers and the relative responsiveness to various kinds of noxious stimuli including chemical irritants (Bessou and Perl, 1969; Burgess and Perl, 1967, 1973; Handwerker, 1976; Kniffki et al., 1976; Perl, 1968, 1984). Recently a case has been made that one particular subset of cutaneous nociceptors is specially, if not uniquely, sensitive to certain algogenic compounds (Szolcsanyi, 1987). Nonetheless, chemically induced responses are not routinely used to evaluate the characteristics of nociceptors.

Cutaneous nociceptors undergo a change in responsiveness, labeled sensitization, which is reflected by an increased activity to repeated stimuli (Bessou and Perl, 1969; Perl, 1972; King et al., 1976; Kumazawa and Perl, 1977). There often is a parallel associated development of background discharge which may not be related to an identical cause. The graphs of Fig. 1 show the successive responses of a cutaneous polymodal nociceptor with a C afferent fiber (CPM) evoked by repeated, identical cycles of stepwise increases in skin temperature to noxious levels; the activity evoked

by the first heating of the skin (A) was substantially less than that produced by the third (B) and fifth (C) repetitions.

The idea that chemical agents act as intermediaries between pain causing stimuli and activation of the sense organs responsible for this sensation is well rooted (Lewis, 1942; Keele and Armstrong, 1964). Classic if not historic observations on human beings suggest that enhanced responsiveness of sense organs may result from agents common to those associated with inflammation.

Our attention was drawn to substance P (SP) for several reasons. SP is reported to be released at peripheral nerve terminals following electrical stimulation of nerves and noxious heating of the skin, an effect partially reduced by denervation (Olgart et al., 1977; Helme et al., 1985). Competitive antagonists for SP infused intra-arterially partially inhibit vasodilation and plasma extravasation produced by antidromic nerve stimulation or by the infusion of substance P itself (Lembeck et al., 1977). While neither SP nor the E-type of prostaglandins (PGEs) are directly algogenic or excitatory for presumed nociceptors (Juan and Lembeck, 1974; Lembeck and Gamse, 1977), these compounds may still be part of processes leading to enhanced responsiveness of 'pain' endings and hyperalgesia (Ferreira and Nakamura, 1979; Ferreira, 1982). Thus, our experiments began with an attempt to evaluate the possible role

---

[*] Current address: Department of Neurosurgery, Johns Hopkins Medical School, 600 N. Wolfe St., Baltimore, MD 21205, USA.

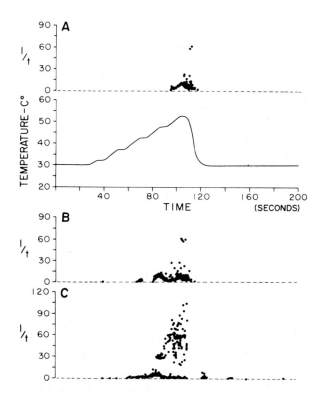

Fig. 1. Responses of a C fiber polymodal nociceptor of monkey skin to repeated heating of the receptive field to noxious levels. Heating was produced by a small contact thermode which went through identical cycles as illustrated in A (lower part) every 200 s. Each dot represents a discharge plotted at time of occurrence (abscissa) at an ordinate position representing the reciprocal of time from the previous impulse. (A) First cycle of heating. (B) Third cycle of heating. (C) Fifth cycle of heating. (Reproduced with permission from Kumazawa and Perl, 1977.)

of SP in the production of enhanced responsiveness of heat-excited skin nociceptors with unmyelinated afferent fibers, most of which are also activated by irritant chemicals (Bessou and Perl, 1969; Szolcsanyi, 1987).

Methods

An innervated in vitro preparation of the rabbit ear was maintained at room temperature by intra-arterial perfusion with oxygenated Krebs – Henseleit solution (King et al., 1976). Recordings were made from single C fiber afferent unitary poten-

tials isolated by the dissection of fine filaments from the great auricular nerve. Unit potentials conducting less than 1 m/s were tested by mechanical stimulation of the skin. Those responding only to strong mechanical stimuli were then subjected to standardized heat stimuli (30 s at 28°C) followed by 2°C increases (1°C/s) at 12-s intervals until 6 – 11 impulses appeared during a single temperature step. When this criterion response was produced, heating ceased and the thermode cooled to the holding temperature. Each unit was subsequently tested at 10-min intervals by a heat sequence identical to that used in the first cycle. Chemical agents were added to perfusing fluid at known concentrations; the perfusate was switched to the tested solution just prior to a 10-min adaptation at the holding temperature.

Results

Under the in vitro conditions, heat-excited, high-threshold cutaneous receptors regularly (21/21) exhibited an enhancement of responsiveness comparable to that seen in vivo including the considerable variability from unit to unit. Fig. 2A compares responses from a control series of units, by arranging them in rank order according to the magnitude of increased response to sequential tests.

Excitation was never observed when the normal Krebs – Henseleit perfusion solution was switched to one containing SP. Units perfused with SP, in concentrations reported to cause fluid extravasation, showed a range of sensitization indistinguishable on statistical grounds from the control population (cf., Fig. 2A, B). Similarly, a SP competitive antagonist in concentrations blocking the effects of SP on fluid extravasation and vasodilation in the rabbit ear (Lembeck et al., 1982) did not significantly modify the spectrum of enhanced responsiveness (Fig. 2B). Since neither the responsiveness nor the evolution of sensitization was affected, it appears unlikely that SP is a chemical intermediary contributing to the enhanced respon-

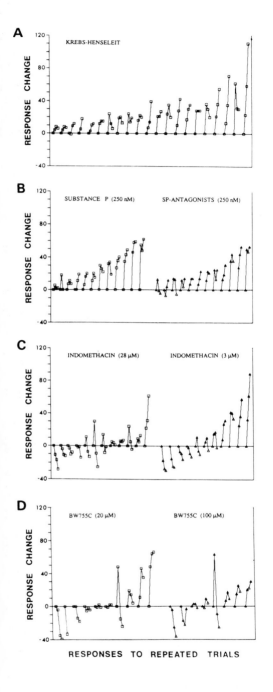

A KREBS-HENSELEIT

B SUBSTANCE P (250 nM)   SP-ANTAGONISTS (250 nM)

C INDOMETHACIN (28 μM)   INDOMETHACIN (3 μM)

D BW755C (20 μM)   BW755C (100 μM)

RESPONSES TO REPEATED TRIALS

Fig. 2. The response of C fiber mechanical heat nociceptors to repeated application of the standardized heat stimulus (see text). The change in each unit in each run relative to that evoked by the first trial is indicated by a series of interconnected squares or triangles. To facilitate comparisons the data for the

siveness of CPMs on repeated exposure to suprathreshold heat stimuli.

After obtaining these negative results with SP we turned our attention to prostaglandins and other derivatives of arachidonic acid metabolism. Prostaglandin E_2 (PGE_2) has been reported to induce hyperalgesia (Ferreira and Nakamura, 1979; Ferreira, 1982). Non-steroidal, anti-inflammatory agents such as aspirin and indometacin are presumed to act by inhibiting prostaglandins produced in the cyclo-oxygenase pathway of arachidonic acid breakdown (Vane, 1971). When indometacin was added to the perfusate solution prior to testing with heat, one half of the tested units failed to show sensitization (Fig. 2C). This division of the population in terms of sensitization by indometacin was not a simple dose effect since the same proportion of units exhibited sensitization when the perfusate contained 1/10th the concentration of indometacin (Fig. 2C).

While indometacin is an effective inhibitor of the cyclo-oxygenase pathway of arachidonic acid metabolism, it not only does not suppress the 5-lipoxygenase chain of products such as leukotrienes but may actually increase their production (Higgs and Vane, 1983). Leukotrienes have been reported to have actions opposing those of prostaglandins (Schweizer et al., 1984). For these reasons we tested a compound reported to inhibit both cyclo-oxygenase and 5-lipoxygenase pathways, BW755C (provided courtesy of the Burroughs-Wellcome Foundation). Adding BW755C to the perfusate gave results essentially identical to those seen with indometacin, approximately one half of the heat responsive C fiber units tested failed to show sensitization comparable to that observed in either the control or SP-treated populations (Fig. 2D). These observations with non-steroidal anti-inflammatory agents, while not

units are presented according to the rank order in the repeated trials of the enhancement of response. Perfusate contents: (A) Control Krebs – Henseleit solution; (B) Substance P (SP) or SP antagonist, 250 nM; (C) Indomethacin, 28 μM or 3 μM; (D) BW755C, 20 μM or 100 μM.

conclusive by themselves, are suggestive of functional differences in the heat sensitive, C fiber cutaneous nociceptor population. One subset of these sense organs appears to have the process leading to enhanced responsiveness on repeated heating dependent upon mechanisms involving prostaglandins or other products which are suppressed by drugs acting on cyclo-oxygenase pathways of arachidonic acid. Sensitization in the other subset of C fiber nociceptors is unaffected by these drugs.

Bradykinin is an algogenic peptide produced in tissue injury and has been implicated as a chemical mediator of the inflammatory process (Keele and Armstrong, 1964; Wilhelm, 1973). Bradykinin does not activate all cutaneous nociceptors (Szolcsanyi, 1987). Given the mixed effect of the non-steroidal anti-inflammatory agents upon the sensitization of the heat-activated nociceptors, we tested the effects of bradykinin and a related peptide, T-kinin (ile-ser-bradykinin) on the C fiber nociceptors in vitro. T-kinin apparently is the principal kinin produced in rat after chemical induc-

tion of inflammation (Barlas et al., 1985). T-kinins and bradykinin were introduced intra-arterially in doses ranging from 1 ng to 3 μg. On first activation, threshold response of heat-sensitive nociceptors to both kinins was a gradual increase in spontaneous activity after 180 s. Subsequent suprathreshold doses initiated responses in less than 30 s. T-kinin proved to be approximately equivalent in potency to bradykinin. C fiber polymodal nociceptors gave a fairly stereotyped response to the kinins: as illustrated in Fig. 3A, after 20 – 30 s a low frequency discharge began which reached a peak rate of under 3 impulses/s some 60 – 180 s after injection. In contrast, in multi-fiber preparations unitary discharges were repeatedly noted that gave quite different responses; some elements produced bursts of activity beginning within a few seconds following the injections and lasting less than a minute, while others showed irregular bursting at high frequencies (Fig. 3B) or continuous discharging lasting for many minutes. The units giving these different responses, i.e., either short in latency and short in

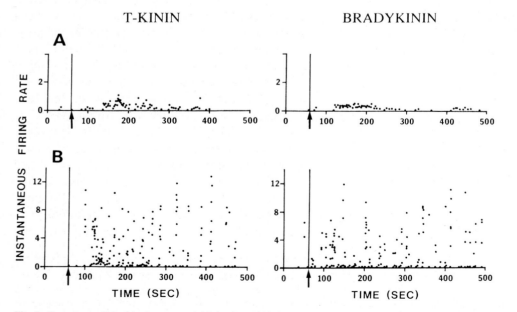

Fig. 3. Responses elicited by intra-arterial injection of kinins. (A) Response of identified C polymodal nociceptors to 1 μg injections. (B) Responses of bursting type units to 0.1 μg injections.

duration or high frequencies of activity, were never identified by eliciting a response with mechanical or temperature stimulation of the skin. Thus, the neural elements producing these short latency or high frequency responses to the kinins represented a population different from those classified as heat-mechanical or polymodal nociceptors. It is conceivable that they could be perivascular nerve terminations.

Comments and summary

Neither SP nor competitive blocking agents for SP were found to modify the responsiveness or changes of responsiveness for heat-sensitive cutaneous nociceptors with C afferent fibers in an in vitro rabbit ear preparation. These results argue against an important part for SP in modifying excitation of such sensory units.

Both a selective cyclo-oxygenase inhibitor (indometacin) and a dual acting cyclo-oxygenase and 5-lipoxygenase inhibitor (BW755C) suppressed the enhanced responsiveness of only a portion of the heat-sensitive C fiber nociceptors tested. The proportion affected by these non-steroidal anti-inflammatory agents was not dose sensitive and stayed the same in several different sets of experiments done on different populations of sense organs. This was taken to indicate diversity in types of mechanical heat nociceptors and in the processes leading to sensitization produced by noxious heat.

Units established to have the characteristics of C fiber polymodal nociceptors in the in vitro rabbit ear preparation gave a consistent delayed onset, low frequency pattern of response to the addition of kinins (bradykinin and T-kinin) to the perfusate. Other units of the same preparations, whose functional properties could not be identified and which were presumed to be high threshold or solely chemically responsive, gave short latency and high frequency responses to the same concentrations of kinins in the perfusing solution.

In addition to providing information on chemical agents associated with changes in responsiveness of cutaneous nociceptors, these observations suggest that the nature of chemical responsiveness should be considered in classifying or describing such sensory units.

Acknowledgements

Supported by Grant NS-10361 from the National Institute of Neurological Communicative Disorders and Stroke, US Public Health Service. R.H.C. was the recipient of a postdoctoral fellowship (NS-07788) from the NINCDS. We thank Ms. Sherry Derr for editorial and bibliographic help.

References

Barlas, A., Sugio, K. and Greenbaum, L.M. (1985) Release of T-kinin and bradykinin in carrageenin induced inflammation in the rat. Fed. Eur. Biochem. Soc., 190: 268 – 270.

Bessou, P. and Perl, E.R. (1969) Response of cutaneous sensory units with unmyelinate fibers to noxious stimuli. J. Neurophysiol., 32: 6.

Burgess, P.R. and Perl, E.R. (1967) Myelinated afferent fibres responding specifically to noxious stimulation of the skin. J. Physiol., 190: 541 – 562.

Burgess, P.R. and Perl, E.R. (1973) Cutaneous mechanoreceptors and nociceptors. In: A. Iggo (Ed.), Handbook of Sensory Physiology, Vol. 2. Somatosensory System. Springer, Berlin, pp. 29 – 78.

Ferreira, S.H. (1982) Prostaglandins, aspirin-like drugs and analgesia. Nature New Biol., 240: 200 – 203.

Ferreira, S.H. and Nakamura, M. (1979) I. Prostanglandin hyperalgesia, a $cAMP^{+2}$ dependent process. Prostanglandins, 18: 179 – 190.

Handwerker, H.O. (1976) Pharmacological modulation of the discharge of nociceptive C fibers. In: Y. Zotterman (Ed.), Sensory Functions of the Skin in Primates. Pergamon, Oxford, pp. 427 – 440.

Helme, R.D., Koschorke, G.M. and Zimmermann, M. (1985) Immunoreactive substance P release from skin nerves in the rat by noxious thermal stimulation. Neurosci. Lett., 63: 295 – 299.

Higgs, G.A. and Vane, J.R. (1983) Inhibition of cyclo-oxygenase and lipoxygenase. Br. Med. Bull., 39: 265 – 270.

Juan, H. and Lembeck, F. (1974) Action of peptides and other algesic agents on paravascular pain receptors of the isolated perfused rabbit ear. Naunyn-Schmiedeberg's Arch. Pharmacol., 282: 151 – 164.

Keele, C.A. and Armstrong, D. (1964) Chemical factors in pain following injury and in inflammation. In: H. Bancroft, H.

206

Davson and W.D.M. Paton (Eds.), *Substances Producing Pain and Itch,* Arnold, London, pp. 268 – 287.

King, J.S., Gallant, P., Myerson, V. and Perl, E.R. (1976) The effects of anti-inflammatory agents on the responses and the sensitization of unmyelinated (C) fiber polymodal nociceptors. In: Y. Zotterman (Ed.), *Sensory Functions of the Skin in Primates.* Pergamon, Oxford, pp. 441 – 454.

Kniffki, K.D., Mense, S. and Schmidt, R.F. (1976) Mechanisms of muscle pain: a comparison with cutaneous nociception. In: Y. Zotterman (Ed.), *Sensory Functions of the Skin in Primates.* Pergamon, Oxford, pp. 463 – 474.

Kumazawa, T. and Perl, E.R. (1977) Primate cutaneous sensory units with unmyelinated (C) afferent fibers. *J. Neurophysiol.,* 40: 1325 – 1338.

Lembeck, F. and Gamse, R. (1977) Lack of algesic effect of substance P on paravascular pain receptors. *Naunyn-Schmiedeberg's Arch. Pharmacol.,* 299: 295 – 303.

Lembeck, F., Gamse, R. and Juan, H. (1977) Substance P and sensory nerve endings. In: U.S. von Euler and B. Pernow (Eds.), *Substance P.* Raven Press, New York, pp. 160 – 181.

Lembeck, F., Donnerer, J. and Barthó, L. (1982) Inhibition of neurogenic vasodilation and plasma extravasation by substance P antagonists, somatostatin and [D-Met^2, Pro^5]-enkephalinamide. *Eur. J. Pharmacol.,* 85: 171 – 176.

Lewis, T. (1942) *Pain.* Macmillan, London.

Olgart, L., Gazelius, B., Brodin, E. and Nilsson, G. (1977) Localization of substance P-like immunoreactivity from dental pulp. *Acta Physiol. Scand.,* 101: 510 – 512.

Perl, E.R. (1968) Myelinated afferent fibres innervating the primate skin and their response to noxious stimuli. *J. Physiol.,* 197: 593 – 615.

Perl, E.R. (1972) Mode of action of nociceptors. In: C. Hirsch and Y. Zotterman (Eds.), *Cervical Pain.* Pergamon, Oxford, pp. 157 – 164.

Perl, E.R. (1984) Characterization of nociceptors and their activation of neurons in the superficial dorsal horn: first steps for the sensation of pain. In: L. Kruger and J.C. Liebeskind (Eds.), *Advances in Pain Research and Therapy,* Vol. 6. Raven Press, New York, pp. 23 – 51.

Schweizer, A., Brom, R., Glatt, M. and Bray, M.A. (1984) Leukotrienes reduce nociceptive responses to bradykinin. *Eur. J. Pharmacol.,* 105: 105 – 112.

Szolcsanyi, J. (1987) Selective responsiveness of cutaneous C-fibre polymodal nociceptors to capsaicin, bradykinin and ultraviolet irradiation. *J. Physiol. (London),* 388: 9 – 23.

Vane, J.R. (1971) Inhibition of prostaglandin synthesis as a mechanism of action for aspirin-like drugs. *Nature New Biol.,* 231: 232 – 235.

Wilhelm, D.L. (1973) Chemical mediators. In: B.W. Zweifach, L. Grant and R.T. McCluskey, (Eds.), *The Inflammatory Process,* 2nd edn. Academic Press, New York, pp. 251 – 301.

W. Hamann and A. Iggo (Eds.)
Progress in Brain Research, Vol. 74
© 1988 Elsevier Science Publishers B.V. (Biomedical Division)

Visceral Receptors, Chemoreceptors and Molecular Aspects of Receptor Function: Summary

A.S. Paintal

In this session essentially two main topics were discussed. These were the structure and responses of possible electroreceptors in the platypus bill and the role of putative chemical transmitters in the initiation and modulation of sensory activity at certain sensory receptors such as cutaneous receptors, arterial chemoreceptors and visceral receptors.

Electroreception(?) in the platypus

At the previous symposium in Hong Kong, Andres and Von Düring (1984) described a complex sensory receptor, located in the platypus bill, in association with the large mucous secretory gland. Since then they have studied the ultrastructure of this receptor further on the one hand and Iggo and his collaborators have examined the physiological responses of the receptor on the other. These complementary studies may shed new light on the actual structural mechanism capable of detecting changes in the electrical field in the fluid environment. As a result of this the interesting possibility has emerged that there may exist two kinds of electroreceptive systems: one derived from hair cells and the other as seen in the platypus bill in which myelinated fibres, after penetrating the gland duct region, break up into small filamentous free terminals ensheathed by the epidermal cells. Andres said that in their first material he could not determine whether there was a gap between the terminal membrane and the epidermal cells. However, from the new material provided by Iggo and his coworkers he could conclude that the very same ter-

minal was ensheathed by the epidermal and specialised dermal cells; every myelinated fibre had its terminal in this sort of specialised arrangement. However, from the responses of these receptors there seems to be some doubt regarding the ability of the receptors of the platypus to detect weak electric fields.

Structure and functions of pulmonary viscero-receptors

Von Düring describing her recent work gave a valuable account of the functional anatomy of sensory receptors in the lungs and airways. She pointed out a hitherto little-known remarkable difference in the ratios of medullated to non-medullated vagal afferent fibres in different animals. For example, in cats and dogs the ratio of medullated to non-medullated fibres is 1:9, while in non-human primates (grass monkey and rhesus monkey), the ratio is 1:3, i.e., in the latter group there are relatively more medullated afferent fibres. She suggested that this fact should be kept in view while looking for an animal model that will shed light on pathophysiological conditions in man. Clearly since the endings of medullated fibres are far less sensitive to chemical substances than the endings of non-medullated fibres (see Paintal, p. 161 in this volume) the above information will be of importance in evaluating the effects of chemical substances such as lobeline injected intravenously in man. In this connection another new noteworthy fact provided by her was that it was not uncommon to find medullated nerve fibres terminating at sensory endings located in the alveolar ducts near the pulmonary capillaries. She confirmed that these endings were probably J receptors. Thus it is clear that in non-human primates (and probably man) the J receptors have both medullated and non-medullated fibres.

Hepatic glucose-sensitive afferent fibres

Niijima gave an account of the effects of glucose and certain gastro-intestinal hormones such as insulin, glucagon and cholecystokinin on certain receptors believed to be located in the wall of the portal vein (or its branches). He believed that these receptors sensed (and possibly monitored) the presence of these hormones in the portal venous blood en route to the liver.

A significant point mentioned by him was that it is very difficult to get a single unit preparation. Therefore, one has to depend on window discriminators for sorting out fibres with particular spike heights. Another disturbing feature was that the concentration of insulin needed for producing an effect on discharge rate was much larger than that which existed in the blood.

Role of chemical transmitters

Apart from exceptions (e.g., see papers by Diamond et al. (p. 51) and Paintal (p. 161)) most of the symposiasts seemed to favour the view that sensory transduction at various sensory receptors involved some kind of chemical transmitter that was released from a receptor cell and which acted on the generator membrane to produce a generator current. Such a role of a chemical was explicitly advanced by Fidone who, in the case of carotid chemoreceptors, suggested that the receptor cell (i.e., type I glomus cell) contained several neuroactive substances such as biogenic amines (dopamine, norepinephrine, and acetylcholine) and neuropeptides (e.g., substance P and enkephalins). These putative transmitters or modulators had a role in initiating and/or

modulating the impulses generated at chemoreceptors, although the precise role of each of them had yet to be demonstrated. In any case an essential requirement for the validity of the above view is that the endings of both medullated and non-medullated fibres should respond in quantitatively the same way to specific chemical substances. This was not so in the case of aortic chemoreceptors; those with medullated fibres were far less sensitive to chemical substances than those with non-medullated fibres (see Paintal, p. 161). New evidence presented by Paintal indicated that the contrary evidence relating to the greater sensitivity of chemoreceptors with medullated fibres obtained by Fidone and Sato (1969) probably arose from gross overestimates of conduction velocities of nerve fibres yielded by the so-called monotopic technique for determining conduction velocities of nerve fibres. This evidence was greatly supported by the recent observations, based on the use of a more conventional approach, of Kirkwood, Nisimaru and Sears (1985). These observations, which were presented at the symposium, showed that the conduction velocities of carotid chemoreceptor fibres were almost entirely below 9 m/s. Fidone suggested that these low values could be due to the slowing of the impulses in the fibre near the soma. However, the conduction velocity of the baroreceptor fibres recorded by Kirkwood et al. (1985) using the same method were 19 – 44 m/s, which is precisely what one would expect from the fibre diameter distribution in the nerve. Thus slowing was an unlikely explanation. Paintal therefore concluded that so far the evidence showed that the endings of non-medullated fibres were decidedly far more sensitive to chemical substances than those with medullated fibres and thus the role of chemical transmitters should be considered with reservations (see also paper by Diamond et al., p. 51 in this volume).

However, Fidone's concept of the role of multiple neuroactive substances acting as transmitters or modulators of neural activity was echoed by Hartschuh and Nohr in the case of the Merkel cell system but here the postulated substances were different. They were certain that the transmitter liberated by the Merkel cell was enkephalin. Hartschuh supported the view that the Merkel cells were members of the diffuse neuroendocrine system (DNES). Using immunocytochemical techniques he showed the presence in the Merkel cell of chromogranin, a marker substance for DNES. The precise role of these substances in mechanoreception, endocrine, paracrine and trophic functions remains to be established. This is particularly relevant to the effects of denervation. In this connection an important point emerged during the discussion regarding the effect of denervation on the Merkel cells. The consensus was that after denervation in both hairy and glabrous skin the Merkel cells definitely did not disappear although there was a variable amount of reduction of Merkel cells after denervation. Some of the variability in the conclusions seems to depend on the interpretation by different investigators of the data obtained by them.

The use of immunohistological techniques, while providing a plethora of new data, seems to have raised far more new questions than provided answers to old ones. For example, one did not seem to be any closer to getting an answer to the mechanisms of the axon reflex following the new information provided by Nohr and his co-workers on the possible existence of several immunoreactive substances in spinal ganglia and peripheral nerves. Nohr suggested that in these tissues there was evidence for the co-existence of excitatory transmitters (e.g., substance P) and opioid peptides which inhibit substance P. However, he also pointed out that there was a problem of cross-reactivity which complicated the interpretation of the results. This has to be kept in mind in studies of this sort.

On the other hand, studying the direct effect of candidate transmitters on the responses of sensory receptors (an approach that has been used for about 50 years) still seems to yield less equivocal conclusions. For example, Perl showed clearly that substance P does not modify the responses of the C cutaneous polymodal nociceptors. He also showed that the response of these nociceptors is not dependent on the formation of prostaglandins. It is still uncertain whether the progressively enhanced effect of repeated noxious stimulation is influenced by substances that inhibit the synthesis of prostaglandin or leukotriene. Bradykinin also seemed to have no definite role in the excitation of C thermal mechanical nociceptors.

In conclusion one got the impression from the proceedings of this and other sessions of the symposium that although some sensory physiologists have been eagerly looking for neurotransmitters or modulators at sensory receptors, they seem to have had little or no luck so far!

Mechanoreceptors and Structural Aspects of Receptor Function

W. Hamann and A. Iggo (Eds.)
Progress in Brain Research, Vol. 74
© 1988 Elsevier Science Publishers B.V. (Biomedical Division)

CHAPTER 23

The cortical lattice: a highly ordered system of subsurface filaments in guinea pig cochlear outer hair cells

L.H. Bannister[1], H.C. Dodson[1], A.R. Astbury[1] and E.E. Douek[2]

[1]*Department of Anatomy, Guy's Campus, United Medical and Dental Schools of Guy's and St. Thomas's Hospitals, London SE1 9RT, UK, and* [2]*E.N.T. Department, Guy's Hospital, London SE1 9RT, UK*

Summary

In the outer hair cells of the guinea pig the subsurface cisternae have been shown previously to be attached to the plasma membrane by rows of tubular pillar-like links. We report that pillars are attached to each other by an ordered lattice of fine (2 – 3 nm thick) interlacing filaments, and that each pillar also possesses a single filament running up its centre. Deeper layers of cisternae are interconnected randomly by thin (3 nm) filaments. The pillars and filament lattice resist disruption by various ototraumatic agents. It is suggested that the subsurface filament – pillar complex stabilises the cell surface during auditory stimulation, and also contains elastic or actively motile components which are involved in acoustically driven changes in cell shape.

Introduction

Tangential sections of outer hair cells (OHCs) show that regular rows of dense particles lie immediately beneath the plasmalemma (see Saito, 1983). Flock et al. (1986) recently studied these and demonstrate that they are links between the plasma membrane and the outermost layer of the membrane-lined sacs, the subsurface cisternae (SSCs) which form a series of layers of smooth endoplasmic reticulum in the cell cortex. They interpreted these connections as tubular structures ('pillars'), and drew attention to their similarity to links between the sarcoplasmic reticulum and transverse tubules in striated muscle (see also Discussion).

In the present paper we have examined the detailed structure of these cortical attachments, and their reactions to cell injury. We show that the SSCs and the plasma membrane are interconnected by a complex three-dimensional network of filaments and pillars which may play a crucial role in maintaining the integrity of the cell during auditory activity.

Materials and methods

Guinea pigs (albinos and pigmented) were used in this study. They were killed by barbiturate overdose, then decapitated and their cochleas exposed. Pieces of cochlear bone were removed to expose the spiral organ, and tissues were fixed by perilymphatic perfusion in 2.5% glutaraldehyde in 0.1 M phosphate buffer of 0.1 M cacodylate buffer (both pH 7.3). In some cases, 1% tannic acid and 0.1 mg/ml saponin were added to the fixative (final pH 7.0). After postfixation in osmium (1% in an

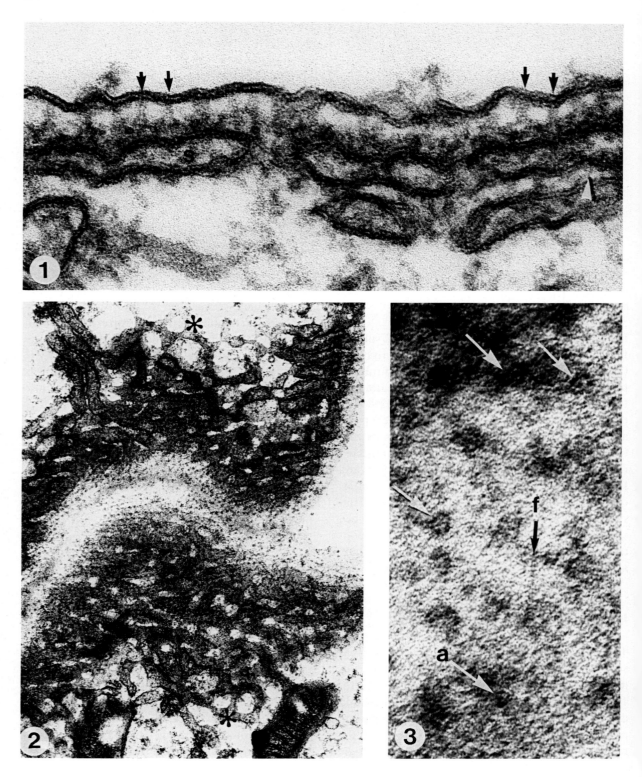

appropriate buffer), some cochleas were stained in 1% aqueous uranyl acetate for 1 h. Specimens were then dehydrated to 70% in an ethanolic series, and half-turns of the spiral organ removed for complete dehydration and embedding in TAAB epoxy resin. Sections were stained with uranyl acetate and lead citrate.

Other (opened) cochleas were treated with 0.3 mg/ml saponin in 0.1 M phosphate buffer (pH 7.3) at room temperature for 10 min before fixation, then fixed in 2.5% glutaraldehyde in phosphate buffer and processed in the same manner as described above.

The structure of the surface regions of OHCs was also examined in electron micrographs from our previously published studies on the effects of ototraumatic agents, including combined gentamicin and sound (Dodson et al., 1982), salicylate (Douek et al., 1983), and electrical stimulation (Dodson et al., 1986). In addition, we examined the effect on the OHC cortex of kanamycin sulphate (a course of 10 days, 400 mg/kg/day, administered intraparenterally, followed by 0 – 6 weeks' survival before microscopic examination).

Results

In guinea pigs, the SSCs are arranged in parallel layers. The stratum closest to the cell surface (Figs. 1, 2), though variable in form, consists mainly of domains of parallel, flattened, anastomotic tubes, each about 40 nm from side to side, running in a predominantly transverse direction around the cell's circumference (see also von Lubitz, 1981), although varying up to 45° from this orientation. In the deeper SSCs, the fenestrations are much wider and the cisternae have no preferred direction.

As described by Flock et al. (1986), pillar-like structures, arranged in parallel rows, link the outer surface of the most superficial SSCs and the plasma membrane (Figs. 1 – 3). The rows, spaced at 27 – 40 nm intervals, are most frequently attached along the edges of the tubular SSCs (see Fig. 3). Pillars are variable in spacing within a row, with a range of 27 – 38 nm.

Sections cut perpendicular to the cell surface (Fig. 1) show a fairly constant gap of about 50 nm between the plasma membrane and the first layer of cisternae. This intermembranous space is divisible into a superficial, electron-lucent zone about 30 nm wide, crossed only by the pillars, and a deeper, denser 20 nm zone overlying the SSC membrane. In tangential sections this deeper zone is seen to include many fine filaments connecting the bases of the pillars in a fairly regular crossed lattice (Figs. 3 – 6), and some amorphous or finely granular material between them. Each filament is 2 – 3 nm thick, and up to 45 nm long. The filamentous links are seen more clearly in saponin-treated cells, where the cytoplasm stains less densely (Fig. 6). In favourable sections, each pillar is seen to radiate up to six filaments; two of these form links to adjacent pillars in its own row, and the other four pass diagonally to pillars of the two neighbouring rows (Fig. 6). The filaments appear to emerge laterally

Fig. 1. Section through the plasma membrane and the first layer of subsurface cisternae (S), showing the complex appearance of the intervening space. Visible are a deep denser zone overlying the cisternae, and the pillar-like attachments crossing the more electron-lucent superficial zone. Examples of pillars are indicated by arrows. × 250 000.

Fig. 2. Oblique tangential section through the surfaces of two adjacent OHCs showing rows of pillars overlying anastomotic, mainly tubular superficial SSCs to which the pillars are attached. Deeper layers of SSCs with larger fenestrations are also visible (asterisks). × 45 000.

Fig. 3. Highly magnified view of a group of pillars, sectioned as in Fig. 2. Note the individual circular cross sections with dense cores in the centres of some examples (white arrows), and faint indications of lattice filaments between (e.g., f). The plane of section is at a shallow angle to the cell surface, and passes through the deeper, dense zone in which the bases of pillars are embedded (at the top of the picture), and through the plasma membrane (at the bottom), where the narrowed tip of a pillar is visible (a). × 500 000.

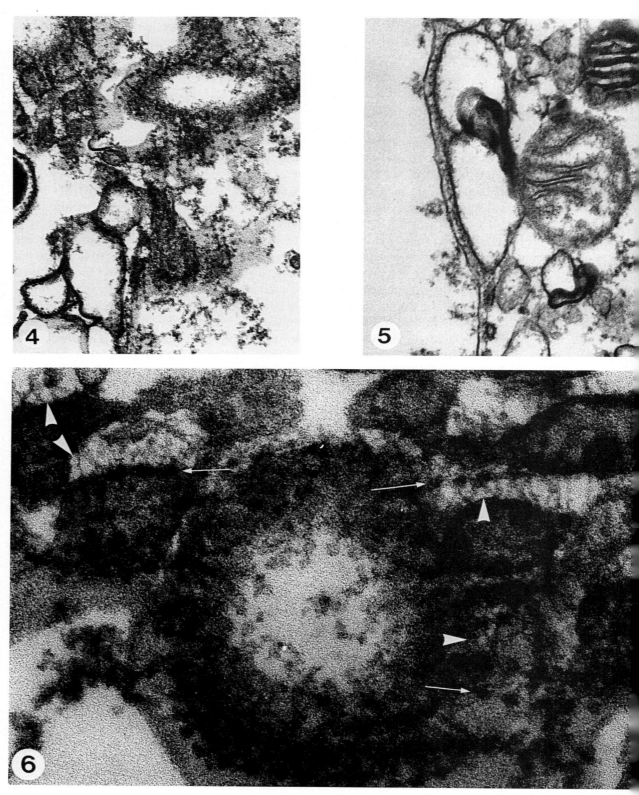

from the pillars near their bases. A diagrammatic three-dimensional schema illustrating this interpretation is shown in Fig. 7.

The pillars themselves are also quite complex in structure, and require further analysis to clarify their detailed form. However, in tangential sections through the OHC surface they are circular in cross section, indicating a tubular organisation, as described by Flock et al. (1986). In tangential sections cut slightly obliquely to the plane of the cell surface, the pillars are sliced through at different levels, providing indications of their cross sectional form at different heights (Fig. 3). The pillars are about 12 nm in diameter for most of their height, tapering at their tips to about 8 nm or less where they contact the plasma membrane. Coatings of dense amorphous material increase the wall thickness of their bases. A dense core, about 2 nm across (Fig. 3), occurs in the centre of most cross sections, interpreted here as a single filament which passes through the centre of the pillar from its base to apex. At the tip of the pillar, small filamentous attachments to the plasma membrane are also often visible.

Close inspection of SSCs shows that the deeper cisternal layers are interconnected by relatively infrequent filaments each 2 – 3 nm thick, arranged apparently at random, spanning distances of 12 – 50 nm. Similar connections also occur between the cisternae of Hensen bodies. All cisternae (both the SSCs and those of Hensen's bodies) contain granular, or occasionally filamentous, material, the granules being about 8 nm in diameter.

All major types of damage that we investigated (see Materials and methods) caused distension of the SSCs and sometimes their lateral fusion (see, e.g., Fig. 5), as well as gross distortions in cell shape and often lysis. However, the first layer of SSCs always remained closely attached at a distance of 50 nm to the plasma membrane by regular rows of pillars, even when the cell lysed.

Discussion

Our structural analysis of the plasma membrane connections generally confirms the findings by Flock et al. (1986), and adds further data: the rows of pillars are found to be interconnected by an elaborate, ordered lattice of filaments, and the pillars themselves appear to have a central axial filament. The connection of the first SSC layer to the plasmalemma is mechanically and metabolically very stable, being unaffected by various injurious agents which otherwise cause major alterations in cell structure, and remaining unchanged when the cell and its cisternae are greatly distorted or lysed.

The highly organised arrangement of cisternae and connecting structures is not shared by inner hair cells (Flock et al., 1986), and is likely to be adaptations to the special circumstances under which OHCs operate. Except at their bases and apices, the OHCs are unsupported, and their walls must withstand considerable tensional and shearing forces during acoustic stimulation. The complex three-dimensional network of cortical fila-

---

Fig. 4. Tangential section through the surface of a saponin-lysed OHC showing several rows of dense particles overlying disrupted SSCs. × 59 000.

Fig. 5. Cross section of the surface region of a saponin-treated OHC. Although considerable swelling and fusion of the SSCs has occurred, the attachment zone with the plasma membrane remains relatively unaltered. × 60 000.

Fig. 6. High power view of the surface of a saponin-treated OHC in tangential section, printed densely to reveal details of the surface lattice. In the central region, a swollen, blister-like SSC has been cut through; around its margins are several rows of pillars seen end-on as densely staining particles (e.g., arrows). A number of areas between the rows show lattices of fine filaments, some of them apparently forming a criss-cross pattern (e.g., arrowheads). The large, dark elliptical masses are slightly swollen portions of superficial SSCs. × 180 000.

ments and pillars would appear to be well suited to strengthen the cell surface, and, in combination with the system of cisternae, to provide additional rigidity to the cortical region.

It must also be borne in mind that OHCs can contract and extend actively (see, e.g., Brownell, 1985; also Ashmore, in this volume), causing significant changes in cell length and diameter. As the diagonal lattice of filaments between adjacent rows is apparently continuous along the sides of the OHC, any change in cell dimensions must be associated with length change in some or all of the lattice components. Certainly the distances between pillars vary considerably, as do the angles at which their filamentous cross links intersect (see, e.g., Fig. 6). Such a system would need to be either elastic or actively motile, or both. An elastic lattice, besides adjusting to the fluctuating geometry of the cell, might also enable it to resonate in response to an oscillating mechanical (or electrochemical) signal. Alternatively (or additionally), such a system could be an active force

generator; the filaments are too narrow (3 nm) for actin (diameter 6 nm), so that some novel contractile – extensile system would presumably be involved.

However, actin has been demonstrated immunochemically by Flock et al. (1986) in the OHC cortex, so it is possible that filaments of this protein are present in some clandestine form, perhaps buried in the dense material between the bases of the pillars, or as short inconspicuous lengths.

Flock et al. (1986; see also this volume) have suggested that the pillars might couple the plasmalemma and the SSCs electrochemically during acoustic stimulation, as also proposed for the tubular links ('feet') between the sarcoplasmic reticulum and transverse tubules of striated muscle (see, e.g., Somlyo, 1979; Franzini-Armstrong, 1980; Eisenberg and Eisenberg, 1982). This suggestion has many attractions in view of the broad similarities in substructure. There are, however, variations of detailed form: the pillars in the OHCs are considerably longer (50 nm) than the triadic

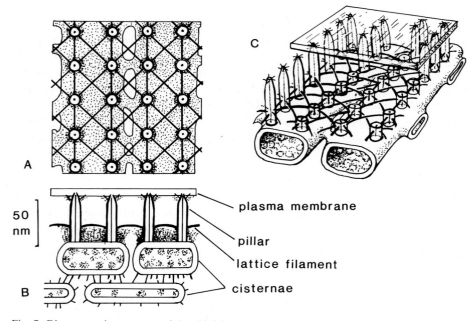

Fig. 7. Diagrammatic summary of the chief findings of this paper, picturing different views of the OHC surface structures. In A the outer layer of cisternae (stippled), attached pillars and lattice filaments are shown in plan view, and B is a cross section. In C a three-dimensional interpretation is presented (in part, cut away to show links).

'feet' (18 nm) of muscle, and are variable in their proximity to each other; they also contain a central filament. Whether or not these are significant differences remains to be seen.

Acknowledgements

This work was supported in part by the Medical Research Council of the UK. The authors also wish to thank Dr. Å. Flock for helpful discussion.

References

Dodson, H.C., Bannister, L.H. and Douek, E.E. (1982) The effects of combined gentamicin and white noise on the spiral organ of young guinea pigs. A structural study. *Acta Otolaryngol. (Stockholm)*, 94: 193 – 202.

Dodson, H.C., Walliker, J., Douek, E.E., Fourcin, A.F. and Bannister, L.H. (1986) Structural alteration of hair cells in the contralateral ear resulting from extracochlear electrical stimulation. *Nature (London)*, 320: 65 – 67.

Douek, E.E., Dodson, H.C. and Bannister, L.H. (1983) The effects of sodium salicylate on the cochlea of guinea pigs. *J. Laryngol. Otol.*, 93: 793 – 799.

Eisenberg, B.R. and Eisenberg, R.S. (1982) The T – SR junction in contracting single skeletal muscle fibres. *J. Gen. Physiol.*, 79: 1 – 19.

Flock, Å., Flock, B. and Ulfendahl, M. (1986) Mechanisms of movement in outer hair cells and a possible structural basis. *Arch. Otorhinolaryngol.*, 243: 83 – 90.

Franzini-Armstrong, C. (1980) Structure of sarcoplasmic reticulum. *Fed. Proc.*, 39: 2403 – 2409.

Saito, K. (1983) Fine structure of the sensory epithelium of guinea-pig organ of Corti: subsurface cisternae and lamellar bodies in the outer hair cells. *Cell Tissue Res.*, 229: 467 – 481.

Somlyo, A.V. (1979) Bridging structures spanning the junctional gap at the triad of skeletal muscle. *J. Cell Biol.*, 80: 743 – 750.

van Lubitz, D. K. J. E. (1981) Subsurface tubular system in the outer sensory cells of the rat cochlea. *Cell Tissue Res.*, 220: 787 – 795.

W. Hamann and A. Iggo (Eds.)
Progress in Brain Research, Vol. 74
© 1988 Elsevier Science Publishers B.V. (Biomedical Division)

CHAPTER 24

Ruffini corpuscle – a stretch receptor in the connective tissue of the skin and locomotion apparatus

Zdenek Halata

Anatomisches Institut der Universität in Hamburg, Abteilung für Funktionelle Anatomie, Martinistrasse 52, D-2000 Hamburg 20, FRG

Summary

This study deals with light and electron microscopical findings of Ruffini corpuscles in hairy and glabrous skin of various mammals and marsupials as well as Ruffini corpuscles in joint capsules of various birds, mammals and marsupials.

In glabrous skin (nasal skin, glans penis, prepuce) Ruffini corpuscles are located in the reticular layer of the dermis. In hairy skin they are located in the reticular layer of the dermis between hair follicles and in the connective tissue capsule of all guard hairs and some vellus hairs as the so-called pilo-Ruffini complex, and also in primate sinus hairs. In joint capsules Ruffini corpuscles are located within the fibrous layer and within the ligaments of the capsule. A Ruffini corpuscle is composed of a myelinated axon with its endings and terminal glial cells. The presence of a capsule depends on the structure of the surrounding tissue. The axon (diameter $4-6$ μm) shows ramifications and thickened nerve endings. They are incompletely ensheathed by terminal Schwann cells. Finger-like protrusions are anchored in the connective tissue belonging to the fibrous layer of the joint capsule or the reticular layer of the dermis. Terminal Schwann cells also cover the nerve terminals and send their slender long protrusions between the bundles of collagenous fibres.

Ruffini corpuscles are classified as typical stretch receptors of the Golgi tendon organ type. Their structure is modified by the connective tissue: in connective tissue with parallel collagenous fibrils they are built like Golgi tendon organs, whereas in loose connective tissue they appear like branched complex free nerve endings. All components of the Ruffini corpuscles can adjust themselves to the surroundings. Changes in the connective tissue evoke modifications in shape of the Ruffini corpuscle. Along with such changes the size of the receptive field may vary however, but the specific function of the Ruffini corpuscle as slowly adapting stretch receptor remains preserved.

Introduction

Our study will concentrate on typical stretch nerve endings of connective tissues, the Ruffini corpuscles (Ruffini, 1893). They are classified as slowly adapting type 2 receptors which respond to stretch in the connective tissue (McCloskey, 1978). Their physiological and electron microscopical features were described in hairy skin of cat (Chambers et al., 1972) and monkey (Biemesderfer et al., 1978). In human skin they were described physiologically by Vallbo et al. (1979) and later electron microscopically by Halata and Munger (1981a,b). In joint capsules Ruffini corpuscles are

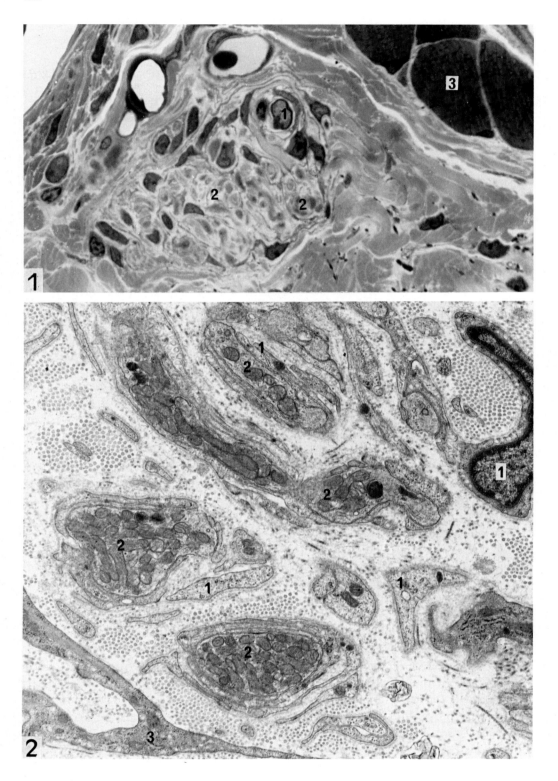

also found with a similar function (Grigg and Hoffman, 1982, 1984).

Materials and methods

The light and electron microscopical studies are based on the following material: hairy and non-hairy areas and sinus hairs from nasal skin of various marsupials (kowari, possum, American opossum, bandicoot) and mammals (rat, cat, mini-pig, monkey), eyelid of monkey and man, scalp of man, skin of the glans and prepuce of the penis of goat and man, joint capsules of various birds (pigeon, duck), marsupials (kowari, monodelphis, possum), mammals (rat, cat, dog, mini-pig, monkey) and man.

Semi-thin sections were taken parallel and perpendicular to the surface of the skin and the joint capsule. Selected material with Ruffini corpuscles was preserved in complete series of alternating semi-thin and ultrathin sections.

Results and discussion

Ruffini corpuscles in non-hairy skin were obtained from pig-nose, prepuce and glans of human penis and glans of goat penis. In pig nose (Figs. 1 and 2) the corpuscles are found in the reticular layer of the deep dermis, usually near the insertion of mimic muscles. They are present with a cylinder-shaped perineural capsule. Both ends of the cylinder are open — whether flat or pointed — and bundles of collagenous fibres form the surrounding tissue entering it on both sides. Inside the capsule nerve terminals are anchored between the collagenous fibres. The afferent axon is myelinated and measures about 5 μm in diameter. Usually each Ruffini corpuscle is supplied by one myelinated axon, but this axon may divide into two inside the cylinder before losing its myelin sheath and forming nerve terminals.

In the glans and the prepuce of human penis (Halata and Munger, 1986) Ruffini corpuscles are found in the deep dermis, in glans of goat penis within dense connective tissue of the tunica albuginea. Corpuscles obtained from human penis were present in two different varieties — those with a perineural capsule and those with a fibroblast capsule. A monolayered perineural capsule belongs to corpuscles in the reticular layer of the deep dermis and near smooth muscle cells. A fibroblast capsule (Fig. 3) often belongs to corpuscles in the dermis of the outer layer of the prepuce (Halata, 1984). Three-dimensional reconstructions of corpuscles in the prepuce have demonstrated that they are usually innervated by one 'parent' axon which before or inside the corpuscle may branch repeatedly into several myelinated axons. Inside the corpuscle the axons measured about 4 μm in diameter.

In the glans and corpus penis of the goat (Fig. 4) Ruffini corpuscles were found along the border between dense connective tissue and the reticular layer of the dermis. They consist of several cylinders formed by perineural cells and arranged parallel to each other and to the long axis of the collagenous fibre bundles. Each cylinder is supplied by one myelinated axon of 5 μm diameter.

Ruffini corpuscles in hairy skin were first described with their physiological and electron microscopical features in the skin of cat (Chambers et al., 1972), later they were observed in human scalp (Halata and Munger, 1981a). Their structure closely resembles that of corpuscles in non-hairy skin and both resemble the Golgi tendon organs (Schoultz and Swett, 1972, 1976) as well as

---

Fig. 1. Light photomicrograph of Ruffini corpuscle from pig snout. One myelinated axon (1) branches in several non-myelinated axons (2). (3) Mimic muscle. × 1000.

Fig. 2. The same Ruffini corpuscle by electron microscopy. (1) Terminal Schwann cell with thin cytoplasmic lamellae. (2) Nerve terminals with mitochondria. (3) Fibroblast. × 14 000.

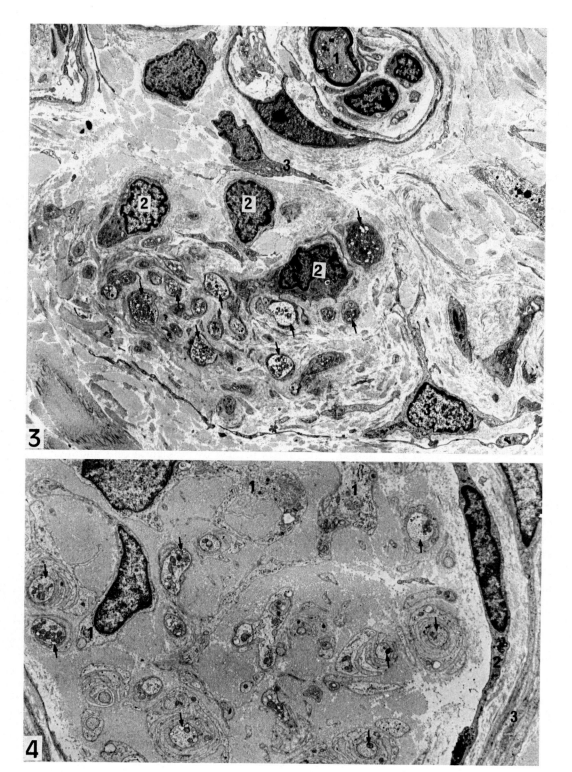

the Ruffini corpuscles in joint capsules. Ruffini corpuscles in hairy skin are supplied by myelinated axons of 4 – 6 μm diameter, their cylinders are orientated with their long axis parallel to the collagenous fibres of the dermis.

The pilo-Ruffini complex (Biemesderfer et al., 1978; Munger and Halata, 1984) is typically associated with the connective tissue capsule of certain types of hair (mainly guard hair, but also vellus hair). It lacks a perineural capsule; the afferent myelinated axon is about 4 μm in diameter and takes a spiral course to approach the hair follicle at a level below the sebaceous gland. After losing the myelin sheath the non-myelinated terminals branch several times and spread between the connective tissue capsule of the hair follicle just below the sebaceous gland (Fig. 5). The nerve terminals resemble those of ordinary Ruffini corpuscles. As they run circularly and thus perpendicularly to the long axis of the hair follicle (Fig. 6) they are also referred to as 'circular lanceolate receptor organs' (Andres and von Düring, 1973). Physiological and morphological studies of Biemesderfer et al. (1978) have proved their function to be similar to that of Ruffini corpuscles in the hairy skin of cat (Chambers et al., 1972). The bending of the hair shaft is the appropriate stimulus.

In sinus hair the Ruffini corpuscles have so far only been found in monkey (Halata and Munger, 1980c). They are flattened, measure approximately 50 μm in diameter and 15 – 20 μm in thickness and are located in the connective tissue capsule of the sinus hair at the level of the entry of the nerve fascicle into blood sinus. A total of 8 – 12 Ruffini corpuscles innervate the sinus hairs in monkey. The afferent axon is myelinated and measures 3 μm in diameter.

Ruffini corpuscles within joint capsules (Figs. 7, 8) were described light microscopically in detail by Polacek (1966) as 'spray-like endings'. The results of electron microscopical studies on joint capsules in mammals (rabbit: Goglia and Sklenska, 1969; cat: Halata, 1977; monkey: Halata et al., 1984; man: Halata et al., 1985), marsupials (Strasmann et al., 1987) and birds (Halata and Munger, 1980b) have simplified the classification. In general there are three types of Ruffini corpuscles: (1) corpuscles without capsule, (2) corpuscles with connective tissue capsule containing perineural derivatives and (3) corpuscles of the Golgi tendon organ type.

All three different types occur within the fibrous layer. Corpuscles of the Golgi tendon organ type are found in those parts of the capsule that are reinforced by ligaments or at least show an arrangement of collagenous fibres similar to ligaments or tendons. The other two types, i.e., corpuscles with and without a connective tissue capsule, are found either on the surface or deep inside the fibrous layer.

Blood vessels are commonly found in the neigbourhood of Ruffini corpuscles. In pilo-Ruffini complexes (Biemesderfer et al., 1978) they usually take a spiral course around the complex thus separating it from the connective tissue of the reticular layer. In the encapsulated Ruffini corpuscles of the pig nose, capillaries can be found

Fig. 3. Electron micrograph of a Ruffini corpuscle from a human prepuce. The afferent axon is myelinated (1). (2) Terminal Schwann cells. (Arrows) Nerve terminals. (3) Fibroblast. × 2400.

Fig. 4. Electron micrograph of a Ruffini corpuscle from a penis of a goat. The corpuscle is encapsulated by perineural cells (3). Between bundles of collagenous fibres there are nerve terminals (arrows). (1) Terminal Schwann cells. (2) Fibroblast. × 4800.

Fig. 5. A pilo-Ruffini complex from hairy skin from the upper lip of kowari. (1) Sebaceous gland. (2) Epithelium of the hair follicle. (3) Myelinated afferent axons. (4) Terminal Schwann cells of the pilo-Ruffini complex. (Arrows) Nerve terminals. × 3000.

Fig. 6. Higher magnification from Fig. 7. Small delicate cytoplasmic processes of a terminal Schwann cell (1) can be seen. In some places the nerve terminals are covered only by a basal lamina (arrows). × 5500.

226

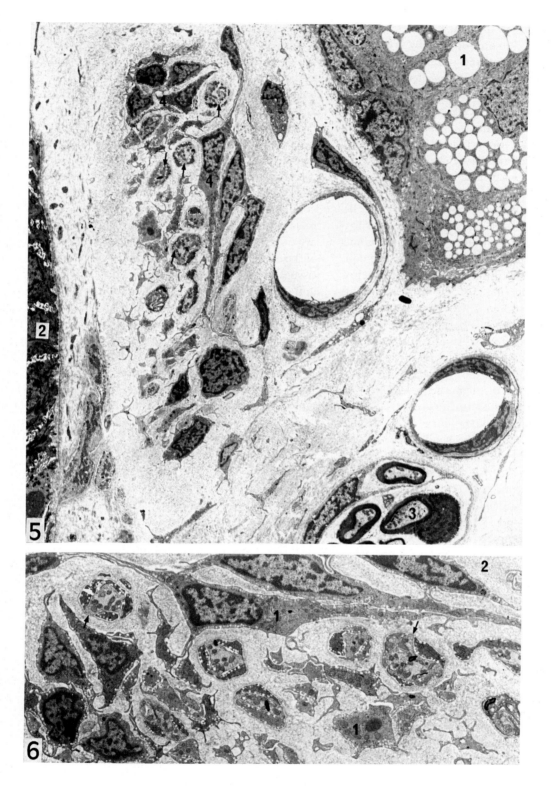

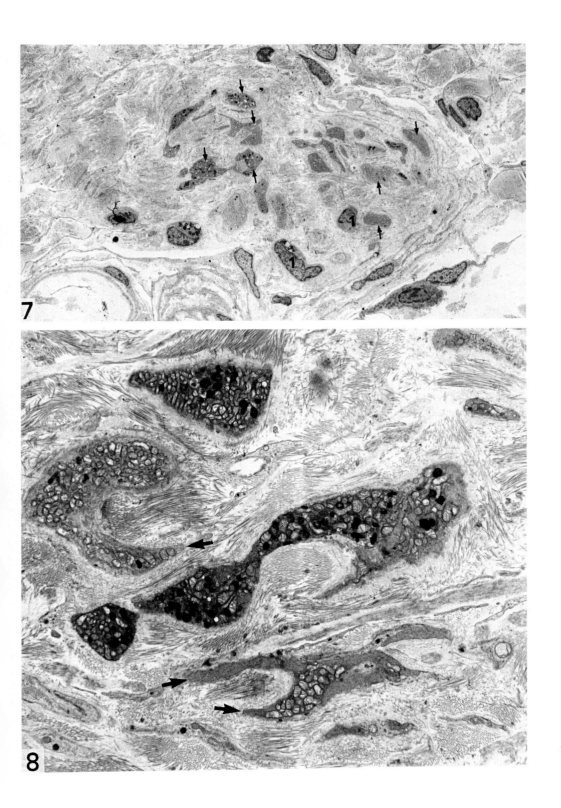

228

between the individual cylinders (Halata et al., 1986) and they are similarly located in the encapsulated corpuscles of joint capsules (Halata et al., 1985). This picture implies a buffer-like function of the capillaries between the cylinders.

Ruffini corpuscles are typical stretch receptors. They are ubiquitous in the musculoskeletal system and the connective tissue of the skin. The nerve terminals always adjust themselves to the structure of the surrounding tissue. Larger accumulations of nerve terminals are often surrounded by a capsule consisting of either fibroblasts or perineural cells. Such a capsule is principally absent in corpuscles associated with hairs (Halata and Munger, 1980a) and in periodontium of teeth (Itoh et al., 1981; Linden, 1984; Byers, 1985). All Ruffini corpuscles belong to the slowly adapting stretch receptors (Chambers et al., 1972; Biemensderfer et al., 1978; McCloskey, 1978; Vallbo et al., 1979). The capsule obviously serves a merely mechanical function; thus absence does not alter the function of the corpuscle, it only decreases the area working as a receptive field for the individual corpuscle. One can presume that structural change in the connective tissue (injuries, malposition of joints, scars, degenerative processes, aging) also leads to change in the Ruffini corpuscles in the sense that they adjust themselves to the new surroundings.

Acknowledgements

The author wishes to thank Prof. Dr. Karl Heinz Höhne and Martin Riemer (IMDM) for the computer facilities to evaluate serial sections, Mrs. T. Coellen and Mrs B. Knutz for their valuable technical assistance and Mrs Dr. med. T. Rettig for translation. Supported in part by the Deutsche Forschungsgemeinschaft (Ha 1194/2-1) and by the Verein zur Förderung der Erforschung und Bekämpfung rheumatischer Erkrankungen e.V. in Bad Bramstedt).

References

Andres, K.H. and von Düring, M. (1973) Morphology of cutaneous receptors. In: H. Autrum, R. Jung, W.R. Loewenstein and D.M. MacKay (Eds.), *Handbook of Sensory Physiology*. Springer, Berlin, pp. 3 – 28.

Biemesderfer, D., Munger, B.L., Binck, J. and Dubner, R. (1978) The pilo-Ruffini complex: a non-sinus hair and associated slowly-adapting mechanoreceptor in primate facial skin. *Brain Res.,* 142: 197 – 222.

Byers, M.R. (1985) Sensory innervation of periodontal ligament of rat molars consists of unencapsulated Ruffini-like mechanoreceptors and free nerve endings. *J. Comp. Neurol.,* 231: 500 – 518.

Chambers, M.R., Andres, K.H., von Düring, M. and Iggo, A. (1972) The structure and function of the slowly adapting type II mechanoreceptor in hairy skin. *Quart. J. Exp. Physiol.,* 57: 417 – 445.

Goglia, G. and Sklenska, A. (1969) Ricerche ultrastrutturali sopra i corpuscoli di Ruffini delle capsule articolari nel coniglio. *Quad. Anat. Prat.,* 25: 14 – 27.

Grigg, P. and Hoffman, A.H. (1982) Properties of Ruffini afferents revealed by stress analysis of isolated sections of knee capsule. *J. Neurophysiol.,* 47: 41 – 54.

Grigg, P. and Hoffman, A.H. (1984) Ruffini mechanoreceptors in isolated joint capsule: response correlated with strain energy density. *Somatosens. Res.,* 2: 149 – 162.

Halata, Z. (1977) The ultrastructure of the sensory nerve endings in the articular capsule of the knee joint of the domestic cat (Ruffini corpuscles and Pacinian corpuscles). *J. Anat.,* 124: 717 – 729.

Halata, Z. (1984) The sensory innervation of the skin of the glans penis in man. (An ultrastructural study). In: W. Hamann and A. Iggo (Eds.), *Sensory Receptor Mechanisms.* World Scientific Publ. Co., Singapore, pp. 67 – 79.

Halata, Z. and Munger, B.L. (1980a) The sensory innervation of primate eyelid. *Anat. Rec.,* 198: 657 – 670.

Halata, Z. and Munger, B.L. (1980b) The ultrastructure of the Ruffini and Herbst corpuscles in the articular capsule of domestic pigeon. *Anat. Rec.,* 198: 681 – 692.

Fig. 7. Electron micrograph of a Ruffini corpuscle from a human knee joint capsule. (1) Terminal Schwann cells. (Arrows) Nerve terminals. × 1400.

Fig. 8. Electron micrograph of a Ruffini corpuscle from a human knee joint capsule. The nerve terminals are incompletely surrounded by terminal Schwann cell lamellae. In some places finger-like protrusions (arrows) have contact with the connective tissue of a corpuscle. × 6400.

Halata, Z. and Munger, B.L. (1980c) Sensory nerve endings in rhesus monkey sinus hairs. *J. Comp. Neurol.*, 192: 645 – 663.

Halata, Z. and Munger, B.L. (1981) Identification of the Ruffini corpuscle in human hairy skin. *Cell Tiss. Res.*, 219: 437 – 440.

Halata, Z. and Munger, B.L. (1986) The neuroanatomical basis for the protopathic sensibility of the human glans penis. *Brain Res.*, 371: 205 – 230.

Halata, Z., Badalamente, M.A., Dee, R. and Propper, M. (1984) Ultrastructure of sensory nerve endings in monkey *(Macaca fascicularis)* knee joint capsule. *J. Orthoped. Res.*, 2: 169 – 176.

Halata, Z., Rettig, T. and Schulze, W. (1985) The ultrastructure of sensory nerve endings in the human knee joint capsule. *Anat. Embryol.*, 172: 265 – 275.

Halata, Z., Schulze, W. and Höhne, K.H. (1986) The ultrastructure and computer-aided three-dimensional aspect of Ruffini corpuscles in human skin of the prepuce and pig skin of the nose. *Anat. Rec.*, 214: 48A.

Itoh, K., Wakita, M. and Kobayashi, S. (1981) Innervation of the periodontium in the monkey. *Arch. Histol. Jap.*, 44: 453 – 466.

Linden, R.W.A. (1984) Periodontal mechanoreceptors. In: W. Hamann and A. Iggo (Eds.), *Sensory Receptor Mechanisms.* World Scientific Publ. Co., Singapore, pp. 179 – 191.

McCloskey, D.I. (1978) Kinesthetic sensibility. *Physiol. Rev.*, 58: 763 – 820.

Munger, B.L. and Halata, Z. (1983) The sensory innervation of the primate facial skin. I. Hairy skin. *Brain Res. Rev.*, 5: 45 – 80.

Munger, B.L. and Halata, Z. (1984) The sensorineural apparatus of the human eyelid. *Am. J. Anat.*, 170: 181 – 204.

Polacek, P. (1966) Receptors of the joints. Their structure, variability and classification. *Acta Fac. Med. Univ. Brunensis*, 23: 1 – 107.

Ruffini, A. (1893) Sur un nouvel organe nerveux terminal et sur la présence des corpuscules Golgi-Mazzoni dans le conjonctif sous-cutané de la pulpe des doigts de l'homme. *Mem. Accad. Lincei*, 249 – 265.

Schoultz, T.W. and Swett, J.E. (1972) Ultrastructural organisation of the sensory fibres innervating the Golgi tendon organ. *J. Neurocytol.*, 1: 1 – 26.

Schoultz, T.W. and Swett, J.E. (1976) Ultrastructural organisation of the sensory fibres innervating the Golgi tendon organ. *Anat. Rec.*, 179: 147 – 162.

Strasmann, T., Halata, Z. and Loo, S.K. (1987) Topography and ultrastructure of sensory nerve endings in the joint capsules of the Kowari *(Dasyuroides byrnei)*, an Australian marsupial. *Anat. Embryol.*, 176: 1 – 12.

Vallbo, A.B., Hagbarth, K.-E., Torebjörk, H.E. and Wallin, B.G. (1979) Somatosensory, proprioceptive, and sympathetic activity in human peripheral nerves. *Physiol. Rev.*, 59: 919 – 957.

W. Hamann and A. Iggo (Eds.)
Progress in Brain Research, Vol. 74
© 1988 Elsevier Science Publishers B.V. (Biomedical Division)

CHAPTER 25

The site and distribution of mechanoreceptors in the periodontal ligament of the cat represented in the mesencephalic nucleus and their possible regeneration following tooth extraction

R.W.A. Linden and B.J.J Scott

Department of Physiology, King's College London, Strand, London WC2R 2LS, UK

Summary

In the first part of the work reported here, receptors represented in the mesencephalic nucleus that respond to a force applied to the mandibular canine tooth of the cat have been located in the periodontal ligament. They were situated in the intermediate area of the ligament between the fulcrum and the apex of the tooth. The receptors appeared to be unevenly distributed around the tooth root. The area of predominant distribution extended from the labial to the mesial aspect of the ligament. In the second part, the fate of these neurones following tooth loss has been investigated. The fibre endings appeared to be situated within the bone itself in the area where the teeth were previously present and did not respond to mechanical stimulation of any oral tissues. In one experiment a unit was found which had reinnervated the skin of the lip. The circumstances under which neurones may reinnervate new sites following tooth loss have yet to be established.

Introduction

When a force is applied to a tooth, receptors in the periodontium are stimulated. The receptors may be situated in any of the tissues that comprise the periodontium, i.e., gingiva, cementum, periodontal ligament and the alveolus (British Standard, 1983), and have been loosely described as 'periodontal mechanoreceptors'. It has been shown by electrophysiological studies in the cat that the cell bodies of these receptors are situated in two anatomically distinct sites: the trigeminal ganglion and the mesencephalic nucleus of the fifth cranial nerve (for review see Linden, 1988).

In 1982 Cash and Linden developed a technique to locate receptors in the periodontal ligament of the mandibular canine tooth of the cat, while recording from functionally single units dissected from the inferior alveolar nerve. In this study the bone overlying the canine tooth root was pared away until a tissue-thin layer was left covering the labial aspect of the periodontal ligament. Receptors in the periodontal ligament could be located using pinpoint mechanical and electrical stimulation. It was found that approximately one quarter of the receptors that responded to mechanical stimulation of the tooth were situated in the labial aspect of the ligament. Since the labial aspect represented approximately one quarter of the total surface area of the ligament, it was suggested that the receptors were distributed evenly around the root of the tooth. However, the central representations of the receptors located in this study were not known. The aim of the first part of the preliminary work reported here was to determine whether receptors represented in the mesencephalic nucleus that respond when a force is applied to the tooth, are situated in the periodontal ligament itself and if so, whether they are distributed evenly around the root of the tooth.

Following loss of the teeth, Heasman (1984) found there was a reduction of approximately 20% of the number of myelinated fibres in the inferior alveolar nerve of human subjects. This is not a very large decrease and suggests that following tooth loss many of the afferent fibres that supplied the teeth and periodontal ligaments are still present within the inferior alveolar nerve. If this is true, it is possible that they may reinnervate new anatomical sites following tooth loss. The mesencephalic nucleus contains the cell bodies of three groups of neurones: (1) periodontal mechanoreceptors, (2) type P mechanoreceptors which respond to mechanical stimulation of any of the maxillary teeth and may be situated in the palatomaxillary suture, and (3) jaw elevator muscle spindles (see Linden, 1988). Within the inferior alveolar nerve, the only neurones present with cell bodies in the mesencephalic nucleus are those of periodontal mechanoreceptors. This situation gives us an opportunity to investigate the fate of these neurones following tooth loss. The aim of the second part of the preliminary work reported here is to determine if following tooth loss, periodontal mechanoreceptor neurones represented in the mesencephalic nucleus are still present in the inferior alveolar nerve, and if so whether they are able to reinnervate new anatomical sites.

Methods

The site and distribution of periodontal mechanoreceptors

In this part of the study anaesthesia was induced in eight adult cats weighing 2.0 – 3.8 kg with ketamine hydrochloride (22 mg/kg). The right femoral vein was cannulated and a loading dose of α-chloralose (50 mg/kg) was given. Thereafter the cats were kept on a continuous infusion of 5 – 20 mg/h of α-chloralose intravenously to maintain anaesthesia. The right femoral artery was cannulated and the blood pressure monitored. A tracheostomy was performed and the animals were artificially ventilated with moistened 40% oxygen in air using a modified Ideal Starling pump. End tidal carbon dioxide was maintained at 3.5 – 4.5%. The body temperature was maintained at 37 ± 0.2°C with a thermostatically controlled electric blanket using feedback from a rectal thermistor probe. Throughout all of the experiments the blood pressure was above 10 kPa.

The external surface of the left side of the mandible was exposed and two small holes about 3 mm apart were made in the bone below the second premolar tooth. Silver wire stimulating ball electrodes of diameter 0.2 mm were placed in contact with the inferior alveolar nerve and were fixed to the adjacent bone of the mandible with dental acrylic (Howmedica Simplex International Ltd). The skin was then closed over.

The head was positioned in a stereotaxic frame using infraorbital bars to fix the cat in a standard stereotaxic position. A bar was cemented with dental acrylic to two screws inserted into the superior wall of the frontal sinus.

A 15-mm square-sided piece of bone was removed from the cranium and the dura reflected back to expose the cerebral cortex on the left side, ipsilateral to the stimulating electrodes. This was covered with agar. In some experiments, the left cerebral cortex was aspirated to expose the superior colliculus just rostral to the bony tentorium. Glass insulated, gold and platinum black-coated tungsten microelectrodes (tip length 10 – 20 μm, impedance 50 kΩ to 1 MΩ at 1 kHz (Merrill and Ainsworth, 1972)) were directed caudally at a 30° angle to the vertical into the mesencephalic nucleus. The whole of the accessible region of the mesencephalic nucleus on the left side of the cat was explored (A4 – P4, 2.3 mm lateral to the midline (Berman, 1968)), while giving square wave pulses (5 V, 0.1 ms duration, 1 Hz) to the inferior alveolar nerve using a constant voltage stimulator (Digitimer). Output from the recording electrodes was amplified through an AC preamplifier and amplifier (Neurolog), and recorded on FM tape. The data were displayed on oscilloscope screens and by a high-speed signal store (Grafitek UK), on a BBC microcomputer.

The skin, mucous membrane and gingivae in the region of the left mandibular canine tooth root were removed and the mental nerves sectioned. The bone overlying the labial aspect of the canine tooth root was pared away under a constant stream of isotonic saline using a large round dental store, until a tissue-paper-thin transparent layer of bone was left covering the periodontal ligament. The receptor sites could be determined by punctate mechanical stimulation, using a hand-held piece of tungsten wire (diameter 127 μm, exerting a force of approximately 40 − 50 mN). Electrical stimulation of the located receptors was carried out with a concentric bipolar stimulating electrode (1 mm diameter) and a constant current stimulator (Neurolog, duration 0.5 − 1 ms). The above technique and determination of the fulcrum of the tooth have been fully described by Cash and Linden (1982).

The effect of tooth extraction

In this series of experiments, four adult cats were anaesthetised with ketamine hydrochloride (22 mg/kg) and the left maxillary and mandibular incisor and canine teeth were extracted. Antibiotics were administered and the animals were allowed to recover.

Terminal experiments were performed at least 6 months after the extractions. The animals were anaesthetised, ventilated and body temperature monitored as in the first series of experiments. Stimulating electrodes were placed in contact with the inferior alveolar nerve on the left side. After positioning the animal in a stereotaxic frame the mesencephalic nucleus was explored. When a unit was found in the inferior alveolar nerve,

mechanical stimulation of the remaining teeth, the edentulous ridge, the oral mucous membrane and the skin of the face was carried out using a glass rod and tungsten wire (diameter 127 μm). Electrical stimulation of these sites was also performed using bipolar stimulating electrodes approximately 2 − 3 mm apart and a constant current stimulator.

At the end of these experiments the mandible was dissected out and radiographs were taken to determine whether any fragments of the extracted teeth were present in the bone of the mandible.

Results

The site and distribution of periodontal mechano-receptors

If identical action potentials were recorded when a force was applied to the tooth and also when the same small area of the periodontal ligament was mechanically and electrically stimulated through the thin layer of bone, it was then possible to identify an area of approximately 1 mm^2 below which a receptor was assumed to be located. In eight cats studied so far, a total of 27 units were found in the mesencephalic nucleus that responded to mechanical stimulation of the mandibular canine tooth. Of these, 11 receptors were situated within the labial aspect of the periodontal ligament where they could be located and their position defined. The receptors were situated in the intermediate area of the periodontal ligament between the fulcrum and the apex of the tooth. No receptors were found in the area close to the fulcrum or close to the apex of the tooth. The site of the receptors in the ligament is shown in Fig. 1.

The located receptors were found to have intermediate adaptation properties. When a force was applied to the crown of the tooth, none of the located receptors were either very slowly adapting or very rapidly adapting. No spontaneously active units were found.

When a force was applied to the tooth, all receptors showed a maximum sensitivity when the force was applied in a certain direction. The direction of

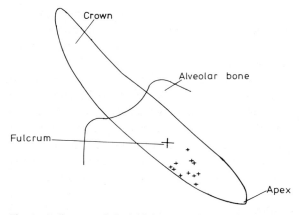

Fig. 1. A diagram of the labial aspect of the periodontal ligament of the left mandibular canine tooth demonstrating the site
of 11 located mechanoreceptors represented in the mesencephalic nucleus of eight cats.

maximum sensitivity for the 11 located receptors
was when a force was applied to the lingual or
disto-lingual surfaces of the crown of the tooth.
The directional sensitivities of the 11 located receptors and the remaining 16 units which were
unlocated indicated that the majority of the units
responded maximally when a force was applied to
the crown of the tooth in the region extending
from the lingual to the distal surface.

The effect of tooth extraction

In four cats studied so far where the teeth have
been extracted, nine units have been found in the
mesencephalic nucleus which responded to electrical stimulation of the inferior alveolar nerve.
These units did not respond to mechanical stimulation of any of the ipsilateral or contralateral mandibular teeth. Of these nine units, eight did not respond to mechanical stimulation of the edentulous
ridge, the adjacent mucous membrane or the skin
of the lip. They could, however, be electrically
stimulated by passing a constant current across the
edentulous ridge. High currents were required
which suggested that the units may have been present in the bone itself. In seven of the units studied
the position of the bipolar electrodes indicated that

they were being stimulated in the area where the
canine tooth was previously present and in one unit
where one of the incisor teeth was previously present.

In one experiment, a unit was found which had
regenerated to the skin of the lower lip. It was
located just on the hairy skin of the lip adjacent to
the edentulous ridge area where the canine tooth
had been previously present. It appeared to be
associated with a vibrissa. The unit had a very low
mechanical threshold; it could be stimulated with
a very fine hair and was not directionally sensitive.

Radiographs of the mandible demonstrated no
evidence of the presence of tooth fragments in the
extraction sockets. No clear outlines of the sockets
of the extracted canine teeth were visible but it appeared that the bone had not yet completely filled
the space.

Discussion

*The site and distribution of periodontal mechano-
receptors*

In this part of the study it has been shown that
receptors represented in the mesencephalic nucleus
that respond when a force is applied to the mandibular canine tooth are situated in the periodontal
ligament itself. They lie in the intermediate area
between the fulcrum and the apex of the tooth. In
peripheral studies where recordings have been
made from functionally single units dissected from
the inferior alveolar nerve, the receptors have been
shown to be distributed in the whole area of the
ligament between the fulcrum and the apex of the
tooth (Cash and Linden, 1982; Linden, 1983,
1984). It appears, however, that receptors represented in the mesencephalic nucleus are not
distributed evenly in the area between the fulcrum
and the apex of the tooth.

The located receptors in the present study were
found to have intermediate adaptation properties.
No very slowly adapting or very rapidly adapting
units were found. Jerge (1963) reported the
absence in the mesencephalic nucleus of any very

slowly adapting mechanoreceptor neurones. Linden (1978) found no periodontal mechanoreceptor units in the mesencephalic nucleus that fired for longer than 10 s to a prolonged 1-N force applied to the canine tooth. The adaptation properties of the units located in the present study are also in agreement with those found in peripheral studies of the properties of receptors related to their position in the periodontal ligament (Linden, 1983, 1984; Linden and Millar, 1985).

The mechanoreceptors located in the present study all responded maximally when the crown of the tooth was pushed in a direction which placed the area of ligament below the fulcrum into tension. This is in agreement with the findings of Cash and Linden (1982). The directional sensitivities of the located receptors and those which could not be located indicate that the majority of receptors (74%) represented in the mesencephalic nucleus respond maximally when a force is applied to the crown of the tooth in the region extending from the lingual to the distal surface. Since the tooth tilts around its fulcrum when a force is applied to the crown, this suggests that the majority of the receptors in the ligament represented in the mesencephalic nucleus are distributed in the region extending from the labial to the mesial surface of the tooth root. These data were further reinforced by a retrospective examination of data collected but not reported in a study by Linden (1978), in which 157 units were recorded in the mesencephalic nucleus that responded to mechanical stimulation of the mandibular canine tooth. The majority of these units (79%) also responded maximally when a force was applied to the crown of the tooth in the region extending from the lingual to the distal surface. The results of the present study and the retrospective data from the previous study suggest that the receptors in the periodontal ligament which are represented in the mesencephalic nucleus are unequally distributed around the tooth. The functional implications of this require further study. In a recent paper published while the present work was in progress, Byers et al. (1986) injected tritiated proline into the mesencephalic nucleus of the cat and looked for labelled structures in the periodontal ligament. Labelled structures were found in the periodontal ligament in the area close to the root apex and mainly on the posterior side of the tooth which as far as can be understood is on the opposite side to where the receptors were located electrophysiologically in the present study. There is no obvious explanation at present for the different findings of these two studies.

Following recordings from single fibres dissected from the inferior alveolar nerve, Cash and Linden (1982) suggested that mechanoreceptors in the periodontal ligament were distributed evenly around the root of the canine tooth. The present study has shown that those represented in the mesencephalic nucleus are unequally distributed. The site and distribution of those receptors represented in the trigeminal ganglion are currently being investigated.

The effect of tooth extraction

Before a study on the effect of tooth extraction on periodontal mechanoreceptors represented in the mesencephalic nucleus could be performed, it was necessary to determine the site of the receptors in the periodontium when the teeth were present. The results from the first part of the present study confirmed that the receptors were located in the periodontal ligament itself. After loss of the teeth, the periodontal ligament is no longer present. If following tooth extraction, a neurone represented in the mesencephalic nucleus was found to be present in the inferior alveolar nerve, provided it did not respond to mechanical stimulation of the remaining teeth, it must have previously innervated the periodontal ligament of one of the extracted teeth.

In the preliminary work so far carried out in which teeth have been extracted, it is apparent that mechanoreceptor fibres which previously had innervated the periodontal ligaments are still present in the inferior alveolar nerve. For the units so far studied it appears that they do not generally reinnervate new anatomical sites. The terminal parts of the fibres appear to be situated in the bone of the mandible itself in the area where the teeth were previously present. Whether these fibres have receptive endings has not been established in this study.

In the one case where a receptor did regenerate it was present on the hairy skin of the lip and appeared to be excited by mechanical stimulation of a vibrissa. In previous electrophysiological studies in which recordings have been made in the mesencephalic nucleus, no receptor has ever been found in the lip (Jerge, 1963; Linden, 1978; Passatore and Filippi, 1983; Passatore et al., 1983). It is possible that in extracting the canine tooth, a small adjacent bundle of lip neurones, not previously represented in the mesencephalic nucleus, were damaged, and a periodontal ligament mechanoreceptor fibre (which would have also been damaged by tooth extraction) was able to enter a new endoneurial tube and regenerate to a new target tissue in the lip.

In conclusion, mechanoreceptors in the periodontal ligament represented in the mesencephalic nucleus are situated in the intermediate area of the ligament between the fulcrum and the apex of the tooth, but are unequally distributed around the tooth root. The area of predominant distribution extends from the labial to the mesial aspect of the ligament. Following tooth loss it appears that mechanoreceptor fibres which previously innervated the periodontal ligament are still present in the bone of the mandible and that the majority do not reinnervate new anatomical sites. Work is currently in progress to determine under what circumstances they may reinnervate new target tissues.

Acknowledgement

This work was supported by a grant from the Medical Research Council of Great Britain.

References

Berman, A.L. (1968) *The Brain Stem of the Cat; A Cytoarchitectonic Atlas with Stereotaxic Coordinates.* University of Wisconsin, Madison, WI.

British Standard Glossary of Dental Terms (1983) *BS 4492, 4-111 Periodontium.* British Standards Institution, London.

Byers, M.R., O'Connor, T.A., Martin, R.F. and Dong, W.K. (1986) Mesencephalic trigeminal sensory neurones of cat: axon pathways and structure of mechanoreceptive endings in periodontal ligament. *J. Comp. Neurol.,* 250: 181 – 191.

Cash, R.M. and Linden, R.W.A. (1982) The distribution of mechanoreceptors in the periodontal ligament of the mandibular canine tooth of the cat. *J. Physiol. (London),* 330: 439 – 447.

Heasman, P.A. (1984) The myelinated fibre content of human inferior alveolar nerves from dentate and edentulous subjects. *J. Dent.,* 12: 283 – 286.

Jerge, C.R. (1963) Organization and function of the trigeminal mesencephalic nucleus. *J. Neurophysiol.,* 26: 379 – 392.

Linden, R.W.A. (1978) Properties of intraoral mechanoreceptors represented in the mesencephalic nucleus of the fifth nerve in the cat. *J. Physiol. (London),* 279: 395 – 408.

Linden, R.W.A. (1983) The relationship between adaptation rate and location of periodontal mechanoreceptors in the cat canine tooth. *J. Physiol. (London),* 345: 20P.

Linden, R.W.A. (1984) Periodontal mechanoreceptors. In: W. Hamann and A. Iggo (Eds.), *Sensory Receptor Mechanisms.* World Scientific Publ. Co., Singapore, pp. 179 – 191.

Linden, R.W.A. (1988) Periodontal receptors and their functions. In: A. Taylor (Ed.), *Neurophysiology of the Jaws.* Macmillan, London, in press.

Linden, R.W.A. and Millar, B.J. (1985) Recent studies on the response characteristics of periodontal mechanoreceptors. In: S.J.W. Lisney and B. Matthews (Eds.), *Current Topics in Oral Biology.* University of Bristol Press, Bristol, pp. 97 – 109.

Merrill, E.G. and Ainsworth, A. (1972) Glass coated platinum plated tungsten microelectrodes. *Med. Biol. Eng.,* 10: 662 – 672.

Passatore, M. and Filippi, G.M. (1983) Sympathetic modulation of periodontal mechanoreceptors. *Arch. Ital. Biol.,* 121: 55 – 65.

Passatore, M., Lucchi, M.L., Filippi, G.M., Manni, E. and Bortolami, R. (1983) Localization of neurons innervating masticatory muscle spindle and periodontal receptors in the mesencephalic trigeminal nucleus and their reflex actions. *Arch. Ital. Biol.,* 121: 117 – 130.

W. Hamann and A. Iggo (Eds.)
Progress in Brain Research, Vol. 74
© 1988 Elsevier Science Publishers B.V. (Biomedical Division)

CHAPTER 26

Functional characteristics of afferent C fibres from tooth pulp and periodontal ligament

E. Jyväsjärvi[1], K.-D. Kniffki[2] and M.K.C. Mengel[2]

[1]*Department of Physiology of the University of Helsinki, Siltavuorenpenger 20 J, SF-00170 Helsinki, Finland, and*
[2]*Physiologisches Institut der Universität Würzburg, Röntgenring 9, D-8700 Würzburg, FRG*

Introduction

Electron microscopic studies have shown that the tooth pulp and the periodontal ligament are innervated by both A-δ and C fibres (cf. Byers, 1984, 1985). The majority of the fibres are C fibres (Johnsen and Karlsson, 1974; Beasley and Holland, 1978; Reader and Foreman, 1981). Some of the pulpal C fibres are postganglionic sympathetic efferent fibres (Pohto, 1972; Arwill et al., 1973; Fehér et al., 1977), and some of the unmyelinated axon profiles may in fact be terminal parts of myelinated A fibres (cf. Byers, 1984). The proportion of afferent C fibres in the dental pulp and the periodontal ligament is unknown.

Electrophysiological recordings from intradental A-δ fibres in animals have demonstrated responses to stimuli applied to the exposed dentine surface which, when applied to human dentine, are capable of evoking a sharp pain sensation (Närhi et al., 1982). Recordings from pulpal C fibres are rare (Wagers and Smith, 1960; Bessou et al., 1970; Anderson and Pearl, 1975; Matthews, 1977; Cadden et al., 1983) and it has been difficult to identify them according to their conduction velocity by stimulating the tooth. Närhi et al. (1982) showed that slowly conducting pulpal nerve fibres in the cat were sensitive to heat stimulation of the tooth crown suggesting an afferent role for them. Jyväsjärvi and Kniffki (in preparation) were able to show by direct stimulation of the nerve trunk that such heat-sensitive slowly conducting nerve fibres in the cat were C fibres and that the same fibres were also excitable by noxious mechanical stimulation of the pulp tissue.

This study was undertaken to obtain more information about the functional properties of afferent C fibres in the dental pulp. In addition, it was aimed at obtaining electrophysiological evidence of periodontal afferent C fibre innervation, which up to now has only been demonstrated morphologically (Byers, 1985).

Methods

The experiments were performed on 92 adult cats (weight: 1.9 – 6.0 kg) with fully developed, intact permanent teeth. The animals were initially anaesthetised with 40 mg/kg i.p. sodium pentobarbital. The right femoral vein was cannulated for subsequent injections of the same anaesthetic and the femoral artery for blood pressure recording. A tracheotomy was performed to allow undisturbed spontaneous ventilation. Body core temperature and mean arterial blood pressure were kept within physiological limits.

The lower margin of the mandible of the left side was exposed and removed between the anterior mental and mandibular foramina to allow access to the inferior alveolar nerve. The nerve was

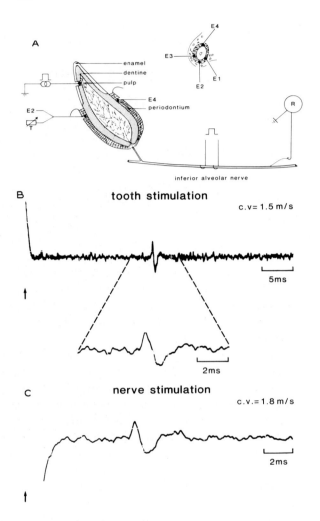

Fig. 1. (A) Schematic drawing showing the experimental set-up for recording functional single fibres in fine filaments split from the cut end of the inferior alveolar nerve. R represents the recording and filter devices. T indicates the measurement of the temperature using a thermistor. Pulpal C fibres were identified by monopolar electrical stimulation of the crown of the tooth and periodontal C fibres were identified by bipolar stimulation of the periodontal tissue using two of the four stimulating electrodes E1 – E4 implanted. In addition, in some experiments the axonal conduction velocity was determined by bipolar stimulation of the nerve trunk with a constant-current stimulator. (B) Example of the identification of a C fibre by electrical stimulation of the crown of the tooth. The conduction velocity (c.v.) was calculated from the conduction distance between the stimulating and recording electrodes and from the shortest latency of the response to a suprathreshold stimulus pulse. In the lower trace of B, the upper sweep is displayed with a faster

carefully dissected free from the connective tissue and cut as far proximally as possible. The cats were then placed on their backs in a recording frame, the jawbones were fixed using a metal bar across the palate. A pool was formed out of the skin flaps and filled with warm paraffin oil subsequently kept above 32°C.

Small holes were cut through the enamel near the tip of the left lower canine tooth and, after removing gingival tissues, also into its periodontal space to insert wire electrodes (diameter: 0.4 mm) for electrical stimulation of the tooth and the periodontal ligament (Fig. 1A). An indifferent electrode was attached to the lower lip. In 20 experiments a pair of platinum hook electrodes were carefully placed distally under the nerve trunk (Fig. 1A) for electrical stimulation of the axons. If, identified by the shape of the action potentials, the unit under investigation was activated by both tooth and nerve stimulation, in most cases occlusion of the electrically evoked action potentials by those evoked by heat or cold stimuli applied to the tooth crown or to the periodontal ligament (see below) was demonstrated. In experiments where thermal stimuli were applied to the tooth or its periodontal ligament a thermistor probe was inserted to measure the temperature of the tooth and the ligament (Fig. 1A).

Fine filaments were then split from the cut end of the nerve and placed on a platinum recording electrode. The neuronal activity of the fibres was amplified, filtered (band pass: 100 Hz – 4 kHz), audiomonitored, displayed on an oscilloscope screen and stored on a magnetic tape.

Functional single fibres originating from the tooth pulp or the periodontal ligament were iden-

sweep velocity to show the form of the extracellularly recorded action potential. The arrow indicates the onset of the cathodic stimulus pulse. (C) Response of the same C fibre as shown in B, to an electrical stimulus pulse applied to the nerve trunk; same time scale as in the lower trace of B. The calculated conduction velocity by using nerve stimulation was greater than by using tooth stimulation; the arrow indicates the onset of the stimulus pulse.

tified by recording single all-or-none action potentials in response to cathodal square-wave constant-current pulses (amplitudes: 0 – 200 μA; duration: 1 – 20 ms) applied monopolarly or bipolarly to the electrodes. Responding fibres were classified according to their conduction velocity calculated from the conduction distance and the shortest response latency to a suprathreshold stimulus: A-δ fibres if their conduction velocity was between 2.6 and 30 m/s, C fibres if the conduction velocity was up to 2.5 m/s. For some fibres with conduction velocities in the C fibre range, the axonal conduction velocity was determined in addition by stimulating the nerve trunk.

After intradental and periodontal fibres had been identified, their responsiveness to stimulation of the tooth and the ligament was tested. Forces of variable intensity and direction were applied manually to the crown of the tooth (see Fig. 4). For thermal stimulation of the tooth crown radiant heat and volatile cold spray were used, and contact heat and cold were applied locally to the periodontal ligament. In some experiments, after thermal stimulation a hole was carefully drilled through enamel and dentine to the pulp chamber and a cannula was fitted and sealed in the hole for pressure application to the pulp. Then the coronal pulp and the periodontal ligament were exposed and mechanically stimulated with a thin probe (dental needle) to determine the receptive fields of the fibres. Finally, saturated KCl solution and/or bradykinin solution (26 μg/ml) was applied on the pulp surface and the exposed periodontal tissue.

Results

Pulpal C fibres

By using electrical current pulses of 1 ms duration applied to the tooth it was possible to excite 175 intradental fibres, which were regarded as C fibres according to their conduction velocity (CV). The distribution (relative frequency) of the conduction velocities of the intradental C fibres is shown in Fig. 2A. The distribution is almost symmetrical;

the mean CV ($\pm$ SD) of the fibres was 1.1 $\pm$ 0.4 m/s ($n = 175$; range 0.4 – 2.5 m/s). The average activation threshold was 96.6 $\pm$ 54.8 μA (range: 32 – 200 μA).

For 25 fibres it was possible to determine in addition the axonal CV by electrical stimulation of the nerve trunk. An example is given in Fig. 1B and 1C. The mean CV for nerve stimulation was 1.7 $\pm$ 0.9 m/s range: 0.6 – 4.0 m/s) whereas the average value for tooth stimulation was 1.4 $\pm$ 0.4 m/s (range: 0.4 – 2.4 m/s). Five of the fibres turned out to be slowly conducting A-δ fibres when classified according to their CV determined by nerve stimulation.

Of the 175 fibres, 74 were tested with radiant heat application to the tooth crown; 65 fibres responded. Fig. 3A shows an example of the heat evoked discharge in C fibres. Typically, a low rate activity started as the temperature reached the threshold, the discharge rate increased with the temperature until the firing pattern changed to

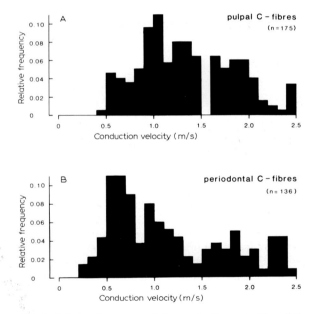

Fig. 2. Relative frequency of the conduction velocities of the recorded 175 intradental C fibres (A) and 136 periodontal C fibres (B). The conduction velocities were calculated from response latencies to electrical stimulation of the tooth or the periodontal tissue.

240

bursts. The evoked activity was present as long as the temperature increased and ceased abruptly as the temperature started to decline. The mean threshold temperature for the first heat stimulus was 41.2 ± 3.7°C ($n = 31$; range: 34.1 – 50.5°C). Repeated heat stimuli with intervals of 10 – 15 min resulted in a gradual elevation of the threshold and a reduction in the response.

Forty-nine of the 56 fibres tested were activated by the application of volatile cold spray to the tooth crown. Thirteen of the 18 fibres tested were also activated by heat stimuli. Fig. 3B shows the regular discharge of a pulpal C fibre starting at an almost static temperature during cold stimulation. The firing was present as long as the temperature gradient remained negative or zero, stopped as the temperature started to increase and did not reappear as the temperature returned to its initial value. The mean temperature threshold was 10.1 ± 3.2°C ($n = 38$; range: 18.4 – 7.2°C). The mean firing rate of the C fibres had a weak linear correlation ($r = 0.6$) with the static tooth temperature

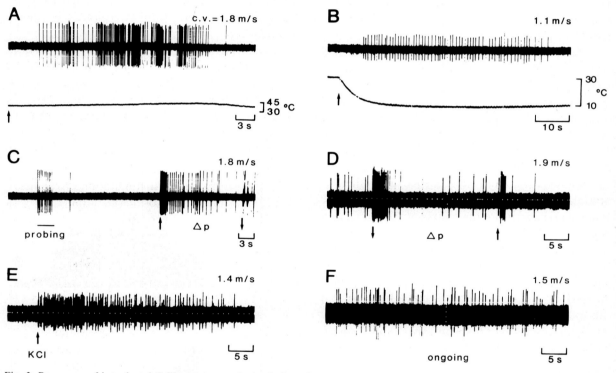

Fig. 3. Responses of intradental C fibres to natural stimulation of the tooth. (A) Response of a C fibre to radiant heat stimulation of the tooth crown. The temperature of the tooth was measured with a thermocouple inserted into a cavity near the pulp in an area isolated from the area of stimulation. The lower trace shows the temperature record. (B) Response of another C fibre to a volatile cold spray application to an isolated stimulation area of the tooth. The temperature recorded near the pulp is shown in the lower trace. (C) The same C fibre as shown in A, responded also to probing with a dental needle of the exposed pulp and to positive pressure application (Δp) to the pulp chamber through a hole drilled to the pulp. (D) Discharge of a pulpal C fibre in response to a negative pressure application (Δp) to the pulp chamber. (E) Firing of a C fibre evoked by topical application of saturated KCl solution on the exposed pulp surface. (F) Ongoing firing of an identified C fibre and an unidentified fibre after thermal stimulation of the tooth and mechanical stimulation of the exposed pulp.

The conduction velocity (c.v.) of the fibres is indicated in the upper right-hand corner of each recording. The duration of probing in C is marked by the solid line under the response. The arrows indicate the onset of stimulation, i.e., pressure application (Δp): arrow upwards in C = positive pressure; arrow downwards in D = negative pressure; second arrow in C and D = offset of stimulation.

achieved. When the end temperature was lower, the mean discharge rate was higher. Repeated applications of the cold stimulus did not alter the response pattern of the fibres.

After thermal stimulation the pulp was exposed (see Methods) in eight experiments and stimulated with positive and negative hydrostatic pressure. Fig. 3C shows a response of a C fibre (same as in Fig. 3A) to probing with a dental needle at the receptive field on the pulp surface under the cut hole for the pressure stimulation cannula (left side of the sweep). A discharge evoked by strong positive pressure application is seen at the right side of the sweep. Eleven fibres of the 21 tested were excited by intense positive (Fig. 3C) or negative (Fig. 3D) pressure stimulation. Of these, five were previously activated by heat, three by cold stimulation and three by both. The response typically was rapidly adapting and the fibres were most sensitive to a change in pressure in the pulp chamber (see Fig. 3D).

The receptive fields of 36 fibres which were sensitive to thermal and/or pressure stimulation were determined by probing of the exposed pulp tissue. The receptive fields were located deep in the pulp, and the fibres required high stimulus intensities to be activated.

After determination of the receptive fields, droplets of saturated KCl solution were applied on the pulp surface in eight experiments. in Fig. 3E a response of a C fibre to KCl application is shown. Nine of the 18 heat, cold and/or pressure sensitive fibres tested responded after a latency, which depended on the distance of the receptive field from the pulp surface, with an initial vigorous discharge, which then decreased and ceased in 0.5 – 2 min. Repeated application resulted in diminishing responses. Three of six fibres also gave a weak response to application of bradykinin (26 μg/ml) to the pulp surface.

In the intact tooth none of the recorded C-fibres had any ongoing activity in the absence of intentional stimulation. However, 25 fibres developed a low rate irregular discharge lasting up to 23 min, especially after repeated heat and mechanical stimuli (example in Fig. 3F).

Periodontal C fibres

One hundred and thirty-six functional single C fibres originating from the periodontal ligament were identified. The distribution of their conduction velocities is shown in Fig. 2B. Compared to the corresponding distribution of the intradental C fibres (Fig. 2A) the distribution of the conduction velocities of the periodontal C fibres is asymmetrical and has its peak at about 0.6 m/s. The mean CV of periodontal C fibres was 1.2 ± 0.6 m/s (range: 0.3 – 2.5 m/s); the mean activation threshold for 200 μA constant-current pulses was 3.0 ± 2.7 ms (range: 1.0 – 20 ms).

Of the 136 C fibres, 127 could not be activated by electrical stimulation of the pulp. The remaining nine fibres were activated by stimulation of the periodontal tissue as well as by stimulation of the pulp. For these nine fibres the conduction velocity determined by pulp stimulation was in the C fibre range.

The axonal conduction velocity was determined for 14 fibres by electrical stimulation of the nerve trunk. The mean CV for nerve stimulation was 1.7 ± 0.8 m/s (range: 0.6 – 3.9 m/s) and for stimulating the periodontal ligament 1.1 ± 0.5 m/s (range: 0.4 – 2.0 m/s). As in the case of pulpal C fibres, some of the fibres ($n = 2$) turned out to be slowly conducting A-δ fibres when classified according to their CV determined by nerve stimulation.

When the periodontal ligament was intact only one of the recorded C fibres showed an ongoing activity without intentional stimulation.

None of the periodontal C fibres could be excited by mechanical stimulation well known to activate periodontal receptors which are associated with large sized myelinated fibres (cf. Cash and Linden, 1982; Karita and Tabata, 1985). For eight out of 12 units tested a response to forces of high intensity manually applied to the crown of the tooth were revealed. As indicated in the middle of Fig. 4 the forces were applied in a horizontal plane in four directions at 90° intervals. The responses were of the slowly adapting type and showed a weak directional sensitivity. This particular unit

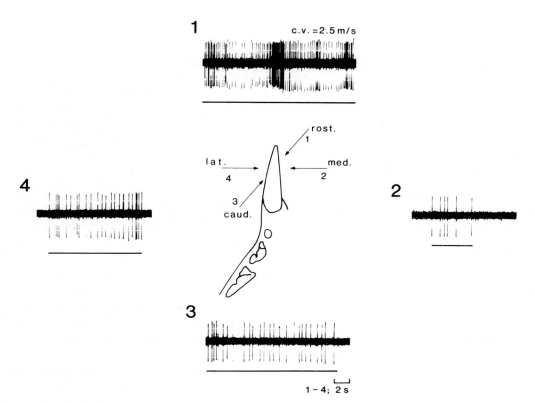

Fig. 4. Responses of a periodontal C fibre (conduction velocity = 2.5 m/s) to sustained manually applied forces of high intensity to the crown of the tooth in a horizontal plane in four directions at 90° intervals. A dorsal view of the lower left canine is indicated. The numbers above the traces indicate the direction of the applied force: 1 = rostrocaudal, 2 = mediolateral, 3 = caudorostral, 4 = lateromedial.

showed the highest mean discharge rate if the force was applied in the rostrocaudal direction (1); the weakest response was evoked when the force was applied in the mediolateral direction (2).

Nine fibres of the 13 tested could be activated by local administration of saturated KCl solution onto the periodontal ligament. The responses were similar to those of pulpal C fibres shown in Fig. 3E, but had a longer latency.

Of the 136 periodontal C fibres, 16 were tested with local contact heat application to the overlying bone of the periodontal tissue; 12 fibres responded to this stimulus. Again the responses were similar to those of pulpal C fibres (e.g., Fig. 3A). Seven of nine fibres tested also responded to local cold application to the bone overlying the periodontal ligament.

In four experiments the periodontal ligament was partially exposed and by probing with a dental needle the receptive field was determined requiring high stimulus intensities. After several trials the fibres showed an ongoing discharge for up to several minutes.

Discussion

The present study provides additional information about the existence of afferent C fibre innervation in the cat's dental pulp and its periodontal ligament, and describes the responses of the C fibres to various stimuli applied to the tooth.

Pulpal C fibres

The existence of afferent C fibres in the dental pulp has been questioned (Matthews, 1977; Cadden et al., 1983) because of the difficulties in determining the conduction velocity according to which the fibres are classified and because of the failure of activating the C fibres by natural stimuli. Indeed, when a tooth is monopolarly electrically stimulated, the actual point of activation remains unknown which results in an uncertainty in the determination of the conduction distance. Furthermore, the conduction velocity of pulpal fibres may increase outside the tooth (Horiuchi, 1965; Lisney, 1978; Jiffry, 1981; Cadden et al., 1982, 1983; Byers, 1984). In the present study the conduction velocity of slowly conducting fibres was additionally determined outside the tooth by using direct bipolar electrical stimulation of the nerve trunk. The results demonstrate that most fibres classified as C fibres by using monopolar tooth stimulation also had their axonal conduction velocity in the C fibre range.

Most of the pulpal C fibres tested were sensitive to radiant heat stimulation of the tooth crown. This is in accordance with the findings of Närhi et al. (1982) and recent studies of Jyväsjärvi and Kniffki (in preparation). The response behaviour and the reduced response to repeated stimulation contradict a thermoreceptive role for the C fibres, the high activation thresholds rather indicate a nociceptive function.

Most of the C fibres recorded in this study were also sensitive to cold stimulation of the tooth. The results are in agreement with those of Jyväsjärvi and Kniffki (1987), but in the present study some fibres were found which were also sensitive to heat stimulation of the tooth. This and the lack of ongoing discharges or dynamic responses to cold stimulation (see Hensel, 1976) does not support the idea that these fibres supply cold receptors, assuming that dental cold receptors would have the same response characteristics as those described for skin and muscle (cf. Jyväsjärvi and Kniffki, 1987).

The observation that after mechanical and pressure stimulation most of the recorded fibres developed an ongoing activity may indicate that this kind of stimulation causes tissue damage to the pulp with a consequent liberation of endogenous pain producing substances (see Olgart, 1979), which sensitises or directly excites the fibre endings.

The findings that a number of C fibres that could be activated by thermal stimuli also responded to direct high intensity probing and pressure stimulation of the pulp tissue, as well as to external application of the pain producing substances KCl and bradykinin, suggest that pulpal C fibres might be polymodal nociceptive fibres. There are, however, some differences to the classical polymodal nociceptors of the skin (Bessou and Perl, 1969). Pulpal C fibres were not sensitised after repeated heat stimulation, but were markedly desensitised. In addition, they responded to cold stimulation. However, if the pulp was additionally injured by probing or pressure stimulation, many C fibres were sensitised and developed an ongoing discharge.

On the basis of these findings, it seems that pulpal C fibres are involved in the mediation of dental pain. It is unlikely, however, that C fibres are responsible for the sharp pain evoked by the manipulation of dentine during treatment (cf. Jyväsjärvi and Kniffki, 1987). The studies of Närhi et al. (1982) suggest that A fibres are involved in dental pain generation due to stimulation of dentine. C fibres, on the other hand, seem to be activated when more intense stimuli affect the pulp. This is of interest since pulp-damaging inflammatory processes often cause a dull aching pain that is poorly localized. In the skin this type of pain is generally associated with the activity of afferent C fibres (see Torebjörk and Hallin, 1974). The often spontaneously occurring pain in pulpal inflammation accompanied by an increase of pressure within the pulp may be explained by the evoked ongoing activity of the C fibres due to damage-induced sensitisation or excitation of C fibres.

Periodontal C fibres

So far electrophysiological studies have not shown the existence of periodontal receptors supplied by afferent C fibres.

The results of the present electrophysiological study demonstrate, in agreement with a recent electron microscopic study (Byers, 1985), the existence of afferent C fibres in the periodontal ligament of teeth.

The classification of the axons recorded from is based on determining the conduction velocity by bipolar electrical stimulation of the periodontal tissue and is supported by the values of the conduction velocities determined by direct stimulation of the nerve trunk. It was observed that the conduction velocities measured by periodontal ligament stimulation were in all but one case lower than those measured by nerve trunk stimulation. This might be due to the slowing of conduction in the terminal parts of the axons. Only two of 14 units were found to be slowly conducting A-δ fibres, which by using stimulation of the periodontal ligament alone would have been classified as C fibres.

As for the periodontal A-δ fibres described by Mei et al. (1977), the periodontal C fibres are insensitive to stimuli which are known to activate periodontal mechanoreceptors supplied by large myelinated fibres (Cash and Linden, 1982; Karita and Tabata, 1985). However, periodontal C fibres were activated by strong mechanical stimuli applied to the ligament. Otherwise their response behaviour was similar to that described for pulpal C fibres.

Based on the current results, periodontal receptors supplied by C fibres can be characterised as polymodal nociceptors involved in nociceptive mechanisms related to the periodontal tissues.

Acknowledgements

The authors express their gratitude to Mrs. Christa Erhard and Mrs. Petra Haumann for competent technical assistance.

The experiments were performed at the Physiologisches Institut der Universität Würzburg with support of the Wilhelm Sander-Stiftung. K.-D. Kniffki was supported by a travel grant from the Deutsche Forschungsgemeinschaft.

References

Anderson, K.V. and Pearl, G.S. (1975) C-fiber activity in feline tooth pulp afferents. *Exp. Neurol.,* 47: 357 – 359.

Arwill, T., Edwall, L., Olgart, L. and Svensson, S.-E. (1973) Ultrastructure of nerves in the dentinal-pulp border zone after sensory and autonomic nerve transection in the cat. *Acta Odont. Scand.,* 31: 273 – 281.

Beasley, W.L. and Holland, G.R. (1978) Quantitative analysis of the innervation of the pulp of the cat's canine tooth. *J. Comp. Neurol.,* 178: 487 – 494.

Bessou, P. and Perl, E. (1969) Response of cutaneous sensory units with unmyelinated fibers to noxious stimuli. *J. Neurophysiol.,* 32: 1025 – 1043.

Bessou, P., Gauthier, J. and Pagès, R. (1970) Mise en évidence de fibres afférentes du groupe C innervant la pulpe de la canine, chez le chat. *C.R. Soc. Biol.,* 164: 1845 – 1850.

Byers, M.R. (1984) Dental sensory receptors, *Int. Rev. Neurobiol.,* 25: 39 – 94.

Byers, M.R. (1985) Sensory innervation of periodontal ligament of rat molars consists of unencapsulated Ruffini-like mechanoreceptors and free nerve endings. *J. Comp. Neurol.,* 231: 500 – 518.

Cadden, S.W., Lisney, S.J.W. and Matthews, B. (1982) A beta-fibre innervation of tooth-pulp in the cat, with a discussion of the functions of nerves supplying tooth-pulp. In: B. Matthews and R.G. Hill (Eds.), *Anatomical, Physiological and Pharmacological Aspects of Trigeminal Pain.* Excerpta Medica, Amsterdam, pp. 41 – 49.

Cadden, S.W., Lisney, S.J.W. and Matthews, B. (1983) Thresholds to electrical stimulation of nerves in cat canine tooth-pulp with A beta-, A delta- and C-fibre conduction velocities. *Brain Res.,* 261: 31 – 41.

Cash, R.M. and Linden, R.W.A. (1982) The distribution of mechanoreceptors in the periodontal ligament of the mandibular canine teeth of the cat. *J. Physiol. (London),* 330: 439 – 447.

Fehér, E., Csanyi, K. and Vajda, J. (1977) Ultrastructure and degeneration analysis of the nerve fibres of the tooth pulp in the cat. *Arch. Oral Biol.,* 22: 699 – 704.

Hensel, H. (1976) Correlations of neural activity and thermal sensation in man. In: Y. Zotterman (Ed.) *Sensory Functions of the Skin in Primates, with Special Reference to Man.* Pergamon Press, Oxford, pp. 331 – 353.

Horiuchi, H. (1965) A study of pulp-nerve excitation through a silver-wire electrode. *J. Dent. Res.,* 44: 1257 – 1263.

Jiffry, M.T.M. (1981) Afferent innervation of the rat incisor pulp. *Exp. Neurol.,* 73: 209 – 218.

Johnsen, D.C. and Karlsson, U.L. (1974) Development of neural elements in apical portions of cat primary and permanent incisor pulps. *Arch. Oral Biol.,* 19: 671 – 678.

Jyväsjärvi, E. and Kniffki, K.-D. (1987) Cold stimulation of teeth: a comparison between the responses of cat intradental Aδ- and C-fibres and human sensation. *J. Physiol. (London),* 391: 193 – 207.

Karita, K. and Tabata, T. (1985) Response fields of the periodontal mechanosensitive units in the superior alveolar nerve of the cat. *Exp. Neurol.,* 90: 558 – 565.

Lisney, S.J.W. (1978) Some anatomical and electrophysiological properties of tooth pulp afferents in the cat. *J. Physiol. (London),* 284: 19 – 36.

Matthews, B. (1977) Responses of intradental nerves to electrical and thermal stimulation of teeth in dogs. *J. Physiol. (London),* 264: 641 – 664.

Matthews, B. (1977) Coupling between nerve terminals in teeth. In: D.J. Anderson and B. Matthews (Eds.), *Pain in the Trigeminal Region.* Elsevier/North-Holland Biomedical Press, Amsterdam, pp. 83 – 93.

Mei, N., Hartmann, F. and Aubert, M. (1977) Periodontal mechanoreceptors involved in pain. In: D.J. Anderson and B. Matthews (Eds.), *Pain in the Trigeminal Region.* Elsevier/North-Holland Biomedical Press, Amsterdam, pp. 103 – 110.

Närhi, M.V.O., Hirvonen, T.J. and Hakumäki, M.O.K. (1982) Activation of intradental nerves in the dog to some stimuli applied to the dentine. *Arch. Oral Biol.,* 27: 1053 – 1058.

Närhi, M., Jyväsjärvi, E., Hirvonen, T. and Huopaniemi, T. (1982) Activation of heat-sensitive nerve fibres in the dental pulp of the cat. *Pain,* 14: 317 – 326.

Olgart, L. (1979) Local mechanisms in dental pain. In: R.F. Beers Jr. and E.G. Bassette (Eds.), *Mechanisms of Pain and Analgesic Compounds.* Raven Press, New York, pp. 285 – 294.

Pohto, P. (1972) Sympathetic adrenergic innervation of permanent teeth in the monkey *(Macaca irus). Acta Odont. Scand.,* 30: 117 – 126.

Reader, A. and Foreman, D.W. (1981) An ultrastructural quantitative investigation of human intradental innervation. *J. Endodont.,* 7: 493 – 499.

Torebjörk, H.E. and Hallin, R.G. (1974) Identification of afferent C units in intact human skin nerves. *Brain Res.,* 67: 387 – 403.

Wagers, P.W. and Smith, C.M. (1960) Responses in dental nerves of dogs to tooth stimulation and the effects of systemically administered procaine, lidocaine and morphine. *J. Pharmacol. Exp. Ther.,* 130: 89 – 105.

W. Hamann and A. Iggo (Eds.)
Progress in Brain Research, Vol. 74
© 1988 Elsevier Science Publishers B.V. (Biomedical Division)

CHAPTER 27

Reinnervation of skin by polymodal nociceptors in rats

Louisa A.M. Bharali and S.J.W. Lisney

Department of Physiology, The Medical School, University Walk, Bristol BS8 1TD, UK

Introduction

Evidence indicates that the largest group of sensory receptors in skin is the polymodal nociceptors, a group of receptors which have unmyelinated axons and which respond to a variety of intense and potentially damaging stimuli. The rat saphenous nerve (a purely cutaneous nerve), for example, contains 5000 or so axons: about 1000 of these are myelinated afferents, about 1000 would be expected to be unmyelinated sympathetic postganglionic efferents, and the remaining 3000 are unmyelinated afferents; of these 3000, 55 – 75% are polymodal nociceptor afferents. Thus of the 4000 sensory axons in the nerve, something like 2000 (50%) are polymodal nociceptor afferents (information from Lynn and Carpenter, 1982; Chad et al., 1983; Fleischer et al., 1983; Lynn, 1984; Peyronnade et al., 1986; Carter and Lisney, 1987).

Their large numbers imply that they are a particularly important group of sensory nerve fibres. Most would accept that impulse traffic in them is usually linked with pain sensations in man and with behaviour indicative of discomfort in animals. Tuckett (1982) has suggested that activation of a subpopulation of polymodal nociceptors may be involved in the feelings of itch and tickle. After peripheral nerve injury and regeneration some people experience disturbances in sensation, including pain and itch, and these could be linked with abnormalities in terms of numbers or properties of these axons and their receptors. At the moment it

is difficult to say how likely this is because very little experimental work has been done on regeneration of unmyelinated axons. The only study in which individual afferents have been investigated is that by Shea and Perl (1985); they compared the properties of normal and regenerated unmyelinated afferents in an isolated rabbit ear preparation. Brenan and Jones (1985) used the technique of antidromic nerve stimulation and plasma extravasation to describe the time course and extent of reinnervation of the rat saphenous nerve field by polymodal nociceptor afferents after nerve crush, and we have used the same method to look at skin reinnervation after nerve transection (Lisney, 1987) and at the effects of age on regeneration.

The technique of antidromic nerve stimulation and plasma extravasation is based on the observation that activation of unmyelinated axons results in an increased vascular permeability in the immediate neighbourhood of the activated axons. A consequence of this is plasma extravasation, and this can be shown up if plasma proteins are labelled with a suitable dye, e.g., Evans' blue. Kenins (1981, 1984) has reported that in normal skin this phenomenon is only associated with activation of polymodal nociceptor afferents and not with activity in other groups of unmyelinated axons. Two possible mechanisms to explain the phenomenon are shown in Fig. 1 and examples of the sorts of results that can be obtained with antidromic nerve stimulation are shown in Fig. 2. In using this technique we have assumed that Kenins'

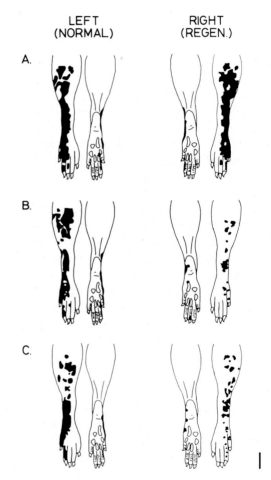

findings for normal skin are correct and, what is more, that they also apply for reinnervated skin. It could be that not all regenerated polymodal nociceptor afferents are capable of bringing about this response, in which case this technique would underestimate the extent of reinnervation. This is a crucial question about the method that needs to be answered one way or the other if we are to con-

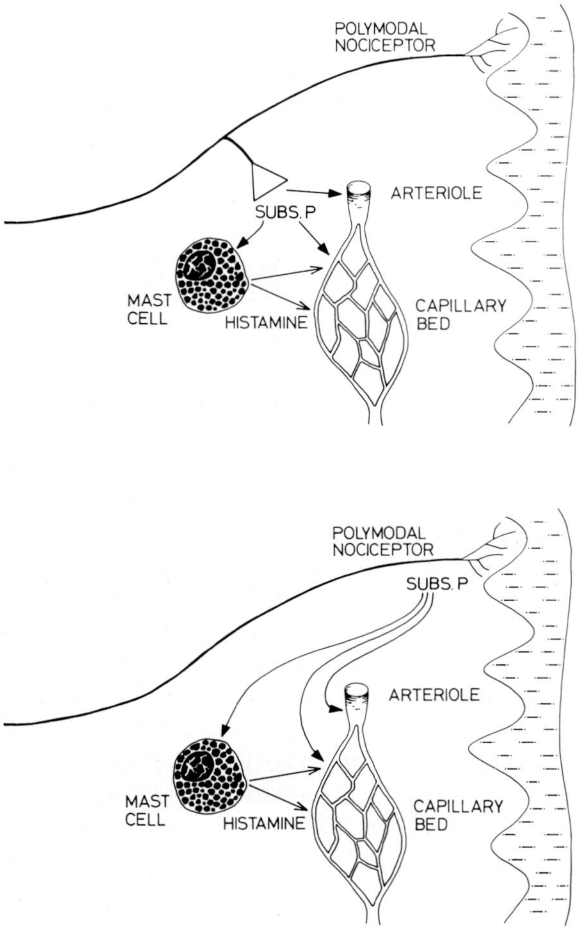

Fig. 1. Diagrams to illustrate possible mechanisms to account for plasma extravasation following activity in polymodal nociceptor afferents. In the scheme shown at the top impulses set up during antidromic nerve stimulation or after activation of the receptor ending are propagated down the branch as well as along the main axon. From here a transmitter substance, possibly substance P, is released which causes arteriolar dilatation and perhaps an increase in capillary permeability as well. In addition, the transmitter substance could act on nearby mast cells to bring about a release of histamine; it is known that histamine causes increased capillary permeability. The combined effects of these vascular changes would be to allow plasma extravasation to take place. The scheme shown at the bottom is similar but instead of the transmitter substance being released from an axon branch it is released from the sensory nerve terminals.

Fig. 2. Examples of the distribution of Evans' blue dye in the skin after antidromic stimulation (12 V, 1.0 ms, 1 i.p.s. for 20 min) of the saphenous nerves in (A) a control rat, (B) a rat in which the right saphenous nerve had been cut 12 weeks before, and (C) a rat in which the nerve had been cut 20 weeks before. The scale bar in the bottom right indicates 10 mm. A full description of these experiments can be found elsewhere (Lisney, 1987).

tinue using it. Here we describe experiments going on at the moment in which we are looking to see if there is the same relationship between antidromic activation of unmyelinated axons and plasma extravasation in reinnervated skin as there is in normal skin.

Methods

The methods used were essentially those described by Kenins (1981). Experiments were carried out on pentobarbital-anaesthetised rats (initially 48 mg/kg i.p., subsequent doses i.v. as required); some of the animals had the right saphenous nerve cut at knee level during a brief operation under pentobarbital anaesthesia about 6 months before. Electrophysiological recordings were made from fine strands dissected from the nerve high in the groin and electrical stimuli (square wave pulses of up to 15 V, 1.0 ms) delivered via more distally placed electrodes to see how many viable axons were present. We selected strands which showed a single all-or-none action potential with a latency to electrical stimulation indicating that it was from an unmyelinated axon. These single units were characterised using the same sort of procedures adopted by others, e.g., stimulation with von Frey hairs, controlled radiant heating where skin temperature was raised by 1°C/s (for details see Kenins, 1981; Lynn and Carpenter, 1982; Fleischer et al., 1983; Shea and Perl, 1985), and the receptive field defined. This testing had to be carried out carefully because the stimuli needed to activate some polymodal nociceptors could be enough to cause plasma extravasation as a consequence of exciting other, neighbouring polymodal nociceptors (Bharali and Lisney, 1987). Once each unit had been classed, Evans' blue solution (50 mg/ml in 0.9% saline) was injected i.v. (50 mg/kg). After a wait of 10 min the leg skin was examined for any signs of plasma extravasation and if there was none the recording strand was stimulated antidromically (for details see Results), the strand being on the anode. After this the skin was re-examined for signs of plasma extravasation and the position of any blue patches that had appeared

were drawn onto a scale figurine of the leg. Between one and four units have been studied in each experiment.

Results

Control animals

The first three polymodal nociceptor afferents we obtained were tested with antidromic stimulation using the parameters given by Kenins (1.0 V, 0.5 ms, 10 i.p.s. for 1 min), but we got no evidence of plasma extravasation in the immediate vicinity of their receptive fields. This could have been because of a difference in our and Kenins' definition of a polymodal nociceptor afferent, or because of some fault with our electrical stimulation procedure. To test the second possibility we took strands in which we knew from orthodromic stimulation that there were several viable unmyelinated axons, and stimulated them antidromically using a variety of stimulation parameters to see what combination of intensity, pulse width, repetition rate, and duration was needed to get plasma extravasation reliably. We found that stimulation at 3.0 V, 1.0 ms, 10 i.p.s. for 3 min brought about plasma extravasation in all the strands tested (6/6) and this regime has been used subsequently.

So far 14 unmyelinated axons have been tested with this modified protocol. Four of them could not be activated from the skin and were assumed to be afferents which had been damaged during the dissection and setting up the pool, or to be sympathetic postganglionic axons. There was no sign of plasma extravasation following antidromic stimulation of any of these units. One of the other axons was from a cooling receptor and there was no sign of plasma extravasation when it was stimulated. The other nine units were classed as polymodal nociceptor afferents, and with five of these we got evidence of plasma extravasation. With two the impulse activity set up by the mechanical stimuli applied when typing the receptor endings was enough to produce extravasation. In both instances discrete blue spots, 1 mm or less in diameter, appeared in the mechanically sensitive areas of skin that made up each receptive field; there were no blue areas in the neighbouring skin. The other three units were characterised without the testing causing plasma extravasation. Antidromic stimulation using the parameters mentioned above produced small areas of extravasation at sites that matched the receptive fields of the units. Thus with these five polymodal nociceptor afferents we have shown a link between impulse activity in their axons and plasma extravasation into small patches of skin corresponding to their receptive fields. We could not show such a link for the other four polymodal nociceptor afferents.

Animals with regenerated nerves

We have tested 16 units from rats with regenerated saphenous nerves. We were unable to find a receptive field for 10 of them and there were no signs of plasma extravasation in the skin when they were stimulated antidromically. These units could have been autonomic efferents, afferents damaged during the experimental preparation, or afferents that had regenerated into the distal stump but which had not gone on to resupply skin. Another of the units was a low-threshold mechanoreceptor afferent and this did not give plasma extravasation on antidromic stimulation either. The remaining five units were identified as polymodal nociceptor afferents. For one of them the impulse activity generated when classifying it was enough to produce plasma extravasation in its receptive field. Three more showed evidence of extravasation following antidromic stimulation and this was within or immediately adjacent to each unit's receptive field. The last afferent did not give signs of extravasation after mechanical and thermal stimulation or after antidromic stimulation.

Discussion

These experiments are still very much in progress and it is too early to draw any firm conclusions. On the basis of what we have seen so far we would agree with Kenins (1981, 1984) to some extent. We seem to be confirming his finding that in normal skin there is no obvious plasma extravasation after activation of unmyelinated axons not associated with polymodal nociceptor endings. It looks as though this is going to be true of reinnervated skin too. We have not been able to confirm that all polymodal nociceptor afferents supplying normal skin bring about changes in the permeability of the adjacent vasculature when activated. We do not believe that this is a failure of our stimulation procedure. It could be because of differences in the criteria used to class unmyelinated afferent receptors. For example, Kenins (1981) tested for responses to heating using hand-held probes at 25, 39 and 50°C whereas others have used more controlled, graded forms of thermal stimulation (Lynn and Carpenter, 1982; Fleischer et al., 1983; Bharali and Lisney, present experiments). According to Kenins' criteria an afferent that responded to 50°C but not to 39°C would have been called a polymodal nociceptor, but one that responded to 50°C and 39°C would not. Lynn and Carpenter (1982) and Fleischer et al. (1983) have described polymodal nociceptor afferents with thresholds to heating below 37°C, so here is a difference in opinion in what to look for in a polymodal nociceptor. Kenins' criteria are such that it seems likely that his sample was biased towards those polymodal nociceptor afferents with the higher thresholds. It is too early to say whether this is the answer to the difference in our results, but if there were two classes of polymodal nociceptors, one that did not produce changes in vascular permeability when activated and perhaps where the receptors had lower thresholds, and a second, higher-threshold group that did cause these changes, then this would explain the difference. On the other hand it could be that threshold has nothing to do with it and that the crucial point is whether or not the polymodal nociceptor being studied contains and/or is capable of releasing the biochemical agent responsible for the vascular changes. A number of substances are associated with unmyelinated afferents but so far none of them has been shown to be in all polymodal nociceptors (for a review see Lynn and Hunt, 1984), so this lends support to this suggestion. Whatever turns out to be the explanation, our findings so far suggest that the technique of antidromic nerve stimulation and plasma extravasation is not a reliable one for demonstrating the total extent of innervation of skin by polymodal nociceptors.

Acknowledgement

This study was supported by the Medical Research Council of the UK.

References

Bharali, L.A.M. and Lisney, S.J.W. (1987) Plasma extravasation after localized skin heating in the rat. *J. Physiol. (London)*, 390: 111P.

Brenan, A. and Jones, L. (1985) Evidence of the regeneration of cutaneous polymodal nociceptor afferents following nerve crush in the rat. *J. Physiol. (London)*, 369: 62P.

Carter, D.A. and Lisney, S.J.W. (1987) The numbers of unmyelinated and myelinated axons in normal and regenerated rat saphenous nerves. *J. Neurol. Sci.*, 80: 163 – 171.

Chad, D., Bradley, W.G., Rasool, C., Good, P., Reichlin, S. and Zivin, J. (1983) Sympathetic postganglionic unmyelinated axons in the rat peripheral nervous system. *Neurology (Cleveland)*, 33: 841 – 847.

Fleischer, E., Handwerker, H.O. and Joukhadar, S. (1983) Unmyelinated nociceptive units in two skin areas of the rat. *Brain Res.*, 267: 81 – 92.

Kenins, P. (1981) Identification of the unmyelinated sensory nerves which evoke plasma extravasation in response to antidromic stimulation. *Neurosci. Lett.*, 25: 137 – 141.

Kenins, P. (1984) Electrophysiological and histological studies on vascular permeability after antidromic sensory nerve stimulation. In: L.A. Chahl, J. Szolcsányi and F. Lembeck (Eds.), *Antidromic Vasodilatation and Neurogenic Inflammation*. Akadémiai Kiadó, Budapest, pp. 175 – 188.

Lisney, S.J.W. (1987) Functional aspects of the regeneration of unmyelinated axons in the rat saphenous nerve. *J. Neurol. Sci.*, 80: 289 – 298.

Lynn, B. (1984) Effect of neonatal treatment with capsaicin on the numbers and properties of cutaneous afferent units from the hairy skin of the rat. *Brain Res.*, 322: 255 – 260.

Lynn, B. and Carpenter, S.E. (1982) Primary afferent units from the hairy skin of the rat hind limb. *Brain Res.*, 238: 29 – 43.

Lynn, B. and Hunt, S.P. (1984) Afferent C-fibres: physiological and biochemical correlations. *Trends Neurosci.*, 7: 186 – 188.

Peyronnade, J.M., Charron, L., Lavoie, J. and Messier, J.P. (1986) Differences in horseradish peroxidase labeling of sensory, motor and sympathetic neurons following chronic axotomy of the rat sural nerve. *Brain Res.*, 364: 137 – 150.

Shea, V.K. and Perl, E.R. (1985) Regeneration of cutaneous afferent unmyelinated (C) fibers after transection. *J. Neurophysiol.*, 54: 502 – 512.

Tuckett, R.P. (1982) Itch evoked by electrical stimulation of the skin. *J. Invest. Dermatol.*, 79: 368 – 373.

W. Hamann and A. Iggo (Eds.)
Progress in Brain Research, Vol. 74
© 1988 Elsevier Science Publishers B.V. (Biomedical Division)

CHAPTER 28

Morphological features of thin sensory afferent fibers: a new interpretation of 'nociceptor' function

Lawrence Kruger

Departments of Anatomy and Anesthesiology and Brain Research Institute, UCLA Center for Health Sciences, Los Angeles, CA 90024, USA

It is generally accepted that nociceptors comprise the simplest, least specialized and most primitive of sensory neurons and that their terminals might best be described as 'free nerve endings'. Sensory thin axons are undoubtedly the least understood of afferent systems and the time is ripe for posing some elementary questions that might lead to a radically different view. This presentation explores the varieties of morphological and related bio-chemical evidence concerning sensory thin fibers, and although more puzzles than answers will emerge, I should like to offer the view that sensory thin fibers probably include the most diverse class of sense organs and that the individual neurons from which they derive are among the most versatile of neuronal populations. If any neuron can qualify for a polyglot status, the several languages by which these extraordinary neural elements communicate via afferent and *efferent* mechanisms may provide some alternative ways of interpreting the role of a putative sense organ consigned to a lifetime of inactivity, excited only by injury or some other rare and pathological event.

The number and distribution of sensory C fibers pose some serious problems. Defense against injury is certainly of crucial biological importance, but would a rarely activated alarm system require more wires than all the other somatic sense organs combined? It can be argued that there are different languages for expressing afferent messages in-

dicating threat of injury, sensitized nociception of 'pain' (Campbell and Meyer, 1986), itch, tickle and thermal sensations. Each class may have developed special dialects and we already recognize that there are several varieties of nociceptors, with 'polymodals' dominant, and of thermosensitive afferents, with cold receptors dominant over warm receptors (Burgess and Perl, 1973). Do the sensory languages of thin fibers require more neurons than the range of exquisite tactile sensitivity and spatial discrimination achieved with the less numerous and highly specialized sensitive mechanoreceptors?

The distribution of a single neuropeptide marker provides some interesting clues and raises some disturbing questions. We have explored the regional innervation patterns of thin axons (mostly unmyelinated) displaying immunoreactivity (IR) for the recently discovered calcitonin gene-related peptide (CGRP) in a variety of specialized tissues. This novel peptide is of special interest because it reveals the largest proportion of peptidergic thin sensory axons (i.e., most of the other neuropeptides are found co-localized within CGRP sub-populations), and its absence in sympathetic ganglia assures its sensory nature. We have also observed that the sensory neurotoxin capsaicin depletes a substantial proportion of thin axons in each structure we have studied to date, although some thin fibers are retained.

An extraordinarily robust and specific antibody

raised by my colleague, Dr. Catia Sternini, has enabled us to study CGRP-IR axons throughout the body, including those in calcified tissues. We have observed CGRP-IR thin fibers in whole mounts of cornea and inner tympanic membrane, in sections of periosteum, and in dental pulp (Colin and Kruger, 1986; Kruger, 1987; Silverman and Kruger, 1987). Excitation of each of these structures with a variety of physical stimuli is known to elicit a sensation of pain. As might be expected, CGRP-IR axons are found in regions of general body sensation associated with various structures, including dermal blood vessels and epidermis similarly to substance P (SP)-IR axons (Kruger et al., 1985), which arise from a subpopulation of those CGRP-IR sensory neurons. It should be noted that the expression of multiple neuropeptides by individual small-medium sensory B ganglion cells is a common feature that we shall return to in the context of the efferent languages of these neurons and their sites of action.

Variation in the density of CGRP-IR axons in different tissues is difficult to explain in terms of a purely sensory role. It is not obvious why the cornea reveals a higher innervation density than the tunica vasculosa of the testis and my colleague Dr. James Silverman has shown an extraordinarily rich supply of CGRP-IR axons in the pulp and dentinal tubules of teeth, with a far greater number in the coronal than the radicular dentin. Vast numbers of fibers are not required for detecting injury, as evidenced by the effectiveness of the small number of testicular afferents in signaling pain. Nor would they be necessary for spatial resolution, especially within a tooth — a structure from which these endings are rarely, if ever, likely to be excited in the course of their life span. Would it not be easier to reconcile the large number of intradental fibers with trophic, regulatory and reparative processes (Silverman and Kruger, 1987), and assume that a sensory role is a rare adjunct to the multifunctional properties of these neurons?

What is the evidence for efferent actions by sensory neurons? 'Axon reflex' mediation of vasodilatation and plasma extravasation has long been known and has been shown to be selectively elicited by nociceptor axons at the single unit level (Kenins, 1981), but a more complete survey of peripheral targets is possible with morphological tools. Although we have successfully traced thin axons, either by horseradish peroxidase transport or by sensory neuropeptide IR labeling, to a wide variety of tissues including blood vessels, mast cells, epithelia, glands and lymphoid tissues, in our experience it is clear that the terminals are 'free' in the sense that they fail to form specialized contacts when studied at the fine structural level. Notwithstanding the restrictions imposed on tracing labeled axons in the electron microscope, it should be noted that target cell contacts have not been demonstrated persuasively. Thus, if substances such as neuropeptides are released from 'sensory' endings in peripheral tissues, they probably would act through broad extracellular diffusion.

An alternative approach has been achieved with remarkable success by my colleague, Dr. Patrick W. Mantyh, who has been studying the specific, high-affinity receptor binding sites of numerous radioligands in brain and peripheral tissues. An aspect of these studies of particular relevance to our thesis is the demonstration of discrete neuropeptide receptor binding sites in specific tissues and cells. One example might demonstrate the general principles underlying the complexity and versatility of neuropeptide actions: thus CGRP receptor binding sites are abundant on smooth muscle cells of blood vessel walls, consistent with the powerful vasodilator action of this peptide (Brain et al., 1985). By contrast, specific intraepidermal binding sites are difficult to identify even with a wide range of radioligands, perhaps reflecting the possibility that epidermal keratinocytes lack receptors for neuropeptides and are unlikely target candidates. It is also quite conceivable that intraepidermal axon terminals may serve a 'sense organ' role.

Returning to effector function, it may prove instructive to speculate on the physiological significance of a single CGRP-IR neuron also expressing other peptides, most notably the tachykinins. It is known that substance P (SP), though less effective a vasodilator than CGRP, plays a role in the plasma extravasation induced by inflammatory processes or 'axon reflex' activation. The expected morphological correlate can be found specific to SP receptor binding sites on small vessel endothelia, unlike CGRP with which it shares vascular smooth muscle binding sites. The roles of the other tachykinins remain to be explored, but the evidence for mitogenicity by substance K (Nilsson et al., 1985) suggests participation in the recovery from injury.

One can speculate further about the functional operations negotiated by each neuropeptide on the basis of location and number of receptor binding sites, but that is too vast a subject to explore in this brief survey. However, before turning to the fine structural features of thin fiber endings, it would be remiss not to include evidence indicating that a large proportion of small sensory ganglion cells display other distinctive biochemical traits, most notably acid phosphatase activity known by the acronym FRAP. The terminal distribution of FRAP positive fibers in the substantia gelatinosa of the dorsal horn is different from that of the neuropeptides just discussed (Hunt and Rossi, 1985) and there is little overlap of FRAP positive cells with those containing CGRP-IR.

FRAP positive small sensory neurons for some time were thought to be an exotic feature of rodents until my colleague, Dr. James D. Silverman, demonstrated and characterized their expression in mammals generally, including primates (Silverman and Kruger, 1988). Other features of FRAP neurons include expression of distinct glycoconjugates characterized by Dodd and Jessell (1985) using monoclonal antibodies. The carbohydrate epitopes of these antibodies thus open new avenues for labeling other non-peptidergic populations of thin sensory axons. The specificity of plant lectin binding to sensory neuron glycoconjugates (Nakagawa et al., 1986) has already enabled Dr. Silverman to find robust lectin markers for presumptive nociceptors. There are other reasons for speculating that these neurons may be

as complex and diverse as their better known peptidergic compatriots (Kruger, 1987; Silverman and Kruger, 1988).

'Polymodal' nociceptors, the largest class of thin fibers (Burgess and Perl, 1973; Kumazawa and Perl, 1977), can be excited by a variety of chemical agents that excite (e.g., bradykinin) or others that 'sensitize' (cf. eicosanoids) selective nociceptor populations (Baccaglini and Hogan, 1983; Kumazawa et al., 1987). These 'chemosensory' properties of single thin afferent fibers may eventually be correlated with the known small sensory cell histochemical markers, drawing upon the finding of CGRP-IR axons in a substantial portion of 'gustatory'-related (Finger, 1986) as well as nociceptor afferents. A new taxonomy based on the distinctive molecular features of individual thin afferent neurons will undoubtedly soon emerge.

Fine structural analysis has been less felicitous than the use of biochemical markers in solving the mysteries of nociceptor axon terminals, and general agreement has not yet been achieved in defining the essence of 'free nerve endings' (Kruger, 1987). Searching for unlabeled axonal endings in the electron microscope may not provide decisive criteria for distinguishing sensory from autonomic axons and the distinctive features of nociceptor terminals are not clearly established, although several authors have published micrographs of axonal profiles containing aggregates of vesicles and mitochondria in regions known to harbor pain endings (e.g., see Yeh and Kruger, 1984).

Another approach is to examine the receptive fields of electrophysiologically characterized nociceptors. This has yielded some success for the sparse myelinated nociceptors of hairy skin (Kruger et al., 1981) and the group III and IV endings associated with articular regions (Andres et al., 1985). We are collaborating with Drs. T. Kumazawa and K. Mizumura who have recently developed an in vitro preparation using canine testis innervated by the small, heavily unmyelinated spermatic nerve (Kumazawa et al., 1987). These experiments have begun only recently and are presented in a preliminary fashion based largely upon the patient efforts of my colleague Yung Yeh in cutting and following serial semi-thin and ultra-thin sections in electrophysiologically characterized and delimited zones surrounded only by fine insect pins inserted after each unit is studied.

One specimen reveals a 'terminal' (i.e., traced to its disappearance) that is 'free' in the sense that it is surrounded by collagenous connective tissue space of the tunica vasculosa, but its ending is totally ensheathed by a narrow Schwann cell process and the axoplasm contains a more luxuriant aggregate of dense bodies than of vesicles and mitochondria. Non-vascular presumptive smooth muscle processes following contours of the ending may be related to its functional role.

Another specimen revealed a small Remak bundle within the receptive field and posed a dilemma by exhibiting several axon profiles containing aggregates of clear spherical vesicles, some far distant from the Schwann cell surface. This feature has often been observed in larger axon bundles and unless they function as nervi nervorum, there is an understandable reluctance to assume that either vesicle or mitochondrial aggregations constitute unimpeachable markers of thin fiber terminals. Single axon profiles emerged within this same receptive field of less than 1 mm, but the putative ending remains thinly surrounded by a Schwann cell and the organelle content is insufficiently distinctive to provide persuasive signatories of a specific 'sense' organ. In each example, nearby profiles of presumptive smooth muscle processes may be targets of a less focal paracrine release of efferent neuroactive substances by these axons. In any case, the findings are decisive of neither sensory nor effector function, and although this zone of very sparsely innervated tissue contains a nociceptor receptive field, there is no way of assuring that a 'free' ending is afferent, efferent or both.

On heuristic grounds, it is difficult to resist the temptation of speculating that the large number of thin sensory axons and their extensive peripheral branching is not required solely for reflex withdrawal from noxious stimuli or providing a sustained warning signal from injured and inflamed tissue. Would it seem too far-fetched to suggest that many, if not all, nociceptor neurons fulfill effector roles and that the signaling of afferent impulses interpreted as pain may constitute a mere adjunct or secondary feature of neurons capable of a vast repertory of chemical expression for tissue maintenance and repair?

In our laboratories we have tentatively agreed to call these neurons 'noceffectors' — a compromise in which the nociceptor-derived prefix takes first place only by historical precedence. In some ways, these neurons are the counterparts of modern human society that sociologists refer to as the 'harried leisure class'. It is difficult to assume that the vast majority of sensory neurons serve the sole function of fortuitous and exceedingly rare excitation informing the central nervous system of noxious stimuli. Fully acknowledging the justifiable prohibitions against proliferating superfluous neologisms, the 'noceffector' can be regarded as a tentative, generalized term subsuming a broad class of sensory neurons. Judging by the number and variety of biochemical markers already assigned to its subpopulations, it is likely that an extensive functional classification will soon emerge for this extraordinarily versatile and varied class of misunderstood sense organs.

Acknowledgements

This essay is based on the research efforts and the exchange of information and ideas with my several colleagues and collaborators, most notably James D. Silverman, Patrick W. Mantyh, Catia Sternini, Nicholas Brecha, Yung Yeh and Samuel Colin. The manuscript was prepared by Anita Roff and the original research reported here was supported by an NIH Javits Award Grant NS-5685 from the US Public Health Service.

References

Andres, K.H., von Düring, M. and Schmidt, R.F. (1985) Sensory innervation of the Achilles tendon by group III and IV afferent fibers. *Anat. Embryol.,* 172: 145 – 156.

Baccaglini, P.I. and Hogan, P.G. (1983) Some rat sensory neurons in culture express characteristics of differentiated pain sensory cells. *Proc. Natl. Acad. Sci. USA,* 80: 594 – 598.

Brain, S.D., Williams, T.J., Tippins, J.R., Morris, H.R. and MacIntyre, I. (1985) Calcitonin gene-related peptide is a potent vasodilator. *Nature (London),* 313: 54 – 56.

Burgess, P.R. and Perl, E.R. (1973) Cutaneous mechanoreceptors and nociceptors. In: A. Iggo (Ed.), *Handbook of Sensory Physiology, Vol. II. Somatosensory System.* Springer-Verlag, New York, pp. 29-78.

Campbell, J.N. and Meyer, R.A. (1986) Primary afferents and hyperalgesia. In: T. Yaksh (Ed.), *Spinal Afferent Processing.* Plenum Press, New York, pp. 59 – 81.

Colin, S. and Kruger, L. (1986) Peptidergic nociceptive axon visualization in whole-mount preparations of cornea and tympanic membrane in rat. *Brain Res.,* 398: 199 – 203.

Dodd, J. and Jessell, T.M. (1985) Lactoseries carbohydrates specify subsets of dorsal root ganglion neurons projecting to the superficial dorsal horn of rat spinal cord. *J. Neurosci.,* 5: 3278 – 3294.

Finger, T.E. (1986) Peptide immunohistochemistry demonstrates multiple classes of perigemmal nerve fibers in the circumvallate papilla of the rat. *Chem. Senses,* 11: 135 – 144.

Hunt, S.P. and Rossi, J. (1985) Peptide- and non-peptide-containing unmyelinated primary afferents: the parallel processing of nociceptive information. *Phil. Trans. R. Soc. London,* 308: 283 – 290.

Kenins, P. (1981) Identification of the unmyelinated sensory nerves which evoke extravasation in response to antidromic stimulation. *Neurosci. Lett.,* 25: 137 – 141.

Kruger, L. (1987) Morphological correlates of 'free' nerve endings: a reappraisal of thin sensory axon classification. In: R.F. Schmidt, H.-G. Schaible and C. Vahle-Hinz (Eds.), *Fine Afferent Nerve Fibers and Pain.* VCH Verlag Chemie, Weinheim, pp. 1 – 13.

Kruger, L, Perl, E.R. and Sedivec, M.J. (1981) Fine structure of myelinated mechanical nociceptor endings in cat hairy skin. *J. Comp. Neurol.,* 198: 137 – 154.

Kruger, L., Sampogna, S.L., Rodin, B.E., Clague, J., Brecha, N. and Yeh, Y. (1985) Thin-fiber cutaneous innervation and its intraepidermal contribution studied by labeling methods and neurotoxin treatment in rats. *Somatosens. Res.,* 2: 335 – 356.

Kumazawa, T. and Perl, E.R. (1977) Primate cutaneous sensory units with unmyelinated (C) afferent fibers. *J. Neurophysiol.,* 40: 1325 – 1338.

Kumazawa, T., Mizumura, K. and Sato, J. (1987) Response properties of polymodal receptors studied using in vitro testis superior spermatic nerve preparations of dogs. *J. Neurophysiol.,* 57: 702 – 711.

Lawson, S.N., Harper, E.T., Harper, A.A., Garson, J.A., Coakham, H.B. and Randle, B.J. (1985) Monoclonal antibody 2C5: a marker for a subpopulation of small neurones in rat dorsal root ganglia. *Neuroscience,* 16: 365 – 374.

Nakagawa, F., Schulte, B.A. and Spicer, S.S. (1986) Lectin cytochemical evaluation of somatosensory neurons and their peripheral and central processes in rat and man. *Cell Tissue Res.,* 245: 579 – 589.

Nilsson, J., von Euler, A.M. and Dalsgaard, C.J. (1985) Stimulation of connective tissue cell growth by substance P and substance K. *Nature (London),* 315: 61 – 63.

Silverman, J.D. and Kruger, L. (1987) An interpretation of dental innervation based upon the pattern of calcitonin gene-related peptide (CGRP) immunoreactive thin sensory axons. *Somatosens. Res.,* 5: 157 – 175.

Silverman, J.D. and Kruger, L. (1988) Acid phosphatase as a selective marker for a class of small sensory ganglion cells in several mammals: spinal cord distribution, histochemical properties and relation to fluoride-resistant acid phosphatase (FRAP) of rodents. *Somatosens. Res.,* 5: 219 – 246.

Yeh, Y and Kruger, L. (1984) Fine structural characterization of the somatic innervation of the tympanic membrane in normal, sympathectomized and neurotoxin-denervated rats. *Somatosens. Res.,* 1: 359 – 378.

W. Hamann and A. Iggo (Eds.)
Progress in Brain Research, Vol. 74
© 1988 Elsevier Science Publishers B.V. (Biomedical Division)

CHAPTER 29

The reinnervation of denervated skin

Bryce L. Munger

Department of Anatomy, The Milton S. Hershey Medical Center, The Pennsylvania State University, P.O. Box 850, Hershey, PA 17033, USA

The regeneration of peripheral nerves in man is frequently associated with undesirable sequelae referred to as paresthesias or dysesthesias as reviewed in detail by Sunderland (1978) and Dellon (1981). Paresthesias and dysesthesias are abnormal sensations in the skin in response to stimuli that ordinarily are not unpleasant. The sensations can involve thermal as well as tactile stimuli and can be quite unpleasant. Individual patients have quite unique responses following nerve regeneration thus precluding a succinct description of the process.

The puzzling process of nerve regeneration prompted Henry Head to perform the heroic experiment on himself of sectioning the two large cutaneous nerves to the dorsum of the hand. Head described his clinical findings on the patient population from the Boer War in 1905 (Head and Sherren, 1905) and had the surgery performed cn himself 2 years before. The final report describing this experiment was authored by Rivers and Head (1908) as Rivers was the psychology professor from Oxford who tested Head on a weekly basis as his cutaneous nerves regenerated. Head also had some unusual sensory responses in the area of regenerating nerves including the persistence of touch in hairs lacking a pain response. This important observation has been correlated with the presence of distinct differences in the sensory terminals on single primate hairs (Munger, 1982) and we can conclude that guard hairs typically have multiple sensory terminals that include lanceolate and Ruffini terminals as well as free nerve endings (FNEs) (Rice and Munger, 1986). Perhaps even more unexpected is the observation that primate guard hairs typically are innervated by more than one spinal segment (Munger, 1984).

Vibrissae are specialized large hairs surrounded by erectile tissue that are innervated by numerous sensory terminals arranged in a pattern that is much more complex than that of guard hairs. As reviewed by Renehan and Munger (1986a) and Rice et al. (1986) vibrissae are innervated by two different nerves that terminate in two separate locations each. The principal sensory nerve or vibrissal nerve as termed by Dorfl (1985) consists of 100 – 150 axons that enter the base of the sinus and terminate as Ruffini terminals and FNEs along the base of the hair follicle as well as provide the principal sensory innervation to the collar of nerve terminals above the ringwulst as lanceolate and Merkel terminals. The other sensory innervation of vibrissae is derived from the superficial dermal nerve plexus and provides the source of nerves innervating the conus region of the sinus (the apex of the sinus) as well as the Merkel rete ridge collar that surrounds the hair as it emerges from the skin surface. The conus innervation consists of lanceolate, Ruffini and FNE terminals.

This brief review is needed to understand the implications of a recent study by Renehan and Munger (1986b) of the process of nerve regeneration in vibrissae. In that study they followed the process of nerve degeneration and regeneration after sectioning the infraorbital nerves in rats. When the axons regenerated the principal sensory nerves did not form sensory terminals restricted to the site they normally innervate but rather entered the conus region in a very complex array of tangled axons. The Merkel terminals were reinnervated to some extent in the sensory collar above the ringwulst but fewer Merkel cells were present and a smaller percentage were innervated than normal. Recently Munger and Renehan (1987) extended these findings to include the guard hairs between the vibrissae and have found that guard hairs are abnormally reinnervated in all cases following nerve transection and in many cases following nerve crush (Table 1).

The following is a preliminary report on the ultrastructural changes seen after nerve regeneration in human biopsies described clinically by Dellon and Munger (1983) and experimental animals from studies by Munger, Ide and Tohyama (unpublished observations). In both cases the skin was prepared for light and electron microscopy with conventional techniques. Serial paraffin sections of skin fixed in 10% neutral buffered formalin were stained with silver using the technique described by Sevier and Munger (1965). The sections were photographed using Kodak Technical Pan film and developed with POTA developer to enhance contrast of blackened axons (Rice and Munger, 1986).

TABLE 1

Percent of guard hairs with typical (complete) piloneural complex

Normal 90% (range 87 – 92%)
After nerve transection 2% (range 1 – 3%)
After nerve crush 31% (range 30 – 35%)

The above percentages and upper and lower limits are derived from only four animals and should not be interpreted as absolute, as errors of evaluation of sensory terminals other than a palisade of lanceolate terminals is extremely subjective. As noted in the text, lanceolate terminals are rarely observed after nerve transection.

In all cases studied to date reinnervated Pacinian corpuscles are abnormal, confirming Zelena's (1984) observations of cat Pacinian corpuscles. The central axon is invariably multiple and in each case only surrounded by a thin layer of inner core cells. Normal human Pacinian corpuscles frequently have multiple axons within the inner core but these are invariably branches of a single parent axon and share a common inner core (Ide et al., 1987). After reinnervation the inner core surrounding the multiple axons is always separate and distinct for each branch. The inner core never regenerates to a structure remotely resembling that of the normal in man or rat (Zelena, 1984).

The other sensory receptors present in glabrous digital skin, namely Meissner corpuscles and Merkel terminals, are also typically abnormal following reinnervation. Meissner corpuscles are in many cases almost normal consisting of numerous thin lamellae and containing robust axons. However, the corpuscles are typically lower in the dermal papillae than normal and often associated with atrophic remnants of former Meissner corpuscles that have small stacks of cells associated with masses of basal lamina. Such atrophic corpuscles can also be identified by light microscopy in both silver- and PAS-stained preparations. In silver-stained preparations the masses of basal lamina appear as homogeneous masses usually lacking signs of an associated axon. The masses of basal lamina are PAS positive appearing as a small scar in the dermal papillae. The position of the corpuscles is perhaps one of the most distinctive features of reinnervated Meissner corpuscles in that normally they are always present at the very top of the dermal papillae and never encountered towards the base of the papillary ridges.

Merkel terminals are also unusual in that many are not reinnervated. When they are reinnervated the axons are expanded to larger than normal and often associated with Schwann cells that have cytoplasmic processes resembling lamellae of Meissner corpuscles. In such cases the Merkel cells are usually multiple and while serial reconstructions were not attempted of the electron microscopic material for quantitative analysis of numbers of Merkel cells, they appeared to be more prominent than normal. The lamellae associated with the reinnervated axons, however, have never been observed in normal human or animal skin.

Recently our studies on peripheral nerve regeneration have been extended to study grafted skin of baboons in a collaborative study with Dykes' group at McGill University and a preliminary account was published with Samulack et al. (1986). This model uses baboons and the entire skin of the digit removed with a neurovascular pedicle. The graft is replaced as a homografted control or the skin grafted onto another animal as an allograft. The animals were treated with cyclosporin for immunosuppression. Samulack and Dykes then studied the single mechanoreceptive afferents in both glabrous and hairy skin of the digit. The animals were perfused following physiologic study and skin processed in the present author's laboratory for both light and electron microscopy. For light microscopy serial sets of sections were stained with the Sevier – Munger silver method. The animals survived for several months to permit regeneration of peripheral nerves.

Upon physiologic evaluation the skin was found to contain both slowly and rapidly adapting receptors but the thresholds were somewhat elevated and the units fatigued easily. Since the animals all had some degree of rejection of the allografts with attendant edema, some of the physiologic findings may have been affected by local changes. But hairy skin was consistently more abnormal than glabrous skin (Samulack et al., 1986).

Upon histologic evaluation all seven animals that have been processed to date were remarkably consistent. In glabrous skin reinnervated Meissner corpuscles could be found, although many were abnormal in location and appearance resembling the human tissue cited above. Only rarely could a normal-appearing Meissner corpuscle be found. Pacinian corpuscles were also reinnervated with the central axon evidencing branching and thus sprouting as described by Zelena (1984).

By electron microscopy we have failed to find Merkel cells in glabrous skin in allografts examined to date. We have also searched our paraffin sections and have not seen intraepidermal axons in the bases of the papillary ridges. Merkel clusters are typically found at the base of the papillary ridges in between successive ducts of the eccrine sweat glands (Dell and Munger, 1986). While this finding is tentative pending confirmation, the absence of Merkel cells, or paucity of same in allografted skin, but the physiologically verified slowly adapting responses would mean that these cells cannot be mechanoelectric transducers. The probability of a trophic function of Merkel cells as proposed when Merkel cells were described by electron microscopy (Munger, 1965) would thus seem more possible.

But even more striking are the changes in allografted hairy skin. In most cases severe to total depilation resulted. Such sites often had remnants of basal lamina that would indicate the presence of former hair follicles, but as in the rat reinnervated skin as described by Munger and Renehan (1987) normal reinnervated hairs are never seen. This again as in glabrous skin must be understood in the context of the presence of rapidly adapting responses, although abnormal in threshold and fatiguability. In this instance at least normal peripheral receptors are not necessary for normal physiological responses.

While the present results have concentrated on the peripheral receptors of regenerated axons, we recognize the fact that the peripheral nerves themselves are also abnormal as reviewed in detail by Sunderland (1978). A consensus can be found in the literature that nerve fiber diameter is smaller and conduction velocity slower following transection as compared to crushing a nerve (Terzis and Dykes, 1980; Dykes and Terzis, 1979; Horch and Lisney, 1981). In nerve transection the continuity of the basal lamina that would act as a guide for regrowing axons is lost (Ide, 1984; Ide et al., 1983). The clinical sequelae encountered when nerves are damaged thus begin at the level of the sensory receptors and include the nerve distal to the damage and central factors that would result from misrouting.

It is important to note that the peripheral abnormalities are diagnostic to the extent that we can always identify reinnervated skin, i.e., these changes in sensory receptors are pathognomic. We propose that the basis for these abnormalities in part is due to the normal ontogeny of cutaneous nerves as described in several studies by the present author (Bressler and Munger, 1983; Dell and Munger, 1986; Rice and Munger, 1986). In these series of studies we conclude that temporal and spatial factors are crucial in the differentiation of skin as well as the sensory nerves innervating skin. Such spatial and temporal factors simply can never be recapitulated during regeneration of nerves. Thus the cells of specialized sensory corpuscles can never redifferentiate normally. The key to understanding the limits of sensory regeneration is thus understanding the process of normal development. The processes of nerve regeneration and nerve development can never be the same.

References

Bressler, M. and Munger, B.L. (1983) Embryonic maturation of sensory terminals of primate facial hairs. *J. Invest. Dermatol.,* 80: 245 – 260.

Dell, D.A. and Munger, B.L. (1986) The early embryogenesis of papillary (sweat duct) ridges in primate glabrous skin: the dermatotopic map of cutaneous mechanoreceptors and dermatoglyphics. *J. Comp. Neurol.,* 244: 511 – 532.

Dellon, A.L. (1981) *Evaluation of Sensibility and Re-education of Sensation in the Hand.* Williams and Wilkins, Baltimore, MD.

Dellon, A.L. and Munger, B.L. (1983) Correlation of histology and sensibility after nerve repair. *J. Hand Surg.,* 8: 871 – 875.

Dorfl, J. (1985) The innervation of the mystacial region of the white mouse. A topographical study. *J. Anat.,* 142: 173 – 184.

Dykes, R.W. and Terzis, J.K. (1979) Reinnervation of glabrous skin in baboons: properties of cutaneous mechanoreceptors subsequent to nerve crush. *J. Neurophysiol.,* 42: 1461 – 1478.

Head, H. and Sherren, J. (1905) The consequences of injury to the peripheral nerves in man. *Brain,* 28: 116 – 338.

Horch, K.W. and Lisney, S.J.W. (1981) On the number and nature of regenerating myelinated axons after lesions of cutaneous nerves in the cat. *J. Physiol. (London),* 313: 275 – 286.

Ide, C. (1984) Nerve regeneration through the basal lamina scaffold of the skeletal muscle. *Neurosci. Res.,* 1: 379 – 391.

Ide, C., Tohyama, K., Yokota, R., Nitatori, T. and Onodera, S. (1983) Schwann cell basal lamina and nerve regeneration. *Brain Res.,* 288: 61 – 75.

Ide, C., Nitatori, T. and Munger, B.L. (1987) The cytology of human Pacinian corpuscles: evidence for sprouting of the central axon. *Arch. Histol. Jap.,* in press.

Munger, B.L. (1965) The intraepidermal innervation of the snout skin of the opossum. A light and electron microscopic study with observations on the nature of Merkel's Tastzellen. *J. Cell Biol.,* 26: 79 – 97.

Munger, B.L. (1982) Multiple afferent innervation of primate facial hairs – Henry Head and Max von Frey revisited. *Brain Res.,* 4: 1 – 43.

Munger, B.L. (1984) Multiple segmental innervation of single primate hairs and rete ridges. *Anat. Rec.,* 205: 137A.

Munger, B.L. and Renehan, W. (1987) Abnormal sensory reinnervation of rat guard hairs following transection or crush of branches of the trigeminal nerve. *J. Comp. Neurol.,* submitted.

Renehan, W. and Munger, B.L. (1986a) Degeneration and regeneration of peripheral nerve in the rat trigeminal system. I. Identification and characterization of the multiple afferent innervation of mystacial vibrissa. *J. Comp. Neurol.,* 246: 129 – 145.

Renehan, W. and Munger, B.L. (1986b) Degeneration and regeneration of peripheral nerve in the rat trigeminal system. II. Acute response to nerve lesion. *J. Comp. Neurol.,* in press.

Rice, F.L., Mance, A. and Munger, B.L. (1986) A comparative light microscopic analysis of the sensory innervation of the mystacial pad in the hamster, mouse, rat, gerbil, rabbit, guinea pig, and cat. I. Innervation of vibrissal follicle-sinus complexes. *J. Comp. Neurol.,* in press.

Rice, F.L. and Munger, B.L. (1986) A comparative light microscopic analysis of the sensory innervation of the mystacial pad in the hamster, mouse, rat, gerbil, rabbit, guinea pig, and cat. II. The common fur between the vibrissae. *J. Comp. Neurol.,* in press.

Rivers, R.H.R. and Head, H. (1908) A human experiment in nerve division. *Brain,* 31: 323 – 450.

Samulack, D.D., Munger, B.L., Dykes, R.W. and Daniel, R.K. (1986) Neuroanatomical evidence of reinnervation in primate allografted (transplanted) skin during cyclosporine immunosuppression. *Neurosci. Lett.,* submitted.

Sevier, E.A. and Munger, B.L. (1965) A silver method for paraffin sections of neural tissue. *J. Neuropathol. Exp. Neurol.,* 24: 130 – 135.

Sunderland, S. (1978) Degeneration of the axon and associated changes. In: *Nerves and Nerve Injuries.* Churchill Livingstone, Edinburgh, pp. 88 – 107.

Terzis, J.K. and Dykes, R.W. (1980) Reinnervation of glabrous skin in baboons: properties of cutaneous mechanoreceptors subsequent to nerve transection. *J. Neurophysiol.,* 44: 1214 – 1225.

Zelena, J. (1984) Multiple axon terminals in reinnervated Pacinian corpuscle of adult rat. *J. Neurocytol.,* 13: 665 – 684.

W. Hamann and A. Iggo (Eds.)
Progress in Brain Research, Vol. 74
© 1988 Elsevier Science Publishers B.V. (Biomedical Division)

CHAPTER 30

Spread of skin deformation and mechanoreceptor discharge

Benjamin H. Pubols Jr.

Neurological Sciences Institute, Good Samaritan Hospital and Medical Center, 1120 N.W. Twentieth Avenue, Portland, OR 97209, USA

Introduction

In their pioneering investigations of the responses of mammalian primary afferent fibers to mechanical stimulation of glabrous skin, Adrian and Zotterman (1926) utilized controlled-force stimuli. Most succeeding studies have used stimuli controlled with respect to stimulus position (indentation or displacement). However, beginning in the late 1970s, a number of laboratories have returned to controlled-force stimuli in order to examine differences in the way in which primary mechanoreceptive afferents respond to controlled-force versus controlled-displacement stimuli (e.g., Petit and Galifret, 1978; Pubols and Maliniak, 1984). Other recent studies have been concerned with responses to spatial and spatiotemporal aspects of mechanical stimulation (e.g., Darian-Smith and Oke, 1980; Phillips and Johnson, 1981; see Darian-Smith, 1984, for a general review).

The availability of a small-motion biological stimulator (Chubbuck, 1966) which allows precise control over either stimulus position or force, and the simultaneous monitoring of both, has made possible new approaches to the study of the role of mechanical properties of skin in determining the responses of glabrous skin mechanoreceptors to tactile stimulation. Results of these experiments have provided new insights into possible contributions of the skin to tactile information processing and perceptual phenomena.

In this review, we shall discuss results from two types of investigation of mammalian glabrous skin and its mechanoreceptors, recently completed in our laboratory. First, we shall review the role of viscoelastic properties of glabrous skin in determining mechanoreceptor discharge. Following this, we shall consider the role of lateral spread of skin indentation in determining the responses of slowly adapting mechanoreceptors to suprathreshold indentations. Sixty-six slowly adapting fibers of the median and ulnar nerves of the raccoon, and 16 single fibers from squirrel monkey median and ulnar nerves contributed data to the studies reviewed here. Viscoelastic properties of forepaw glabrous skin were studied at an additional 12 sites in raccoons, two in squirrel monkeys, and seven in domestic cats. All animals were anesthetized with pentobarbital sodium, and single fiber isolation was achieved by microdissection. Further details regarding the experimental preparations may be found in previously published reports (Pubols, 1982, 1987; Pubols and Benkich, 1986).

Mechanical factors affecting responses to vertical indentation of skin

For these studies, one stimulus probe, a Plexiglas cone tapering to a 1 mm diameter cylinder, was used to vertically indent the glabrous skin of the hand or forepaw. Feedback-controlled displacements up to 1000 μm and controlled forces up to

20 g were superimposed on small resting forces between 40 and 200 mg. Responses of both skin and mechanoreceptors were examined as a function of stimulation time and stimulus intensity.

Effects over time

Glabrous skin displays the viscoelastic properties of stress relaxation (when a constant indentation is applied to the skin, reactive force first peaks and then gradually decays over time) and creep (when a constant force is applied, in order for that force to be maintained, the skin continues to indent over time). Both of these features are illustrated in Fig. 1, which also illustrates the contrasting effects of constant-force versus constant-displacement stimulation on rates of mechanoreceptor adaptation. In these studies, stimulus parameters are adjusted to yield discharge rates that are comparable at the onset of constant stimulation. Because rates of adaptation have been shown to be more rapid the faster the stimulus onset velocity (Pubols and Pubols, 1976), it is also necessary to take this factor into account (Pubols and Benkich, 1986). In the great majority of cases, as illustrated in Fig. 1, discharge rate declines more rapidly (i.e., adaptation is faster) during controlled-displacement than during controlled-force stimulation. Even though both stress and discharge rate appear to decline together when displacement-controlled stimuli are used, they do not do so in a strictly parallel fashion. Further, regardless of whether displacement or force is controlled, displacement grows progressively relative to force. Thus, one cannot infer from these data a greater role for either force or displacement in determining mechanoreceptor discharge level at any instant in time.

Effects of stimulus magnitude

Effects of stimulus force on skin displacement were systematically examined at seven different skin loci on the squirrel monkey hand, three on digital pads and four on palm pads. The forces used ranged between 0.5 g and 8 – 15 g. To allow comparisons with earlier findings in the raccoon, measurements of skin displacement were obtained at the onset of static force, and at 300 ms and 20 s after static force onset. At all seven loci, the

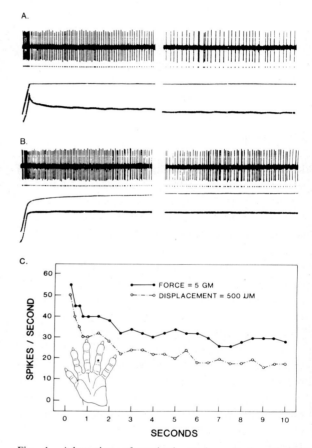

Fig. 1. Adaptation of squirrel monkey slowly adapting mechanoreceptor during (A) constant displacement (500 μm; ramp velocity, 5.0 μm/ms) versus (B) constant force (5 g; dynamic force, 50 mg/ms, corresponding to 4.8 μm/ms displacement velocity) stimulation. Left half shows discharge during first 2 s of constant stimulation; right half shows discharge during s 9 – 10 of constant stimulation. (A and B) Upper trace is of unit spikes, second trace is of output of spike amplitude discriminator, third trace is of voltage analog of skin displacement, and fourth trace is of voltage analog of force. Resting level, 40 mg. (C) Adaptation over full 10 s of stimulation. Each curve represents one trial. Inset in C shows location of RF on middle phalanx of fourth digit of left hand. (Modified from Pubols and Benkich, 1986, reproduced with permission.)

following features were revealed: (a) for any given applied force, displacement increases over time (creep); (b) displacement is an increasing, monotonic function of applied force, the function asymptoting at approximately 10 g; (c) on double logarithmic coordinates, between values of approximately 1 g and 10 g, there is a straight-line relationship between applied force and reactive displacement; and (d) the slope of this function decreases over time.

Over the force range 1 – 10 g, power functions were fit to each of the 21 sets of data (seven stimulating loci, three measurement times). The means (and ranges in parentheses) of the power function exponents *(b)* at each of the three measurement times were 1.17 (0.98 – 1.41) at static stimulus onset, 0.78 (0.60 – 0.98) at 300 ms, and 0.53 (0.41 – 0.67) at 20 s. At static force onset, the mean value of *b* did not differ significantly from 1.00 (*t* test), while mean exponents were significantly less than 1.00 at both 300 ms post

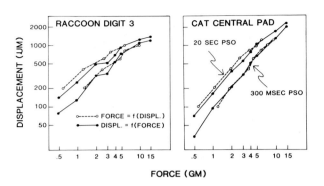

Fig. 3. Reactive force as a function of applied indentation contrasted with reactive indentation as a function of applied force, at two times following onset of maintained stimulation: 300 ms post plateau onset, and 20 s post plateau onset. Left: raccoon digit 3; right: cat central pad. Forces or indentations superimposed on resting levels of 200 mg. Double logarithmic coordinates. Over the ranges of force and displacement common to the two stimulating conditions, there is close agreement between pairs of corresponding curves.

static force onset (*P* <0.01), and 20 s post static force onset (*P* <0.001). Fitted power functions are illustrated in Fig. 2 for one digital stimulating locus and one palm pad locus. Since a power function with an exponent of 1.00 is equivalent to a linear function, skin displacement may be said to increase linearly with increasing force at the onset of static force. Over time, however (at least up to 20 s), the relationship becomes progressively negatively accelerated. All product – moment correlation coefficients *(r)* were 0.96 or higher. These results in squirrel monkey are similar to those found earlier in raccoon glabrous skin (Pubols, 1982).

The above data raise the interesting question of whether or not the effect of applied displacement on reactive force can be predicted from knowledge of the effect of applied force on reactive displacement. Data from raccoon and cat glabrous skin indicate that this is in fact possible. Fig. 3 shows plots of displacement as a function of force and force as a function of displacement, at two times following onset of static stimulation (300 ms and 20 s), at stimulating loci on a raccoon forepaw

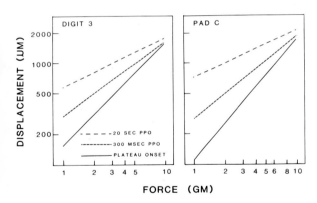

Fig. 2. Skin displacement as a function of applied force at each of three times following onset of static forces achieved at a rate of 10 mg/ms (static force, or plateau, onset; 300 ms post plateau onset; 20 s post plateau onset), over the range 1 – 10 g at each of two squirrel monkey stimulating loci, the distal pad of digit 3 (left) and the central pad (pad C, right). Indicated forces were superimposed on resting levels of 200 mg. Double logarithmic coordinates. The lines represent the best-fitting power functions (method of least squares) according to the equation, Displacement = a · Force^b. With time into the plateau, the value of *a* increases and the value of *b* decreases.

digit and the central pad of a cat's forepaw. In each of the four comparisons, the curves are nearly identical.

In the earlier study of raccoon glabrous skin mechanoreceptors (Pubols, 1982), discharge rates of 12 slowly adapting units during ms 100 – 500 of static stimulation were plotted as a function of constant force (range, 0.5 – 20.0 g), and as a function of displacements at 300 ms post static stimulation onset (the temporal midpoint of the spike discharge frequency measurement period). Linear, logarithmic, and power functions were fit to each of the 24 sets of data. There was no one best-fitting function, although a logarithmic function provided the best fit in the majority of cases. Reliability of the relationships between discharge rate and force versus displacement (sign tests) were not significantly different (Pubols, 1982).

Effects of mechanical stimulus spread

For studies of lateral spread of mechanical stimulation and its effect on mechanoreceptor discharge, two stimulus probes were used. The tip of each was again 1 mm in diameter. One probe, the stimulus probe, was used in the controlled-displacement mode, to indent the skin to known depths at constant-ramp velocities, while the other probe, the monitor, was used in the controlled-force mode, to track vertical movements of the skin at a distance from the stimulus. The position of the monitor remained fixed, while that of the stimulus was systematically moved various distances and directions from the monitor locus. When the activity of a primary mechanoreceptive afferent fiber was simultaneously being recorded, the monitor probe was positioned over the threshold receptive field (RF) of that unit. In the text and figures which follow, all distances are expressed in terms of the center-to-center separation of the two probes. At a center-to-center separation of zero (i.e., when the monitor site was being stimulated), the same probe served as both stimulus and monitor.

In order to ensure that the monitor probe re-

mained in contact with the skin at all times, several conditions had to be met. Thus, it was necessary to use a sufficiently high resting or tracking force (usually 400 mg), and a sufficiently low stimulus indentation velocity (either 5 or 10 µm/ms). Contact of the monitor probe with the skin was visually monitored by the experimenter, and all trials in which contact was not maintained throughout were discarded.

The results revealed a monotonic decline in both the depth and velocity of skin indentation with increasing distance of the stimulus probe from the monitor probe; as distance increased, velocity declined more rapidly than did indentation depth. These decreases varied with skin topography, animal species, and stimulus indentation velocity.

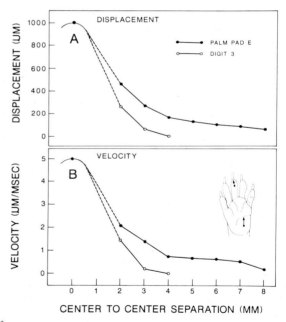

Fig. 4. Comparison of spread of indentation from distal stimulation sites to more proximally located monitor site on raccoon distal digit 3 versus palm pad E. (A) Effects on indentation depth. (B) Effects on indentation velocity. Resting force, 400 mg; stimulus indentation depth, 1000 µm; stimulus indentation velocity, 5 µm/ms. Inset in B: solid circles, monitor loci; arrows, direction and extent of stimulating locus sites distal to monitor loci.

Role of skin topography

The degree of decline in both indentation depth and indentation velocity depends upon the size, shape, and curvature of the digital or palm pad stimulated, as well as on the compliance of skin and subjacent tissues. Thus, spread of indentation is more restricted on digital pads than on palm pads, and is more restricted when the stimulus is applied over a bony prominence than when applied over the center of a pad. Because skin curvature acts as a major factor limiting the spread of indentation (Pubols, 1987), the data which follow were obtained from relatively flat skin surfaces.

Fig. 4 illustrates the more restricted spread of

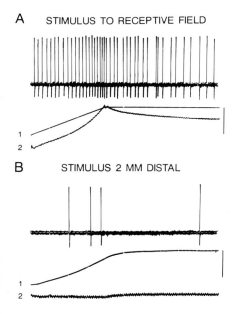

Fig. 5. Comparison of responses to stimulation of digit 3 RF (A) versus stimulation 2 mm distal to RF (B). Resting force, 400 mg; stimulus probe indentation depth, 1000 μm; indentation velocity, 5 μm/ms. Gain of displacement stimulus monitor in B is five times that of displacement monitor in A; therefore, indentation depth at RF is 250 μm; indentation velocity is 1.2 μm/ms. Total sweep, 500 ms. Trace 1: monitor displacement (stimulus displacement in A); trace 2: monitor force (stimulus force in A). Displacement calibration bar, 1000 μm in A, 200 μm in B.

stimulation on digital as opposed to palmar skin. In this example, in which the stimulus was moved progressively distal to the monitor on either a digital or a palm pad, both indentation depth and velocity dropped to zero within 4 mm on the digital pad, while some indentation of the palm pad occurred as far away as 8 mm. As would be expected, decline in discharge rate of slowly adapting mechanoreceptors occurs more rapidly with distance of the stimulus from the unit's RF when the stimulus is applied to digital than to palmar skin. In fact, in many instances, few or no spikes were elicited when the stimulus was as little as 2 mm away from the RF. Fig. 5 illustrates the sharp decline in discharge rate when an otherwise identical stimulus is delivered 2 mm away from the digital RF of a slowly adapting mechanoreceptor (same as unit with digital RF in Fig. 4). When the stimulus (indentation depth, 1000 μm; indentation velocity, 5 μm/ms) was applied to the RF, 22 spikes were elicited during the 200 ms rise time and 20 spikes were elicited during the first 300 ms of static indentation. When the same stimulus was applied 2 mm distal to the RF, the indentation depth at the RF declined to approximately 250 μm, and the indentation velocity declined to 1.2 μm/ms; the number of spikes elicited during the ramp phase of stimulation dropped to three, and only one spike occurred during the first 300 ms of static indentation.

In a sample of nine raccoon units with digital RFs and nine with palmar RFs (indentation depth, 1000 μm; indentation velocity, either 5 or 10 μm/ms), indentation depth, indentation velocity, the number of spikes occurring during ramp stimulation, and the number of spikes occurring during the first 500 ms of static indentation when the stimulus was applied 2 mm away from the RF were all expressed as percentages of values obtained when the stimulus was applied directly to the RF. Scores were uniformly lower for all four variables, and significantly so ($P < 0.05$, or better) for all variables except indentation velocity when the RF was on a digital pad as opposed to a palm pad (Pubols, 1987).

Species differences

For homotopic glabrous skin regions, spread of indentation is more restricted across squirrel monkey hand than across raccoon forepaw, and spread across raccoon forepaw is more restricted than spread across cat forepaw. These statements hold true for both digital and palmar sites, and are manifest as differences in decline with distance in both indentation depth and indentation velocity. A comparison of spread across the central pad of the cat's forepaw with spread across the central pad of the raccoon's forepaw is illustrated in Fig. 6. This figure also illustrates (as does Fig. 4) that velocity declines with distance more rapidly than does indentation depth.

Role of mechanical stimulus velocity

Spread of indentation, expressed in terms of either indentation depth or velocity, appears to be af-

fected only minimally by the magnitude of skin indentation. Similarly, indentation velocity does not appear to affect the spread of indentation depth. However, the greater the stimulus velocity, the more rapidly the velocity declines with distance. This is true for both variations in velocity of linearly rising displacement ramps and for variations in sine wave frequency (Pubols, 1987). Vigor of spike discharge also declines more rapidly with distance the greater the stimulus velocity.

Fig. 7 illustrates skin indentation at the RF center and slowly adapting mechanoreceptive afferent fiber discharge when a 1000 μm stimulus indentation is applied at each of two velocities, 10 μm/ms and 2 μm/ms, either to the threshold RF of the unit or 2 mm distal to the RF. The decline in indentation depth at the RF when the stimulus was applied 2 mm distal was approximately the same at both velocities. However, the relative decline in indentation velocity at the RF when the stimulus was applied 2 mm distal was greater with the faster of the two velocities. The relative decline in spike discharge activity when the stimulus probe was applied 2 mm distal to the RF rather than directly to it was also greater when the higher velocity stimulus was applied. This was true during both ramp and early static phases of stimulation.

In many instances, spike discharge ceased when the stimulus was applied within a short distance of the RF even though there was still an appreciable indentation at the RF, well above the absolute indentation threshold for the unit in question. It was noted above, and illustrated in Figs. 4 and 6, that indentation velocity declines with distance at a faster rate than does indentation depth. Thus, the hypothesis was proposed, and evidence has been presented (Pubols, 1987), that indentation velocity and indentation depth jointly contribute to the size of a suprathreshold RF when the stimulus is delivered some distance from the center of the threshold RF. In order for there to be a spike discharge, the indentation depth at the center of the RF must equal or exceed that at which the first spike occurs when a stimulus of that velocity is applied directly to the RF center.

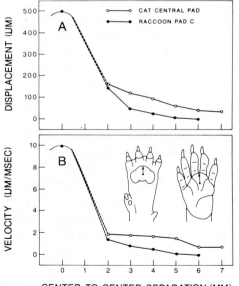

Fig. 6. Comparison of stimulus spread across central pad of cat paw with spread across pad C of raccoon paw. (A) Effect on indentation depth. (B) Effect on indentation velocity. Resting force, 400 mg; stimulus indentation depth, 500 μm; indentation velocity, 10 μm/ms. Inset diagrams as in Fig. 4.

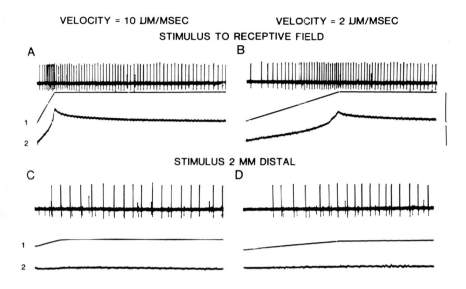

Fig. 7. Comparison of indentation and spike discharge when RF was stimulated versus stimulation 2 mm distal to RF (located on distal phalanx of raccoon digit 3). Stimulus velocities and loci indicated in figure. Resting force, 400 mg; stimulus probe indentation depth, 1000 μm. Total sweep = 1 s. Traces as in Fig. 5. In A – D, displacement calibration bar, 1000 μm; force calibration bar, 4 g. (Modified from Pubols, 1987, reproduced with permission.)

Conclusions

The results of the studies reported here have a number of general implications for tactile information processing and tactile perceptual phenomena (Pubols, 1987). First, they suggest that many 'higher-order' neural and perceptual phenomena usually attributed to central mechanisms of afferent inhibition (Mountcastle, 1984) may be due, at least partially, to mechanical properties of the skin which provide a focusing or sharpening mechanism, operating prior to mechanoreceptor transduction. Second, the results suggest that regional variations in the two-point limen may be associated with variations in spread of mechanical stimulation, as well as with variations in peripheral receptor innervation density. Third, the findings with respect to the effect of stimulus velocity on spread of indentation suggest that high-frequency stimuli, because they remain more spatially localized, should be more efficacious than low-frequency stimuli in tactile pattern perception.

Finally, the results emphasize the importance of viewing the skin and subjacent tissues, along with tactile receptors, as forming a tactile organ system, the starting point for all tactile information processing and perception.

Acknowledgement

This work was supported in part by Research Grants NS-17425 and NS-19487 from the USPHS.

References

Adrian, E.D. and Zotterman, Y. (1926) The nerve impulses produced by sensory nerve endings. Part 3. Impulses set up by touch and pressure. *J. Physiol. (London)*, 61: 465 – 483.

Chubbuck, J.G. (1966) Small motion biological stimulator. *APL Tech. Digest,* 5: 18 – 23.

Darian-Smith, I. (1984) The sense of touch: performance and peripheral neural processes. In: J.M. Brookhart, V.B. Mountcastle and I. Darian-Smith (Eds.), *Handbook of Physiology, Section I, The Nervous System, Vol. 3, Sensory Processes.* American Physiological Society, Bethesda, MD, pp. 739 – 788.

Darian-Smith, I. and Oke, L.E. (1980) Peripheral neural representation of the spatial frequency of a grating moving across the monkey's finger pad. *J. Physiol. (London),* 309: 117 – 133.

Mountcastle, V.B. (1984) Central nervous mechanisms in mechanoreceptive sensibility. In: J.M. Brookhart, V.B. Mountcastle and I. Darian-Smith (Eds.), *Handbook of Physiology, Section I, The Nervous System, Vol. 3, Sensory Processes.* American Physiological Society, Bethesda, MD, pp. 789 – 878.

Petit, H. and Galifret, Y. (1978) Sensory coupling function and the mechanical properties of the skin. In: G. Gordon (Ed.), *Active Touch: The Mechanism of Recognition of Objects by Manipulation.* Pergamon Press, Oxford, pp. 19 – 27.

Phillips, J.R. and Johnson, K.O. (1981) Tactile spatial resolution: II. Neural representation of bars, edges, and gratings in monkey primary afferents. *J. Neurophysiol.,* 46: 1192 – 1203.

Pubols, B.H. (1982) Factors affecting cutaneous mechanoreceptor response: I. Constant-force versus constant-displacement stimulation. *J. Neurophysiol.,* 47: 515 – 529.

Pubols, B.H. (1987) Effect of mechanical stimulus spread across glabrous skin of raccoon and squirrel monkey hand on tactile primary afferent fiber discharge. *Somatosens. Res.,* 4: 273 – 308.

Pubols, B.H. and Pubols, L.M. (1976) Coding of mechanical stimulus velocity and indentation depth by squirrel monkey and raccoon glabrous skin mechanoreceptors. *J. Neurophysiol.,* 39: 773 – 787.

Pubols, B.H. and Maliniak, C.H. (1984) The role of skin mechanics in tactile receptor discharge. In: W. Hamann and A. Iggo (Eds.), *Sensory Receptor Mechanisms.* World Scientific Publ. Co., Singapore, pp. 157 – 166.

Pubols, B.H. and Benkich, M.E. (1986) Relations between stimulus force, skin displacement, and discharge characteristics of slowly adapting Type I cutaneous mechanoreceptors in glabrous skin of squirrel monkey hand. *Somatosens. Res.,* 4: 111 – 125.

W. Hamann and A. Iggo (Eds.)
Progress in Brain Research, Vol. 74
© 1988 Elsevier Science Publishers B.V. (Biomedical Division)

CHAPTER 31

Sensory receptors in a mammalian skin – nerve in vitro preparation

Peter W. Reeh*

II. Physiologisches Institut der Universität Heidelberg, Neuenheimer Feld 326, D-6900 Heidelberg, FRG

Introduction

Recently, a preparation has been published which provides single fiber recording from sensory afferents of excised rat skin kept 'outside down' under superfusion in an organ bath (Reeh, 1986). Like other in vitro techniques in somatosensory research, it improves experimental control over the environmental conditions in the tissue (King et al., 1976; Kumazawa and Mizumura, 1983; Kieschke and Mense, 1984; Sharkey and Cervero, 1986). In addition, the exposure of the corium side of the skin gives direct access to the nerve fibers and endings avoiding the diffusion barriers of epidermis or vascular walls. This aroused new interest in the chemical excitability of sensory and especially of nociceptive endings.

However, preserving the innervation, skin can only be subcutaneously dissected producing a tissue layer of considerable thickness. The long diffusion distances could impair the oxygen supply of superficially or even intraepidermally located endings. Moreover, the surgical trauma of the skin excision could pathologically change the receptive properties. This was to be feared since a partial isolation of skin flaps has been reported to induce excessive activity and sensitization to heat in the C fibers (Perl, 1976). To dispel such doubts, comparisons were drawn between in vitro and previous in vivo findings of our group with regard to mechano – heat-sensitive ('polymodal') C fibers (Fleischer et al., 1983; Reeh et al., 1986, 1987; Handwerker et al., 1987; Kocher et al., 1987).

Methods

The methods of the skin – nerve in vitro preparation and examination have previously been described in detail and will only briefly be summarized here (Reeh, 1986).

The rat saphenous nerve and hind paw skin innervated by that nerve were subcutaneously excised and mounted 'outside down' in an organ bath. This was perfused with carbogen-saturated 'synthetic interstitial fluid' (SIF, Bretag, 1969) at a temperature of 32°C; 36°C was only used in experiments involving bradykinin (according to Kumazawa and Mizumura, 1983; Kumazawa et al., 1987). Natural and electrical stimulations were applied to single fiber receptive fields localized in the exposed corium side of the skin. This involved probing with a blunt glass rod for delineation of the receptive fields and probing with calibrated von Frey bristles for determination of the mechanical thresholds. Controlled radiant heat stimulation with a halogen lamp was applied using a perspex cone for heat transduction across the aqueous layer over the skin. For cold and chemical stimulation metal rings were placed on the recep-

---

* Present address: Institut für Physiologie und Biokybernetik, Universitätsstr. 17, D-8520 Erlangen, FRG.

tive fields ('RF chamber') and filled with defined test solutions. In the bradykinin (BKN) experiments these RF chambers were separately perfused with gassed SIF and, once in 10 min, this perfusion was switched for 1 min to nano- or micromolar BKN solutions. In some experiments the BKN solutions were stained with Evans blue (0.1%) and light extinction across the RF chamber was measured with a photodiode to establish the time course of the BKN concentration change (see Fig. 3).

Further methodical details are reported in the Results section where needed.

Results

A random sample ($n = 24$) of mechano–heat-sensitive C fibers (MH-C) was taken from previous in vivo experiments on saphenous afferents in order to compare with in vitro data from fibers ($n = 24$) of the same sensory category.

In both types of experiments the *conduction velocities* were measured in the same part of the saphenous nerve. They ranged between 0.6 and 1.3 m/s in vivo (mean 0.9 m/s) and between 0.45 and 0.8 m/s in vitro (mean 0.66 m/s); both distributions were approximately gaussian. The slower

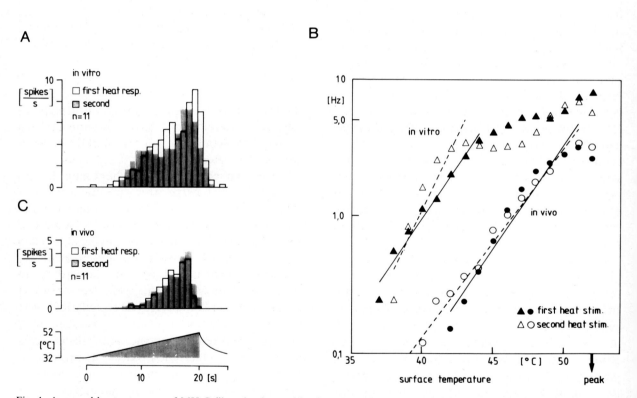

Fig. 1. Averaged heat responses of MH-C fibers in vivo and in vitro. In each part of the figure responses to first and second heat stimulation (5 min later) are compared. (A) Radiant heat was applied and controlled at the corium side of the saphenous skin in vitro; average spike density histograms. (B) Spike rate (log)-to-temperature function as derived from histograms in A and C treated by a 'running average' procedure. Regression lines are computed from thresholds to peak discharge in vivo respectively to a comparable spike rate in vitro. (C) Radiant heat was applied and controlled at the epidermal surface of the saphenous skin in vivo; average spike density histograms.

mean conduction in vitro may be due to a lower temperature and to a certain shrinkage of the excised nerve which leads to an underestimation of its actual length.

The *mechanical (von Frey) thresholds* ranged from 3 to 160 mN in vivo (mean 22.7 mN) and from 1 to 40 mN in vitro (mean 24.9 mN). The threshold distributions were almost congruent though the variability was much less in vitro than in vivo; about 70% of the MH-C fibers in vitro had von Frey thresholds of 20 or 40 mN. This is probably due to the homogeneous support of the skin flap (silicon rubber) in contrast to the inhomogeneity of underlying tissue in vivo (bone, tendon, muscle, fat).

None of the 24 MH-C fibers in both samples initially showed *ongoing activity*. After strong mechanical probing or constant pressure stimulation 10 fibers in vitro and eight fibers in vivo developed irregular firing which did not exceed 20 spikes/min and ceased within 3 min. Also heat stimulation occasionally induced transient low-frequency discharges in vivo as well as in vitro.

The comparison between the *heat responses* of the MH-C fibers was complicated by the fact that higher intracutaneous temperatures were reached in vitro than in vivo, although the radiant heat stimulation was the same, a ramp-shaped heating from 32 to 52°C in 20 s. In vitro, these temperatures were actually reached inside the skin where the thermocouple for feedback control was located, whereas in vivo the stimulus temperature was measured and controlled at the epidermal surface, being actually much lower inside the skin (Reeh, 1986). This led, on average, to a considerably stronger heat response in vitro than in vivo (Fig. 1): the number of spikes per heat stimulus and the maximal discharge rate were higher and the threshold was lower. Nevertheless, on average, there were no typical signs of sensitization to heat which would be a peak discharge at lower than maximal stimulus temperature (as shown in Fig. 2) and a change in slope of the log spike rate-to-temperature function (Reeh et al., 1986; Kocher et al., 1987). In a comparable range

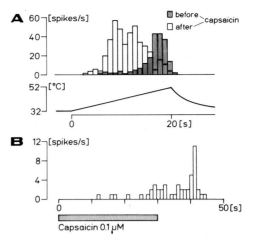

Fig. 2. MH-C fiber sensitization to heat by capsaicin in vitro. (A) Single fiber responses to radiant heat stimulation before and 4 min after capsaicin application; spike density histograms. (B) Single fiber response to application of capsaicin (in SIF) at threshold concentration into the 'receptive field chamber'. The dilution was made from a stock solution of 1% (32.74 mM) capsaicin (Merck) and 1% ethanol in SIF.

of mean discharge rates this slope was almost the same in vitro as in vivo (Fig. 1B), and the maximal mean firing frequency coincided with the peak temperature. A further similarity between the MH-C fibers in vivo and in vitro can be seen in the fact that, on average, there was no change in heat responsiveness from the first heat stimulation to the second (Fig. 1) which is typical for the rat (Lynn and Carpenter, 1982; Fleischer et al., 1983).

In contrast to heat, *chemical excitation* by bradykinin or capsaicin (Fig. 2) regularly produced a prominent sensitization to heat in vitro. Vice versa, heat stimulation produced a sensitization to bradykinin (BKN) in MH-C fibers (Fig. 3). This effect cannot be related to the temperature dependency of the BKN sensitivity shown in visceral nociceptors (Kumazawa and Mizumura, 1983; Kumazawa et al., 1987), since the short heat stimulation in our experiments was applied at least 3 min before the subsequent BKN superfusion. Noxious heat stimulation might, however, release prostaglandins and serotonin. These substances were shown to exist in human burn blister fluid

274

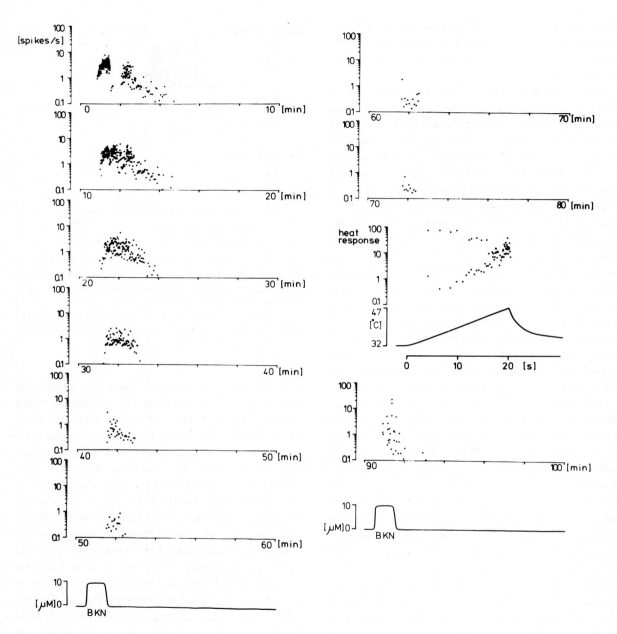

Fig. 3. MH-C fiber responses to bradykinin and sensitization by heat. Nine consecutive single fiber responses to perfusion of the 'receptive field chamber' with bradykinin (BKN – 2HCl in SIF) demonstrating the typical tachyphylaxis which was partially reversed by heat stimulation (at 82 min). Note the log instantaneous discharge frequency plot which displays the linear increase of the spike rate during the rise of intracutaneous temperature and the high intra-burst firing frequency of the fiber. Radiant heat stimulation in this experiment was applied to the epidermal side of the receptive field but controlled at the corium side.

(Johansson, 1960; Arturson et al., 1973).

In a recent series of in vitro experiments we examined the *interaction of BKN* with other hormones by superfusing the receptive fields of MH-C fibers with them at the end of the washing period between two consecutive BKN applications. Noradrenaline (0.1 μM for 2 min) was ineffective, prostaglandin E_2 (1 μM for 5 min) weakly effective and serotonin (1 μM for 2 min), like heat stimulation, was highly effective in increasing the subsequent responses to BKN. In these experiments only serotonin was able to excite some of the MH-C fibers; its sensitizing action, however, also occurred without a prior excitatory effect. As shown for example in Fig. 3, the sensitization was not sufficient to compensate for the regular tachyphylaxis to repeated BKN stimulation. This led to a progressive — on average exponential — loss of response magnitude and to a prolongation of the latency. Even 30 min of washout did not let the BKN excitability recover.

Discussion

Regarding MH-C fibers, polymodal nociceptors, cutaneous sensory afferents in vitro displayed all properties of their receptor class known from single fiber studies in the intact animal. They conducted action potentials in a comparable range of velocities, they had similar mechanical (von Frey) thresholds and they showed a fundamentally similar heat sensitivity in spite of some complication in comparing in vivo with in vitro findings. It is mainly the heat responsiveness which verifies the competence of polymodal nerve fibers in nociception since only these afferents are able to encode tissue-damaging temperatures (Beck et al., 1974). In vitro, the discharge frequencies of MH-C fibers followed an intracutaneous temperature increase up to 52°C which corresponds to an epidermal temperature close to 60°C (Reeh, 1986). The related logarithmic temperature function (Fig. 1B) showed a distinct bend between 44 and 45°C (intracutaneous) approaching the peak temperature with a smaller slope. Such a bend has not been

reported from rabbit experiments in vivo employing epidermal peak temperatures up to 60°C (Lynn, 1979). This range had not yet been investigated in the rat.

Ongoing activity without prior stimulation to the receptive field and a progressive loss of physical excitability in cutaneous sensory afferents have been reported to indicate the time-dependent limits of another in vitro preparation, the isolated perfused rabbit ear (King et al., 1976; Perl, 1976). In our superfused skin preparation such limits became apparent about 8 – 9 h after excision if the organ bath was kept at 36°C; they were not reached within up to 12 h if the temperature was 32°C.

Ongoing activity and abnormally low heat thresholds in MH-C fibers have been reported to occur in partially isolated skin flaps and even when a nick injury was applied close to receptive fields (Perl, 1976; Fitzgerald, 1979). These and other signs of sensitization did not occur in completely isolated skin under superfusion in the organ bath. It is generally accepted that nociceptor sensitization is due to a number of yet incompletely known, diffusible substances which are locally released from nerve endings and from damaged cells and which enter injured tissue by plasma extravasation and immigration of blood cells. After complete isolation of the skin, blood flow and cell destruction stop and accumulated sensitizing agents could be washed out by the superfusion. By that, posttraumatic sensitization could subside until the first single fiber of the experiment is on the recording electrode.

One more argument for a normal and not pathologically increased sensitivity of polymodal nociceptors in vitro is derived from the finding that appropriate chemicals, capsaicin and bradykinin, could induce a marked sensitization to heat, as they do in intact skin (Handwerker, 1976; Kenins, 1982). This and related previous evidence gradually gives an understanding of the thermal hyperalgesia in inflamed or injured tissue (see Campbell and Meyer, 1986 for review; Reeh et al., 1986; Kumazawa et al., 1987). Still there is, however, no clue as to the biochemical mechanism of the even more prominent mechanical hyperalgesia, a probable source of chronic pain. In vitro techniques in nociceptor physiology might help to overcome this lack of knowledge.

Acknowledgements

I gratefully acknowledge the cooperation of J. Cop, Dr. E. Lang and A. Novak and I thank Prof. H.O. Handwerker for many valuable discussions. This research was supported by DFG Grants HA 831/9-3 and -4.

References

Arturson, G., Hamberg, M. and Jonnson, C. (1973) Prostaglandins in human burn blister fluid. *Acta Physiol. Scand.*, 87: 270–276.

Beck, P.W., Handwerker, H.O. and Zimmermann, M. (1974) Neuronal outflow from the cat's foot during noxious radiant heat stimulation. *Brain Res.*, 67: 373–386.

Bretag, A. (1969) Synthetic interstitial fluid for isolated mammalian tissue. *Life Sci.*, 8: 319–329.

Campbell, J.N. and Meyer, R.A. (1986) Primary afferents and hyperalgesia. In: T.L. Yaksh (Ed.), *Spinal Afferent Processing*. Plenum, New York, pp. 59–81.

Fitzgerald, M. (1979) The spread of sensitization of polymodal nociceptors in the rabbit from nearby injury and by antidromic stimulation. *J. Physiol. (London)*, 297: 207–216.

Fleischer, E., Handwerker, H.O. and Joukhadar, S. (1983) Unmyelinated nociceptive units in two skin areas of the rat. *Brain Res.*, 267: 81–92.

Handwerker, H.O. (1976) Influences of algogenic substances and prostaglandins on the discharges of unmyelinated cutaneous nerve fibers identified as nociceptors. In: J.J. Bonica and D. Albe-Fessard (Eds.), *Advances in Pain Research and Therapy*. Raven Press, New York, pp. 41–45.

Handwerker, H.O., Anton, F. and Reeh, P.W. (1987) Discharge patterns of afferent cutaneous nerve fibers from the rat's tail during prolonged noxious mechanical stimulation. *Exp. Brain Res.*, 65: 493–504.

Johansson, S.A. (1960) 5-Hydroxytryptamine in burns. *Acta Physiol. Scand.*, 48: 126–131.

Kenins, P. (1982) Responses of single nerve fibres to capsaicin applied to the skin. *Neurosci. Lett.*, 29: 83–88.

Kieschke, J. and Mense, S. (1984) The use of a nerve-muscle preparation for studying nociceptors in vitro. *Pain*, Suppl. 2: 6.

King, J.S., Gallant, P., Myerson, V. and Perl, E.R. (1976) The effects of anti-inflammatory agents on the responses and the sensitization of unmyelinated (C) fiber polymodal nociceptors. In: Y. Zotterman (Ed.), *Sensory Functions of the Skin in Primates*. Pergamon Press, Oxford, pp. 441–454.

Kocher, L., Anton, F., Reeh, P.W. and Handwerker, H.O. (1987) The effect of carrageenan-induced inflammation on the excitability of unmyelinated skin nociceptors in the rat. *Pain*, 29: 363–373.

Kumazawa, T. and Mizumura, K. (1983) Temperature dependency of the chemical responses of the polymodal receptor units in vitro. *Brain Res.*, 278: 305–307.

Kumazawa, T., Mizumura, K. and Sato, J. (1987) Thermally potentiated responses to algesic substances of visceral nociceptors. *Pain*, 28: 255–264.

Lynn, B. (1979) The heat sensitization of polymodal nociceptors in the rabbit and its independence of the local blood flow. *J. Physiol. (London)*, 287: 493–507.

Lynn, B. and Carpenter, S.E. (1982) Primary afferent units from the hairy skin of the rat hind limb. *Brain Res.*, 238: 29–45.

Perl, E.R. (1976) Sensitization of nociceptors and its relation to sensation. In: J.J. Bonica and D. Albe-Fessard (Eds.), *Advances in Pain Research and Therapy*. Raven Press, New York, pp. 17–28.

Reeh, P.W. (1986) Sensory receptors in mammalian skin in an in vitro preparation. *Neurosci. Lett.*, 66: 141–146.

Reeh, P.W., Kocher, L. and Jung, S. (1986) Does neurogenic inflammation alter the sensitivity of unmyelinated nociceptors in the rat? *Brain Res.*, 384: 42–50.

Reeh, P.W., Bayer, J., Kocher, L. and Handwerker, H.O. (1987) Sensitization of nociceptive cutaneous nerve fibers from the rat's tail by noxious mechanical stimulation. *Exp. Brain Res.*, 65: 505–512.

Sharkey, K.A. and Cervero, F. (1986) An in vitro method for recording single unit afferent activity from mesenteric nerves innervating isolated segments of rat ileum. *J. Neurosci. Methods*, 16: 149–156.

W. Hamann and A. Iggo (Eds.)
Progress in Brain Research, Vol. 74
© 1988 Elsevier Science Publishers B.V. (Biomedical Division)

CHAPTER 32

Regeneration of retinal ganglion cell axons in adult mammals

Kwok-Fai So

Department of Anatomy, Faculty of Medicine, University of Hong Kong, Hong Kong

Introduction

In lower vertebrates including goldfish (Grafstein, 1986) and amphibians (Sperry, 1944), the axons of retinal ganglion cells regerenate vigorously after damage. Regrowth of optic axons across a lesion site has also been observed after damaging these axons in early postnatal hamsters (So et al., 1981; Schneider et al., 1985) or young rats (Gan and Harvey, 1986; Harvey et al., 1986). The situation is, however, quite different for adult mammals. For example, transection of the optic nerve (Kiernan, 1985a; Richardson et al., 1982) or optic tract (Yu et al., 1987) in adult rodents led to retrograde degeneration of optic axons (Kiernan, 1985a; Richardson et al., 1982) and cell death in retinal ganglion cell layers (Grafstein and Ingoglia, 1982; Misantone et al., 1984). The RNA content of axotomized neurons in the rat fell after optic nerve or tract lesion (Barron et al., 1985). Some of the cut axons display an abortive regenerative response before retrograde degeneration (Kiernan, 1985a; Ramón y Cajal, 1928; Richardson et al., 1982). But no optic axon has been observed to cross the lesion site and a conditioning lesion does not apparently induce regeneration of these axons (Kiernan, 1985b). However, limited regrowth of retinal axons has been observed within the adult mouse retina after discrete damage in the retina (McConnell and Berry, 1982; Goldberg and Frank, 1980).

Since the retinal projection is especially suited for anatomic, physiologic and molecular studies of central nervous system (CNS) regeneration, we are interested to find out if this failure of regeneration of retinal ganglion cell axons in adult mammals is due to an intrinsic inability of the cell to regenerate extensively in response to damage or is due to some other extrinsic factors. For example, the CNS environment might not be favorable for the regeneration of retinal axons. In order to test this hypothesis, we have carried out a series of experiments in which a new external environment is provided to the damaged optic axons by transplanting segments of peripheral nerve into the eye of adult rats (So and Aguayo, 1985) or hamsters (So et al., 1986).

Our results show that the peripheral nerve system (PNS) environment is favorable for supporting extensive regrowth of axons from retinal ganglion cells which had been axotomized. Undamaged ganglion cells do not seem to sprout into the graft. In addition to supporting the growth of the retinal axons, the peripheral nerve grafts seem to play an active role in attracting and/or guiding the damaged ganglion cell axons to grow into them. The fastest regrowing axons are found to grow into the graft about 4 days after transplantation and they regenerate at about 2 mm/day in the graft. Electrophysiological studies indicate that some of these retinal axons in the graft appear, at least temporarily, to maintain or resume ability to respond to light. We shall elaborate on these points in the following sections of this paper.

Extensive regrowth of axons into PNS graft from axotomized retinal ganglion cells

The new environment for the optic axons is provided by transplanting a segment of autologous sciatic nerve of about 2 cm length into the retina via a lesion made in the superior temporal quadrant of the eye of adult rats or hamsters (Fig. 1). The remainder of the graft is blind-ended and laid subcutaneously over the skull. One month later, horseradish peroxidase (HRP) is applied to the stump (Fig. 2A) to retrogradely label neurons which have extended axons into the graft (rat: So and Aguayo, 1985; hamster: So et al., 1986; Xiao and So, 1986). The labelled cells are all retinal ganglion cells and they are distributed within pie-shaped areas peripheral to the sites of grafting (Fig. 2B), their number being greater for grafts near the optic disc than for those in the outer portions of the retina. Other types of neurons in the retina do not seem to send axons into the graft, suggesting that different types of retinal neurons might react differently to PNS grafts.

To establish whether the fibers in the graft represent regenerative outgrowth from axotomized neurons or collateral sprouts from uninjured neurons which still retain their axons in the optic tract, we have traced the cells of origin of the retinal projections to the graft and to the optic tract, with two different fluorescent retrograde labels. If the axons in the graft are collateral sprouts from uninjured neurons which still retain their axons in the optic tract, we should be able to detect double labelled neurons after application of the cytoplasmic label True Blue (TB) to the graft and Nuclear Yellow (NY) to the contralateral or ipsilateral optic tract. In all our experiments in rats (So and Aguayo, 1985) or hamsters (Xiao and So, 1986), we have not observed any cell containing both fluorescent dyes suggesting that the axons in the graft orginate from neurons whose axons have been damaged.

The demonstration that damage of CNS fibers seems to be a prerequisite for graft innervation might explain why only ganglion cells in the retina send axons into the graft since the other types of cells in the retina do not possess an axon and therefore would not be axotomized by the grafting procedure. The finding that only axotomized neurons send axons into the graft might also ex-

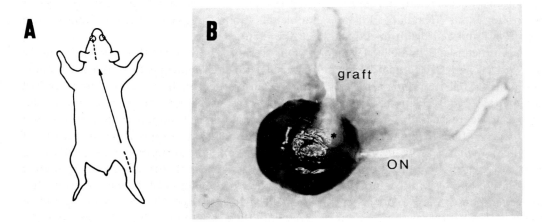

Fig. 1. (A) Schematic diagram illustrating the experimental paradigm of transplantation of a segment of sciatic nerve into the retina. (B) Photograph of an eye from a hamster showing the optic nerve (ON) and the graft. The star (*) denotes the insertion site of the graft. (From So et al., 1986.)

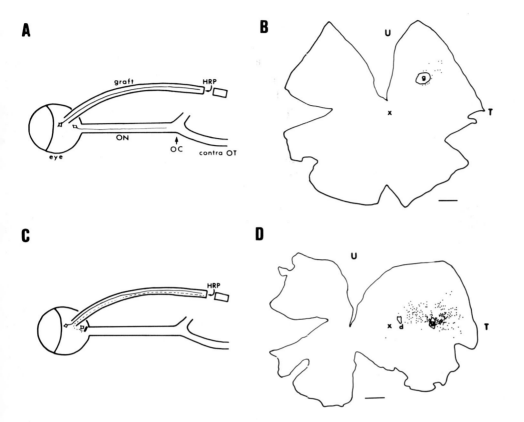

Fig. 2. (A) Schematic diagram illustrating a retrograde horseradish peroxidase (HRP) labelling experiment in animals with a segment of sciatic nerve transplanted to the left eye. ON, optic nerve; OC, optic chiasm; contra OT, contralateral optic tract. (B) Diagram of retinal whole mount of a hamster from the experiment illustrated in A. Black dots are HRP-labelled neurons; g, graft; U, upper retina; T, temporal retina; x, optic disk. Scale bar, 1 mm. (C) Schematic diagram illustrating retrograde HRP labelling experiment in animal with PNS graft plus additional damage (black bar) in the retina. (D) Diagram of a retinal whole mount of a hamster from the experiment illustrated in C. d, additional damage in the retina. Other abbreviations as in B. Note the HRP-labelled neurons (black dots) are also found in areas of the retina between the graft and optic disk. Scale bar, 1 mm. (From So et al., 1986.)

plain in part why in previous experiments many of the neurons regenerating axons into the peripheral nerves grafted into other parts of the CNS are located in areas that their axons pass through or in areas that are close to the site of graft transplantation (Aguayo, 1986).

Retinal ganglion cells of different sizes are capable of regenerating axons into the graft (Fig. 3). In addition, there is evidence suggesting that there is an increase in cell diameter (So and Aguayo, 1985) or area (Xiao and So, 1986) of these regenerating neurons (Fig. 3B), a phenomenon which has been observed in the retinal ganglion cells of fish after axotomy (Grafstein, 1986).

Using the HRP retrograde labelling method, we have studied the rate of regrowth of retinal ganglion cell axons regenerating in PNS graft (Cho and So, 1987). Our results show that the fastest regrowing retinal axons grow into the peripheral nerve about 4 days after grafting and their rate of regeneration in the graft is about 2 mm/day. This rate is similar to the growth rate of developing retinal axons in prenatal rats (1.9 – 2.4 mm/day, Lund and Bunt, 1976) and hamsters (1.4 – 1.9

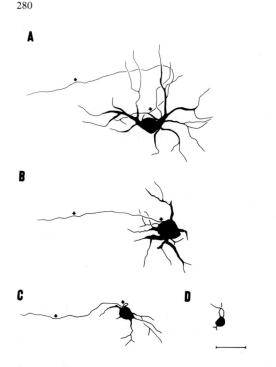

Fig. 3. Morphology of four HRP-labelled retinal ganglion cells which have sent axons into the graft in a hamster. A is a large, C medium, and D small neuron. B is a retinal ganglion cell with an extra-large soma. Arrows point to axons. Scale bar, 50 μm.

mm/day, Jhaveri et al., 1983) but is much slower than the rate of regenerating peripheral axons in adult mammals (4.4 ± 0.2 mm/day, Forman and Berenberg, 1978). This suggests that the intrinsic factors operating in the retinal ganglion cell bodies might be important in controlling the rate of regrowth of axons.

Active role of the PNS graft in attracting and/or guiding damaged ganglion cell axons

The graft in the retina seems to play an active role in attracting and/or guiding the regenerating axons to grow into it rather than playing a passive role in the sense that it intercepts cut ganglion cell axons located peripheral to the graft which are trying to grow towards the direction of the optic disc. We reach this conclusion after studying the response of ganglion cells whose axons would not normally be

intercepted by the graft (So et al., 1986). At the same time as the transplantation of the graft into the eye, an additional lesion is placed in the retina between the location of the insertion of the graft and the optic disc (Fig. 2C). The results of retrograde HRP labelling experiments show that, in addition to the labelled cells situated peripheral to the graft, a population of labelled neurons located between the graft and the optic disc is also observed (Fig. 2D). The positive effect is demonstrated if the lesion is placed at 1.5 mm from the site of grafting. There is no effect if the lesion is placed 3 mm away suggesting that it is a distance-dependent phenomenon. The mechanisms underlying the attracting and/or guiding role of the grafted peripheral nerve are not clear at the moment. The PNS nerve could secrete a diffusible chemical into the environment to attract the damaged axons (Richardson and Ebendal, 1982; Skene and Shooter, 1983). On the other hand, it is also possible that Schwann cells and/or other types of cells might migrate from the graft into the retina thus providing a substrate to guide the axons to grow into the graft (Williams et al., 1983). Our recent in vitro experiments of co-culturing a segment of PNS nerve and a strip of retina from adult hamsters seem to suggest that a diffusible substance is being released by the PNS nerve to modify the direction of growth of the regenerating axons from the ganglion cells (Liu and So, unpublished experiments). However, we cannot rule out the possibility that Schwann or other types of cells might still play a guiding role in the in vivo situation.

In in vivo experiments, only a small population of retinal ganglion cells grows into the graft. The maximum number of cells observed is about 15% of the axotomized neurons (So and Aguayo, 1985). Thus, the trophic substance released from the PNS graft does not seem to affect the whole population of axotomized retinal ganglion cells in the same way. Or alternatively, most of the damaged axons have retracted too far away from the site of injury and grafting and therefore would not be influenced by the trophic substance released from the graft.

Functional properties of regenerating retinal ganglion cell axons

After discovering that damaged retinal axons regenerate extensively in PNS graft, it is important to find out what are their functional properties. Thus, we have carried out physiologic experiments to study the responses to light of injured regenerated retinal neurons by recording the unitary electrical activity of their axons in blind-ended peripheral nerve graft in rats (Keirstead et al., 1985) and hamsters (Diao et al., 1986). Light-responsive units are observed and some of them have discharge properties very similar to those of normal animals (Diao et al., 1986; Keirstead et al., 1985). For example, 'on', 'off' and 'on – off' units have all been encountered (Keirstead et al., 1985). However, in the rat, in which the response of the regenerating retinal ganglion cell axons has been monitored for 9 – 48 weeks post grafting, it is discovered that the number of light-responsive units declined over time suggesting perhaps that the PNS environment cannot maintain the functional integrity of these regenerating axons forever (Keirstead et al., 1985). This might be due to a gradual dying of retinal axons in the graft or a gradual disruption of the local circuitry of the regenerating ganglion cells in the retina.

Units with abnormally large receptive fields have also been observed (Diao et al., 1986; Keirstead et al., 1985). This might suggest that there is a reorganization or disorganization of local circuitry of the regenerating ganglion cells with the other types of neurons in the retina.

The ability of regenerating retinal ganglion cell axons to enter and form synaptic connections in target sites

In order to investigate if regenerating retinal axons can enter and form synaptic connections with their normal targets, the PNS graft is used to connect the retina and superior colliculus (SC). Two months after grafting a PNS nerve of 4 cm length into the retina of the rat, the ipsilateral optic tract is completely transected and the other end of the graft is inserted into the ipsilateral SC. One month later HRP is injected into the grafted eye to trace the growth of the regenerating fibers. Labelled axons are observed to grow the entire length of the graft but they stop growing at the interface of the graft and SC. Thus, no labelled axon has been observed to terminate in the SC (So, unpublished experiments). However, after inserting the PNS graft into the optic disk, more axons have been observed to regenerate into the graft and when the other end of this graft is inserted into the SC in the rat (Vidal-Sanz et al., 1987), a few labelled axons have been observed to grow up to 0.5 mm beyond the graft – target interface and labelled synaptic contacts in the SC have also been found. However, it is important to rule out the possibility that these labelled axons might have come from other sources, e.g., ciliary ganglion cells. The axons of these PNS neurons might have grown into the graft and entered the SC since they might have been damaged at the time of grafting. These PNS cells can take up HRP which might have been leaked from the eye during or after HRP injection. Further work is needed to clarify this issue.

General comments

Our results seem to suggest that the external environment surrounding the axons of the damaged retinal ganglion cells is important in determining whether the injured axons would regenerate or not. Abortive sprouting is observed after retinal axons are damaged in matured animals (Kiernan, 1985a, b; Richardson et al., 1982). The ability of this sprouting response to develop into an extensive regrowth might depend on a critical balance of facilitatory and inhibitory factors in the local environment of the CNS.

The facilitatory factors could be the nerve growth factor (Levi-Montalcini, 1983) or other growth-related substances (Richardson and Ebendal, 1982; Skene and Shooter, 1983; Varon et al., 1983) and the degenerating CNS myelin might contribute to the inhibitory factors (Berry, 1982).

Thus, the peripheral nerve seems to be able to provide the damaged retinal axons with facilitatory growth factors (Liu and So, unpublished experiments; Richardson and Ebendal, 1982; Skene and Shooter, 1983). However, after extensive regrowth in this conducive environment, the retinal axons are not able to reinnervate the targets in matured mammals which presumably have more inhibitory than facilitatory growth factors. Thus, the identification of these factors and the use of them to promote extensive but appropriate reconnection of damaged CNS axons of adult mammals remain challenging problems in neurology.

Acknowledgements

The research of the author is supported by grants from the Croucher Foundation and the University of Hong Kong.

References

Aguayo, A.J. (1986) Regenerative capacities of nerve cells in the central nervous system. In: A.K. Asbury, G.M. McKhann and W.I. McDonald (Eds.), *Diseases of the Nervous System. Clinical Neurobiology, Volume 1.* Heinemann Medical, London, pp. 98 – 108.

Barron, K.D., McGuinness, C.M., Misantone, L.J., Zanakis, M.F., Grafstein, B. and Murray, M. (1985) RNA content of normal and axotomized retinal ganglion cells of rat and goldfish. *J. Comp. Neurol.,* 236: 265 – 273.

Berry, M. (1982) Post-injury myelin-breakdown products inhibit axonal growth: an hypothesis to explain the failure of axonal regeneration in the mammalian central nervous system. In: M. Berry (Ed.), *Bibliotheca Anatomica No. 23, Growth and Regeneration of Axons in the Nervous System.* Karger, Basel, pp. 1 – 11.

Cho, E.Y.P. and So, K.-F. (1987) Rate of regrowth of retinal ganglion cell axons regeneration in a peripheral nerve graft in adult hamsters. *Brain Res.,* 419: 369 – 374.

Diao, Y.-C., Xiao, Y.-M. and So, K.-F. (1986) Retinal ganglion cells regenerating axons into peripheral nerve graft in adult hamsters can respond to light. *Science Bull.,* 16: 1280.

Forman, D.S. and Berenberg, R.A. (1978) Regeneration of motor axons in the rat sciatic nerve studied by labelling with axonally transported radioactive proteins. *Brain Res.,* 156: 213 – 225.

Gan, S.K. and Harvey, A.R. (1986) Lack of ingrowth of retinal axons into the visually deafferented superior colliculus in young rats: a horseradish peroxidase study. *Neurosci. Lett.,* 70: 10 – 16.

Goldberg, S. and Frank, B. (1980) Will central nervous systems in the adult mammal regenerate after bypassing a lesion? A study in the mouse and chick visual systems. *Exp. Neurol.,* 70: 675 – 689.

Grafstein, B. (1986) The retina as a regenerating organ. In: R. Adler and D.B. Farber (Eds.), *The Retina: A Model for Cell Biology Studies, Part II.* Academic Press, New York, pp. 275 – 335.

Grafstein, B. and Ingoglia, N.A. (1982) Intracranial transection of the optic nerve in adult mice: preliminary observations. *Exp. Neurol.,* 76: 318 – 330.

Harvey, A.R., Gan, S.K. and Dyson, S.E. (1986) Regrowth of retinal axons after lesions of the brachium and pretectal region in the rat. *Brain Res.,* 368: 141 – 147.

Jhaveri, S., Edwards, M. and Schneider, G. (1983) Relation of lateral geniculate neuron migration to stages of optic tract growth in the hamster. *Soc. Neurosci. Abstr.,* 9: 702.

Keirstead, S.A., Vidal-Sanz, M., Rasminsky, M., Aguayo, A.J., Levesque, M. and So, K.-F. (1985) Responses to light of retinal neurons regenerating axons into peripheral nerve grafts in the rat. *Brain Res.,* 359: 402 – 406.

Kiernan, J.A. (1985a) Axonal and vascular changes following injury to the rat's optic nerve. *J. Anat.,* 141: 139 – 154.

Kiernan, J.A. (1985b) A conditioning lesion does not induce axonal regeneration in the optic nerve of the rat. *Exp. Neurol.,* 87: 181 – 184.

Levi-Montalcini, R. (1983) The nerve growth factor-target cells interaction: a model system for the study of directed axonal growth and regeneration. In: A. Giuffrida-Stella, R. Perez-Polo and B. Haber (Eds.), *Birth Defects: Original Article Series,* Vol. 19, No. 4. Alan R. Liss, New York, pp. 3 – 22.

Lund, R.D. and Bunt, A.H. (1976) Prenatal development of central optic pathways in albino rats. *J. Comp. Neurol.,* 165: 247 – 264.

McConnell, P. and Berry, M. (1982) Regeneration of ganglion cell axons in the adult mouse retina. *Brain Res.,* 241: 362 – 365.

Misantone, L.J., Gershenbaum, M. and Murray, M. (1984) Viability of retinal ganglion cells after optic nerve crush in adult rats. *J. Neurocytol.,* 13: 449 – 465.

Ramón y Cajal, S. (1928) *Degeneration and Regeneration of the Nervous System* (R.M. May, Trans.). Hafner Press, New York, reprint 1957.

Richardson, P.M. and Ebendal, T. (1982) Nerve growth activities in rat peripheral nerve. *Brain Res.,* 246: 57 – 64.

Richardson, P.M., Issa, V.M.K. and Shemie, S. (1982) Regeneration and retrograde degeneration of axons in the rat optic nerve. *J. Neurocytol.,* 11: 949 – 966.

Schneider, G.E., Jhaveri, S., Edwards, M.A. and So, K.-F. (1985) Regeneration, re-routing, and redistribution of axons after early lesions: changes with age, and functional impact. In: J. Eccles and M.R. Dimitrijevic (Eds.), *Recent Achieve-*

ment in Restorative Neurology 1: Upper Motor Neuron Functions and Dysfunctions. Karger, Basel, pp. 291 – 310.

Skene, P.J.H. and Shooter, E.M. (1983) Denervated sheath cells secrete a new protein after nerve injury. *Proc. Natl. Acad. Sci. USA,* 80: 4169 – 4173.

So, K.-F. and Aguayo, A.J. (1985) Lengthy regrowth of cut axons from ganglion cells after peripheral nerve transplantation into the retina of adult rats. *Brain Res.,* 328: 349 – 354.

So, K.-F., Schneider, G.E. and Ayres, S. (1981) Lesions of the brachium of the superior colliculus in neonate hamsters: correlation of anatomy with behavior. *Exp. Neurol.,* 72: 379 – 400.

So, K.-F., Xiao, Y.-M. and Diao, Y.-C. (1986) Effects on the growth of damaged ganglion cell axons after peripheral nerve transplantation in adult hamsters. *Brain Res.,* 377: 168 – 172.

Sperry, R.W. (1944) Optic nerve regeneration with return of vision in anurans. *J. Neurophysiol.,* 7: 57 – 69.

Varon, S., Manthorpe, M., Longo, F.M. and Williams, L.R. (1983) Growth factors in regeneration of neural tissues. In: F.J. Seil (Ed.), *Nerve, Organ and Tissue Regeneration: Research Perspectives.* Academic Press, New York, pp. 127 – 156.

Vidal-Sanz, M., Bray, G.M., Villegas-Perez, M.P., Thanos, S. and Aguayo, A.J. (1987) Axonal regeneration and synapse formation in the superior colliculus by retinal ganglion cells in the adult rat. *J. Neurosci.,* 7: 2894 – 2909.

Williams, L.R., Longo, F.M., Powell, H.C., Lunborg, G. and Varon, S. (1983) Spatial-temporal progress of peripheral nerve regeneration within a silicone chamber: parameters for a bioassay. *J. Comp. Neurol.,* 218: 460 – 470.

Xiao, Y.-M. and So, K.-F. (1986) Ganglion cells regenerating axons into peripheral nerve graft transplanted into the retina of adult hamsters. *Neurosci. Lett.,* Suppl., 25: S21.

Yu, E., So, K.-F. and Tay, D. (1987) Retrograde degeneration of the optic fibres following axotomy in the optic tract in the hamster. *Neurosci. Lett.,* Suppl., 28: S33.

W. Hamann and A. Iggo (Eds.)
Progress in Brain Research, Vol. 74
© 1988 Elsevier Science Publishers B.V. (Biomedical Division)

CHAPTER 33

Morphology and response characteristics of the cercus-to-giant interneuron system in locusts to low-frequency sound

Shen Jun-Xian and Xu Zhi-Min

Institute of Biophysics, Academia Sinica, Beijing, People's Republic of China

Summary

This study, using intracellular recording and injection with the Lucifer Yellow technique, reveals the morphology of the cercus-to-giant interneuron system and response characteristics to low-frequency sound in *Locusta migratoria*. The system consists of four bilateral pairs of identifiable giant interneurons (GIs $1-4$), which receive inputs from the mechanoreceptive hair sensilla on the cerci. We describe here the dendritic branching pattern of each GI, the pattern of projection of the cercal sensory nerve, and the overlap of the cercal projections with the dendrites of the GIs. The position of the soma and the locations and orientations of the major processes are characteristic for each GI. The cercal sensory afferents respond with tonic firing to sound stimuli. The GIs show different patterns of spike discharge by sound stimulation. The GIs 1 and 4 display phasic responses and fire only one spike to each sound stimulus. The lowest thresholds of GI1 and GI4 in terms of air particle displacement are ca. 0.15 μm and 0.4 μm respectively. GI2 is excited with tonic firing by low-frequency sound and has a frequency − threshold relationship like that of the cercal sensory nerve. Spike count of GI2 per stimulus is related to stimulus cycle, intensity and duration. These results indicate that the GIs in the
locust play a role in information processing and transmission of low-frequency sound.

Introduction

Many investigations on the cercus-to-giant interneuron system in insects have suggested that the system can mediate, at least in part, three behavioral complexes: (1) presence of a predator (escape reaction of cockroaches, Camhi et al., 1978; Camhi, 1980); (2) flight activity (Ritzmann et al., 1980, 1982); (3) intraspecific communication (Kämper and Dambach, 1979).

Recent advances in single cell staining and recording techniques have made the extensive study of the system unusually accessible (Mendenhall and Murphey, 1974; Murphey et al., 1977; Daley et al., 1981; Shen, 1983), and the analysis of the functional role of the system in animal behavior at the cellular level possible (Ritzmann and Camhi, 1978; Westin and Ritzmann, 1982; Comer, 1985; Kämper, 1985; Ritzmann and Pollack, 1986).

However, a detailed description of the morphology of all four pairs of giant interneurons (GIs) in the terminal abdominal ganglion of the locust does not exist (Cook, 1951; Seabrook, 1971; Boyan et al., 1986). This morphological information would be particularly useful. Thus, the aim of our study is to explore the anatomical organization

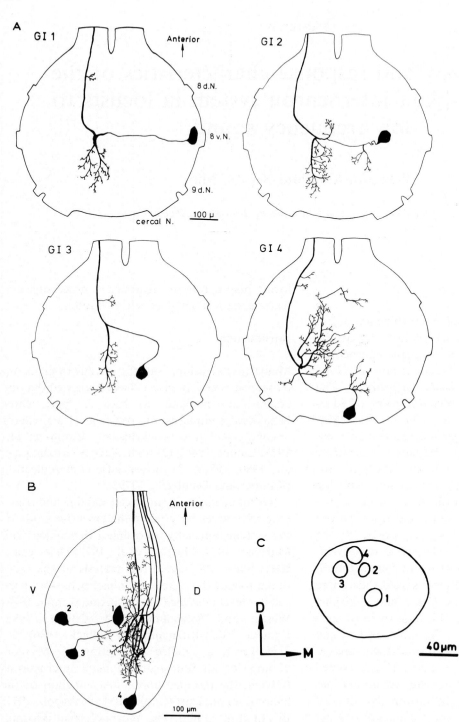

Fig. 1. Morphology of GIs 1 – 4 in the terminal abdominal ganglion. Each cell is represented in whole mount. Camera lucida drawings based on 24 preparations. (A) GIs viewed dorsally, anterior is at the top. (B) Drawing of left GIs viewed from the right side. D, dorsal; V, ventral. (C) Diagram of a cross section of the one-side connective anterior to the terminal ganglion showing characteristic positions and numbering of the GIs. D, dorsal; M, medial.

of the cercus-to-giant interneuron system, the overlap of projections of cercal nerve with the dendritic fields of the GIs, and the basic principles of information processing and transmission in the GIs. In this paper we describe the morphology of the system in the locust *Locusta migratoria* and response characteristics to low-frequency sound

Materials and methods

Intracellular recordings and stainings were obtained from the single GIs and cercal sensory afferents in the terminal abdominal ganglion of adult males or females of *Locusta migratoria* L.

The methods used throughout this paper were the same as those used in our previous study (Shen, 1983).

Results

The morphology of the giant interneurons

Visualization of the GIs and cercal sensory afferent projection was accomplished by intracellular iontophoretic injection with Lucifer Yellow after collecting physiological data from the identified neurons. An extracellular axonal backfilling with cobalt was used to compare the spatial organization of the GIs with that revealed by Lucifer Yellow filling.

Fig. 1A illustrates the dorsal views of the structure of the left GIs 1 – 4 in the terminal abdominal ganglion, which are reconstructed from a total of 24 whole mount preparations with a camera lucida. The left GIs are defined as those whose axons run in the left connectives of the ventral nerve cord. Fig. 1B shows the right-side view of the organization of the left four GIs.

Each GI arises from a single cell body. Comparisons of the same GI in different preparations show that the position of the soma and the locations and orientations of the major processes are characteristic for each GI. All the somata of the GIs are contralateral to their ascending axons. The soma of GI1 (ca. 35 μm in diameter) is located far

to the side of the ganglion contralateral to its axon and lies midway between the dorsal and ventral surfaces of the ganglion close to the root of ventral nerve 8. The somata of GIs 2 and 3 (ca. 35 – 40 μm in diameter) are located close to the ventral surface of the ganglion. From dorsal views, the soma of GI2 is located in the middle of the equator of the right half of the ganglion, whereas the soma of GI3 is located near the middle of the posterior contralateral quadrant of the ganglion. The soma of GI4 (ca. 40 μm in diameter) is situated more medially and along the posterior edge (see also Fig. 1B for soma positions of all GIs).

GIs 2 and 4 have relatively small contralateral branches and these are located on the initial process. Each of the GIs 1, 2 and 3 has a major ipsilateral process directed posteriorly and large dendritic arborization, whereas GI4 has two major ipsilateral processes directed anteriorly and larger dendritic arborization, even projecting across the midline of the ganglion and into the contralateral neuropil. In contrast, we have seen no branches extending from the dendritic field of GIs 1, 2 or 3 over the contralateral side of the ganglion. All the dendritic arborizations of the GIs lie dorsally in the ganglion (Fig. 1B). In addition, GIs, 1, 3 and 4 have medially directed axon collaterals, which are well anterior to the large dendritic fields, whereas GI2 has no collaterals in this region.

In the cord, the ascending axons of GIs 2, 3 and 4 (ca. 10 μm for GI2, ca. 15 μm for GIs 3 and 4 in diameter) constitute the dorsal group of the giant fibers, whereas the axon of the GI1 (ca. 18 μm in diameter) is located in the middle of the connective, as viewed from cross section of the connective on leaving the terminal ganglion (Fig. 1C).

The projections of the cercal nerve

The projections of the cercal sensory afferents were investigated with intracellular recording and staining techniques. One example of a single cercal sensory axon, which responds to low-frequency sound with tonic burst discharge, is shown in Fig. 2A. The cercal afferent, as a discrete fiber, enters

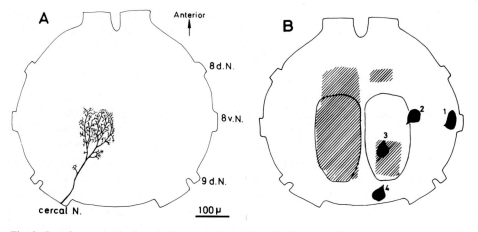

Fig. 2. Cercal nerve projections in the terminal ganglion. (A) Drawing of the projection of a single cercal sensory afferent fiber made from the negatives. (B) Overlap between cercal nerve projections and the dendritic fields of the GIs. Outlined areas: left and right cercal projections shown by drawing oulines of a left cercal field and its mirror image. Slanted areas: ipsilateral and contralateral dendritic fields of left GIs are from the morphological drawings of identified GIs. Soma positions of left GIs are shown.

medially-directed the terminal ganglion and forms a large but well-defined ipsilateral arborization. By cobalt backfilling the projections of the unilateral cercal nerve within the terminal ganglion were investigated and the gross outline of the projections is shown in Fig. 2B in solid line. There is a high degree of overlap between the cercal sensory afferent projections (left and right) and both ipsi- and contralateral dendritic fields of the left GIs.

Response characteristics of the GIs to sound

The responses of identified giant interneurons, which receive inputs from mechanoreceptive hair sensilla on the cerci, studied by intracellular recording during stimulation of the cerci with low-frequency sound, reveal basic principles of information processing and transmission of the GI system in the locust.

On the basis of the time course of discharges in the responses of the GIs to low-frequency sound stimulation, the identified cells fall grossly into two types: tonic and phasic. Tonic firing describes the discharge of a burst of spikes with a duration equal to the stimulus duration or longer, in response to stimulus application. Phasic firing

means that usually only one spike, rarely two, is excited by each stimulus. In this study, we have found that GIs 1 and 4 and, with qualifications, GI3 in the locust respond with a phasic pattern of spike discharge to sound stimulation. GI2 is excited with tonic firing by low-frequency sound.

The frequency – threshold relationships of GIs 1, 2 and 4 and of the cercal sensory afferents are demonstrated in Fig. 3. GIs 1 and 4 have

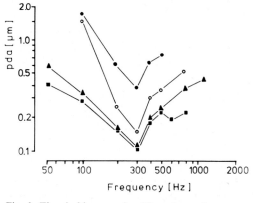

Fig. 3. Threshold curves for GIs and cercal sensory nerve. Ordinate: air particle displacement amplitude (pda) (in μm). Abscissa: sound frequency (in Hz). Open circles: GI1; filled triangles: GI2; filled circles: GI4; filled squares: cercal sensory nerve.

characteristic filter properties and show a clear maximum of sensitivity at 300 Hz with the lowest threshold of 0.15 μm and 0.4 μm, respectively. The effectively responding frequency range is 100 – 800 Hz for GI1 and 100 – 500 Hz for GI4. GI2 has a broad-band characteristic curve, like that of the cercal sensory nerve, and is sensitive to sound stimulation in the range between 50 and 800 Hz. The maximum of sensitivity for GI2 is also at 300 Hz with threshold of ca. 0.1 μm.

When different frequencies of sound stimulation (e.g., 50, 80, 100 and 200 Hz) with the same duration and displacement amplitude were used to the cerci, GI2 discharged frequency-dependent spikes: the spike count excited at lower frequency is always less than that at higher frequency. The intervals between consecutive spikes reproduce the stimulus cycle (Fig. 4A). It appears that there is a certain coupling of spikes of GI2 to stimulus cycle. Furthermore, GI2 discharges increasing spike numbers per stimulus as the stimulus intensity in-

creases (Fig. 4B). It shows an approximately linear relationship between particle displacement amplitude and spikes per stimulus.

Discussion

The morphology of the cercus-to-giant interneuron system in the locust has been described by intracellular injection with Lucifer Yellow and axonal backfilling with cobalt. The anatomical description provides a detailed map of the dendritic fields and soma positions of the GIs within the terminal ganglion. Many of the response properties of the system to low-frequency sound have been determined.

The present finding indicates that all the GIs have extensive ipsilateral dendritic fields and some GIs have relatively small contralateral branches as well. The ipsilateral overlap between the dendritic fields of GIs and projections of the cercal nerve is larger than the contralateral overlap. All the morphological arrangements show that the GIs receive stronger excitatory inputs from the ipsilateral cercus than from the contralateral cercus. Thus, the morphology of the GIs agrees well with the physiologically observed laterality of excitatory inputs (also see Boyan et al., 1986).

The GIs of the locust are here classified as tonic or phasic type in terms of their characteristic pattern of spike discharge to sound stimulation. But the response pattern of some GIs could be varied under certain particular conditions. For instance, we have observed that the phasic interneuron (GI1 or GI4) is able to discharge some more spikes with a limited duration instead of one or two spikes per stimulus, when sound intensity increases greatly or when a short sound pulse is replaced by a long and strong puff of wind. The alternation of discharge pattern of the GI may result from the temporal and spatial integration of excitatory inputs in the GI.

As mentioned above, the responses of the tonic interneuron reflect not only stimulus frequency and duration with interspike intervals and firing duration, but also stimulus intensity with spike count per stimulus. Therefore, the tonic in-

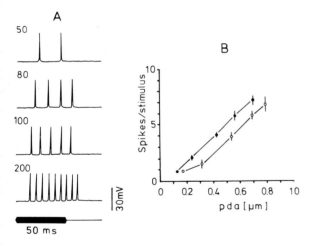

Fig. 4. Frequency and intensity characteristics for tonic interneuron GI2. (A) Responses of GI 2 to stimuli at four frequencies. For 50, 80 and 100 Hz spike intervals correspond to stimulus cycle. The number on the left of each record is stimulus frequency in Hz. (B) Intensity characteristic for GI2. Ordinate: spikes per sound stimulus. Abscissa: air particle displacement amplitude (pda). Filled circles: at 300 Hz; open circles; at 200 Hz. Mean and standard deviations; $n = 5$.

terneuron is well suited to transmit information on sound frequency, intensity and duration. The phasic interneuron may play a role in signalling the onset of sound stimulation (e.g., the approach of a predator) and in transferring information on amplitude-modulated organization of sound (e.g., species-specific song).

It appears from the frequency – threshold relationships of the GIs that the GIs have low-frequency bandpass properties with high sensitivity. But it is quite mysterious that some GIs are most sensitive to sound around 300 Hz. To date the importance of such a spectral component in insect behaviour is still unknown.

Acknowledgements

This work was supported by the Ministerium für Wissenschaft und Forschung, NordRhein-Westfalen, FRG (Heinrich-Hertz-Stiftung B 42 264/80 and 365/81) and by Sonderforschungsbereich 'Bionach SFB 114'.

References

Boyan, G.S., Ashman, S. and Ball, E.E. (1986) Initiation and modulation of flight by a single giant interneuron in the cercal system of the locust. *Naturwissenschaften,* 73: 272 – 274.

Camhi, J.M. (1980) The escape system of the cockroach. *Sci. Am.,* 243: 158 – 172.

Camhi, J.M., Tom, W. and Volman, S. (1978) The escape behavior of the cockroach *Periplaneta americana.* II. Detection of natural predators by air displacement. *J. Comp. Physiol.,* 128: 203 – 212.

Comer, C.M. (1985) Analyzing cockroach escape behavior with lesions of individual giant interneurons. *Brain Res.,* 335: 342 – 346.

Cook, P.M. (1951) Observations on the giant fibres of the nervous system of *Locusta migratoria.* Q. J. Microsc. Sci., 92: 297 – 305.

Daley, D.L., Vardi, N., Appignani, B. and Camhi, J.M. (1981) Morphology of the giant interneurons and cercal nerve projections of the American cockroach. *J. Comp. Neurol.,* 196: 41 – 52.

Kämper, G. (1985) Processing of species-specific low-frequency song components by interneurons in crickets. In: K. Kalmring and N. Elsner (Eds.), *Acoustic and Vibrational Communication in Insects.* Paul Parey, Berlin, pp. 169 – 176.

Kämper, G. and Dambach, M. (1979) Communication by infrasound in a non-stridulating cricket. *Naturwissenschaften,* 66: 530.

Mendenhall, B. and Murphey, R.K. (1974) The morphology of cricket giant interneurons. *J. Neurobiol.,* 5: 565 – 580.

Murphey, R.K., Palka, J. and Hustert, R. (1977) The cercus-to-giant interneuron system of crickets. II. Response characteristics of two giant interneurons. *J. Comp. Physiol.,* 119: 285 – 300.

Ritzmann, R.E. and Camhi, J.M. (1978) Excitation of leg motor neurons by giant interneurons in the cockroach *Periplaneta americana. J. Comp. Physiol.,* 125: 305 – 316.

Ritzmann, R.E. and Pollack, A.J. (1986) Identification of thoracic interneurons that mediate giant interneuron-to-motor pathways in the cockroach. *J. Comp. Physiol.,* 159: 639 – 654.

Ritzmann, R.E., Tobias, M.L. and Fourtner, C.R. (1980) Flight activity initiated via giant interneurons of the cockroach: evidence for bifunctional trigger interneurons. *Science,* 210: 443 – 445.

Ritzmann, R.E., Pollack, A.J. and Tobias, M.L. (1982) Flight activity mediated by intracellular stimulation of dorsal giant interneurons of the cockroach *Periplaneta americana. J. Comp. Physiol.,* 147: 761 – 781.

Seabrook, W.D. (1971) An electrophysiological study of the giant fiber system of the locust *Schistocerca gregaria. Can. J. Zool.,* 49: 555 – 560.

Shen, J.-X. (1983) The cercus-to-giant interneuron system in the bushcricket *Tettigonia cantans:* morphology and response to low-frequency sound. *J. Comp. Physiol.,* 151: 449 – 459.

Westin, J. and Ritzmann, R.E. (1982) The effect of single giant interneuron lesions on wind-evoked motor responses in the cockroach, *Periplaneta americana. J. Neurobiol.,* 13: 127 – 139.

W. Hamann and A. Iggo (Eds.)
Progress in Brain Research, Vol. 74
© 1988 Elsevier Science Publishers B.V. (Biomedical Division)

Mechanoreceptors and Structural Aspects of Receptor Function: Summary

L. Kruger

Dr. Bannister's account of the fine structure of cochlear outer hair cells and their response to injury elicited comments largely focused on the subcisternal membrane complex, which was compared (by Dr. Flock) to the T tubule-sarcoplasmic reticulum of muscle. The crucial role of calcium in regulating phosphatidyl inositol metabolism in motile cells raised questions related to other models of cell injury, including the mitochondrial changes seen in Merkel cells subjected to antibiotic damage and concomitant changes in organelle density and the number of presumed calcium particles.

Dr. Halata's presentation of electron micrographs of Ruffini endings from a wide variety of tissues and species raised a question concerning the definition of Ruffini endings and whether it was now being extended beyond its original definition. Dr. Halata indicated that the definition was indeed based upon the fine structure of Ruffini terminals, according to the suggestions of Dr. Munger and his colleagues, and did not refer to the corpuscles of the original descriptions by Ruffini. Although there undoubtedly are species differences, such as the hair bending slowly adapting type 2 (SA2) discharge associated with Ruffini endings in primates (noted by Dr. Iggo), the differences appear to be basically in number and in size, at least in those species examined by Dr. Halata (mainly cat, pig, monkey and man), and the range of findings is consistent with the description in cat dermis by Chambers et al. An explanation of the orientation-specific stretch sensitivity of SA2 (i.e., Ruffini) endings was offered in terms of orienta-

tion asymmetry in corpuscles, but Dr. Halata felt that the 'polarization' problem raised could not be accounted for by mechanical properties of a collagen collar that is essentially unstretchable.

Dr. Linden's presentation, dealing with sensitive mechanoreceptor innervation of the periodontal ligament and the perturbations resulting from tooth removal and/or bone damage, was discussed principally in terms of technical factors relevant to sample size in such nerve recordings or to accidental nerve damage in such surgical procedures. The suggestion by Dr. W. Hamann that the innervation patterns might be determined by horseradish peroxidase transport is currently under active investigation in Dr. Linden's laboratory.

Tooth innervation by intrapulpal thin sensory fibers was presented by Dr. Kniffki and questions were raised concerning their spectrum. Dr. Munger reported Turner's unpublished observations on monkey tooth revealing that unmyelinated (C) fibers were largely absent except for some vascular endings. It was also suggested that there may be two classes of C fibers, including a range with a conduction velocity of $1.2 - 3$ m/s that might be thinly myelinated, but this would not fit with the distinct unimodal distribution noted by Dr. Kniffki. Technical factors of monopolar C fiber stimulation were discussed in relation to some apparently discrepant findings.

Dr. Lisney's presentation on reinnervation patterns of polymodal nociceptors revealed by dye-labeled plasma extravasation patterns elicited questions concerning the categories of thin fibers that might be implicated in plasma extravasation, especially whether nociceptors other than 'polymodals' are involved. He emphasized that a sample of one fiber per experiment precluded facile generalization. Dr. Diamond reported his experience that in reinnervation, the expansion of receptive fields for heat nociceptors and the zone of plasma dye extravasation matched nicely. The role of anesthesia, mast cell granule depletion, the number of thin fibers lacking substance P, and the specialization of vascular peptide receptor binding sites were discussed as relevant factors in relating electrophysiological properties to vascular response.

This was followed by a broader discussion of thin sensory fiber patterns, presented by Dr. Kruger, in relation to sites with specialized nociceptor innervation. Arguments concerning the nature of the non-peptidergic axons labeled for fluoride-resistant acid phosphatase (FRAP) by an indirect method centered on the large number of such small sensory ganglion cells and their purported selective dorsal horn localization pattern, which is not easily reconciled with patterns of dorsal horn selectivity revealed by electrophysiological studies. The selection of specific regions of low innervation density for precise morphological identification of physiologically characterized receptive fields will probably prove an important factor in future fine structural studies. Dr. B. Matthews offered support for the hypothesis that nerve exerts a trophic effect on dentine formation, although this need not implicate the calcitonin gene-related peptide (CGRP) immunoreactive axons shown in dentinal tubules. A question concerning the CGRP efferents to the temporal bone elicited a brief account of findings by Dr. J. Silverman in Dr. Kruger's laboratory who, in addition to large motor fibers to stapedius and tensor tympani muscles, found thin sensory fibers to both inner and outer rows of hair cells and to vestibular epithelia. Some of these fibers can be traced from the lateral superior olivary complex.

Dr. Munger's presentation on the abnormalities of reinnervation, especially in primate skin, raised questions of how this can be reconciled with the highly differentiated patterns reported earlier by Burgess and Horch. This elicited comments based on personal experience by Dr. A. Iggo concerning the sequence of events, after crush injury, in reestablishing an SA type 1 response in reinnervated Merkel cell complexes, and a similar account by Dr. E. Perl of the remarkable recovery of C fiber innervation patterns. Dr. Munger indicated that while many aspects of reinnervation might be indistinguishable from normal, especially if sufficient time were allowed for recovery, there were distinct morphological alterations in reinnervation patterns. In the primate allografts, it was nevertheless striking that physiologically specialized afferent units could be detected in the absence of concomitant morphological specialization.

A provocative account of the importance of viscoelastic properties of the skin as a continuous sheet, in contrast to a discrete distribution of sense organs displaying regional variation, was presented by Dr. B.H. Pubols and was followed by a discussion restricted to technical factors in traveling waves and the application of two perpendicular adjacent controlled stimuli at small distances.

Dr. Reeh's account of an in vitro skin — nerve preparation raised numerous questions related to sensitization, principally the prominent heat sensitization of A-δ (but not C) fibers in rat, the possible effects of calcium antagonists, and whether the absence of effect by prostaglandin E_2 in such preparations might be explained by use of low concentrations or short exposure, although this does not appear likely from Dr. Reeh's findings to date. The relationship between calcium concentration and bradykinin elicited response was discussed by several workers. Clearly, further experiments will prove useful.

The discussion of Dr. So's presentation on retinal ganglion cell regeneration centered on the suggested use of specific fetal tissues for rescuing the graft.

Dr. Shen's presentation on the locust cercal organ led to a discussion of the possible functional role of a system tuned to a 300 Hz best frequency, and it was noted that each species possesses a distinctive tuning pattern, probably a crucial factor in mating calls. Dr. Hashimoto noted that workers in his laboratory found that the interneurons described by Dr. Shen served to sharpen the tuning curves.

Modulation and Efferent Control of Transduction

W. Hamann and A. Iggo (Eds.)
Progress in Brain Research, Vol. 74
© 1988 Elsevier Science Publishers B.V. (Biomedical Division)

CHAPTER 34

Do sensory cells in the ear have a motile function?

Åke Flock

Department of Physiology, Karolinska Institute, S-104 01 Stockholm, Sweden

Summary

In recent years auditory physiology has seen a number of challenging results which cast doubt on the traditional view of the inner ear as a passive signal analyzer.

It has been demonstrated at the light microscopic level that the apical region of cochlear hair cells contains contractile proteins. Actin has now been identified and localized by antibody labelling techniques at the electron microscopical level. Actin is found to be present also along the wall of outer hair cells, between the plasma membrane and the fenestrated cisternae, which are present here. This was confirmed by labelling with myosin S1 fragments, which further showed a circular spiralling orientation of the actin filaments. In order to investigate if outer hair cells show some form of contractile response, isolated cells were subjected to media that would induce relaxation or contraction in muscle cells. In response to Ca^{2+} + ATP, hair cells showed a significant shortening and a narrowing of diameter. These experiments were performed on cells demembranated by detergent. In intact cells electron microscopy showed that the plasma membrane is intimately associated with subsurface cisternae by membrane associated rodlets that remind of the connection between the transverse tubule system and the sarcoplasmic reticulum in skeletal muscle fibers. In muscle, the sarcoplasmic reticulum is electrically excited by the action potential to release Ca^{2+} which triggers the contractile event.

The above results lead to the following hypothesis for the function of outer hair cells in the organ of Corti: outer hair cells possess voltage-sensitive channels in the hair cell plasma membrane which interact with subsurface fenestrated cisternae. These possess a calcium release and uptake mechanism which controls the contractile state of the outer hair cells. It is suggested that outer hair cells can exhibit motor activity, which is integrated in the electro-mechanical function of the organ of Corti. Inner hair cells, lacking submembraneous actin, are suggested to have a mainly sensory function.

Introduction

In recent years general agreement has arisen that in the organ of Corti a mechanism exists which in an active mechanical way enhances the sensibility of the ear at low sound levels (Davis, 1983). Several observed phenomena have led to this conclusion. One of these is the so-called oto-acoustic emission, discovered by Kemp (1978), which is generated from the inner ear in response to a click stimulus. The nature of this emission will be more thoroughly described further on in the article. Also, Zurek (1981) has shown that 50% of the normal hearing population spontaneously produce a tone from the inner ear, which can be measured by a sensitive microphone in the external auditory meatus.

It has been shown that the muscles of the middle ear are not involved. There are, instead, indications that the generator is to be found in the organ of Corti and is an important and vulnerable part of the sensory system. It seems to be of significance for the very fine frequency selectivity in the auditory organ.

Frequency selectivity in the auditory nerve fibers is established by the mechanics of the hearing organ

In Fig. 1 a number of curves of frequency selectivity in the mechanical basilar membrane vibration pattern, when determined at rather high intensity, are compared with the sensitivity curves of individual nerve fibers. The downward sharp curves show neural data, the broad ones mechanical sen-

sitivity. An enhanced frequency selectivity is seen in the nerve fibers compared to the mechanical tuning. It was long believed that the increase was due to neural properties. However, intracellularly recordings made from inner hair cells by Russell and Sellick (1978) show a sensitivity curve strikingly similar to that of the neural data (Fig. 2).

Recordings of mechanical movements of the basilar membrane have mostly been performed at high intensities. By modern methods such recordings have been carried out at much lower sound pressure (Fig. 3). It is found that the basilar membrane selectivity is actually sharper at low intensities than at high and will decrease if the sound pressure is increased (Sellick et al., 1982). This illustrates a non-linearity in the response of the organ to mechanical stimulation. This region of most sensitive frequency selectivity is dependent on the biological situation of the organ, e.g., blood supply and normal voltage gradients within the organ of Corti. It is vulnerable and can be traumatized by noise, ototoxic antibiotics, etc. The

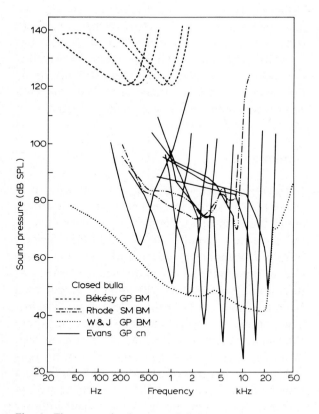

Fig. 1. The curves in the upper left hand corner show the mechanical vibration pattern of the basilar membrane. The frequency selectivity of the auditory nerve fibers is seen below (Wilson and Johnstone, 1975).

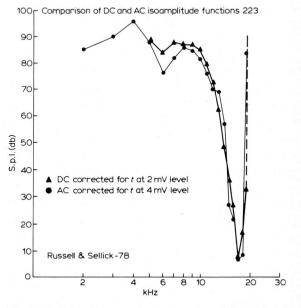

Fig. 2. The electrical response from an inner hair cell of the organ of Corti shows a very sharp frequency selectivity (Russell and Sellick, 1978).

responsible mechanism is probably also controlling the phenomenon next to be described.

Kemp's oto-acoustic emissions

Kemp (1978) described an oto-acoustic 'echo', a generated mechanical response within the organ of

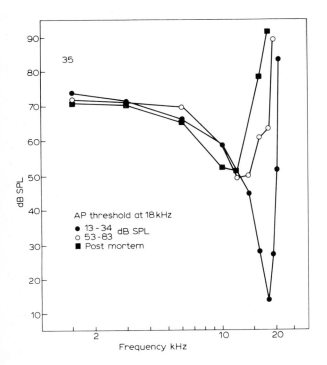

Fig. 3. At low sound pressure (13 – 34 dB) even the basilar membrane shows a sharp frequency selectivity which decreases at higher intensities (53 – 83 dB).

Corti. The experimental set-up is illustrated in Fig. 4. A click sound is delivered from a sound source in the external auditory meatus and simultaneously the sound pressure is recorded by a sensitive microphone. Fig. 5 shows to the left a recording on a model, where the tone pulse is seen followed by single resonance. To the right is a recording from a human ear showing a late reflected sound, amplified below. This sound is missing in persons with neuronal hearing loss, is unilateral and cannot be attributed to the muscles of the middle ear. The oto-acoustic emission exists also in experimental animals and shows the same non-linearity and biological sensitivity for, e.g., oxygen deficiency as the sharp frequency selectivity in the mechanical vibration pattern and in nerve fibers. Kemp suggests that the phenomenon originates from a mechanical generator in the organ of Corti, which is physiologically controlled. The activity of the mechanical generator is evidently fed back to the basilar membrane and is emitted via the acoustic ossicles and the tympanic membrane. The responsible structure is assumed to be able to produce mechanical work.

Structure of the sensory hairs

Each hair cell is equipped with approximately 100 sensory hairs, named stereocilia. We have found that they are built by the protein actin, which is also found in the muscle cells where it takes part in muscle contraction together with other proteins

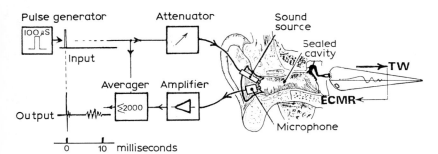

Fig. 4. Illustration of the recording principles of Kemp's oto-acoustic emission (Kemp, 1978).

300

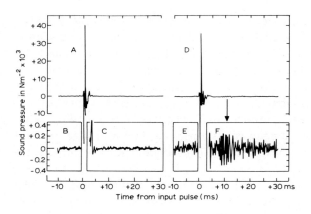

Fig. 5. To the left oto-acoustic emissions are seen in D and in high amplification in F. The measurements to the left are controls from a dummy ear (Kemp, 1978).

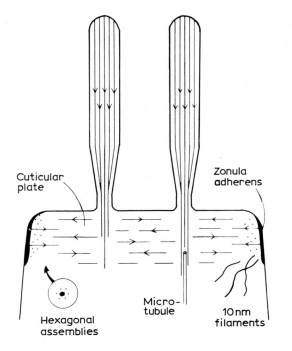

Fig. 6. The muscle protein actin is present in the apical region of hair cells. The arrows indicate their functional orientation (Flock et al., 1981).

(Flock et al., 1981). Fig. 6 shows the organization of the actin filaments as determined by electron microscopy. The filaments run parallel within the stereocilia and have rootlets extending into a plate under the cell surface, the cuticular plate. In the cuticular plate actin filaments are also present. By means of immunological methods myosin, the second filament participating in muscle contraction, has also been demonstrated. It is located in the cuticular plate.

In experiments on hair cells of the crista ampullaris of the semicircular canal we have demonstrated that the movements of the sensory hairs are slowed down in an environment that would have caused muscle contraction, while in a milieu which causes muscle relaxation the movement is unrestricted (Orman and Flock, 1983). This response may have a counterpart in the organ of Corti.

The sensory hairs of the hearing organ offer 'resistance'

By means of a thin filament made of quartz glass the stiffness of the sensory hairs of the organ of Corti has been measured (Strelioff and Flock, 1984) (Figs. 7, 8). Stiffness values were found to vary with position along the coils in accordance with frequency location. Also, measures were obtained in two opposite directions; on the one hand in the direction giving increased impulse activity in the auditory nerve fibers, on the other hand in the opposite inhibitory direction. It was found, surprisingly, that the sensory hairs offer twice the resistance to displacement in the excitatory direction. This can be interpreted as if the sensory hairs offer 'resistance', maybe as a result of an active muscle-like mechanism. Possibly, the sensory hairs can 'kick back' in synchrony with a tone, as if pushing the swinging pendulum of a clock. Such a mechanism may amplify the mechanical movements of the organ of Corti at low sound pressures and also be responsible for Kemp's 'echo'. This hypothesis meets a difficulty in that it is hard to understand how such a mechanism could work synchronously at such high frequencies as are required in the hearing organ. However, it is known that flight muscles of insects can work at several thousand Hz; hair cells can of course have access to a private type of rapid 'muscle'.

It is thus possible that the active mechanism in the inner ear is located in the sensory hairs and in their capacity for mechanical work. If so, we should look at the sensory hairs for the sensitive link which is vulnerable and can be damaged in

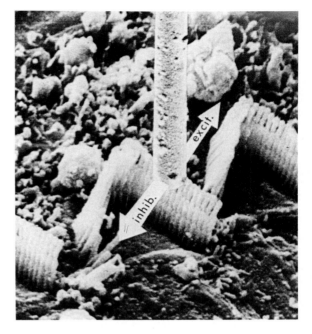

Fig. 8. The filament is 1 μm thick and is pushed against the parallel rows of sensory hairs in the excitatory or inhibitory direction.

connection with certain types of hearing impairment.

Contractility in the outer hair cells

In experiments already mentioned light microscopy was used to identify contractile proteins. Labelling techniques for identification at the electron microscopical level have now also been used (Flock et al., 1986). Actin was found to be present not only in the sensory hair region but also along the wall of the outer hair cells, between the plasma membrane and fenestrated cisternae, which are present here (Figs. 9, 10).

In order to investigate if outer hair cells also show some form of contractile response involving the sensory hairs, isolated cells were subjected to media that would induce relaxation or contraction in muscle cells. In response to Ca^{2+} + ATP, hair cells showed, much to our surprise, a significant shortening and a narrowing of diameter (Flock et

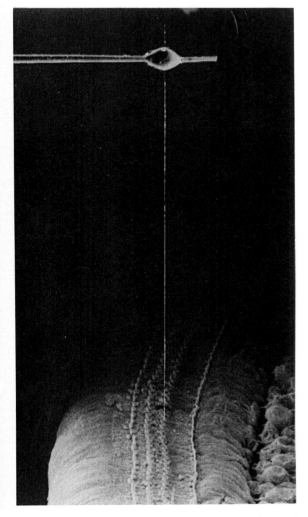

Fig. 7. The mechanical properties of the sensory hairs can be measured by a thin filament of quartz glass which is pressed against the hairs displacing them 1 μm. The bending of the filament is a measure of hair stiffness (Strelioff and Flock, 1984).

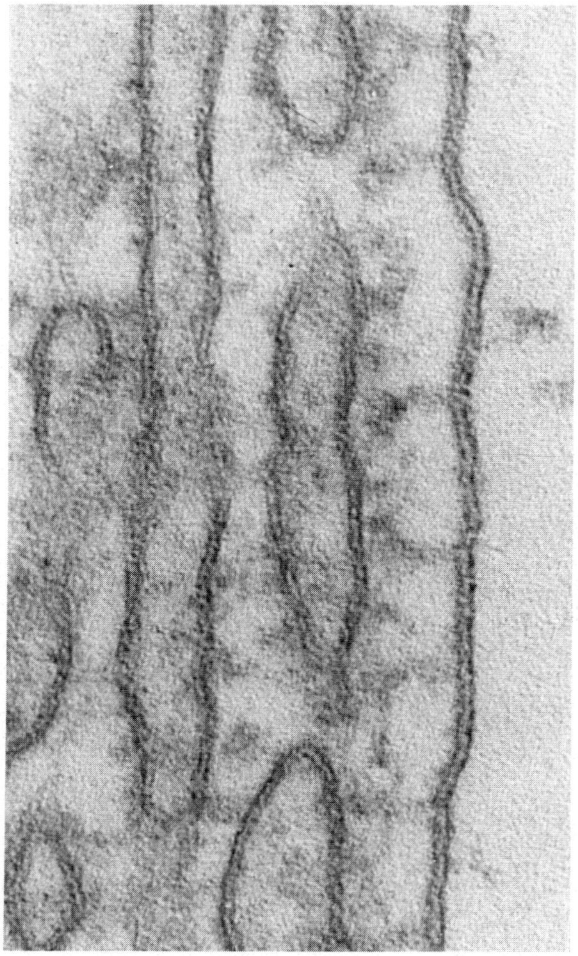

Hair cells can also respond to electrical current applied extra- or intracellularly (Brownell et al., 1985). This movement is fast and can follow several thousand Hz (Ashmore, 1987). It therefore seems that outer hair cells can exhibit different forms of motor activity, which is integrated in the electro-mechanical function of the organ of Corti. Inner hair cells, lacking submembraneous actin, are suggested to have a mainly sensory function.

Fig. 9. Membrane-bound cisternae are present beneath the outer hair cell membrane. They are connected to the cell membrane by pillar-like structures (Flock et al., 1986).

al., 1986) (Fig. 11). These experiments were performed on cells demembranated by detergent. In intact cells electron microscopy showed that the plasma membrane is intimately associated with subsurface cisternae by membrane associated rodlets that remind of the connection between the transverse tubule system and the sarcoplasmic reticulum in skeletal muscle fibers (Fig. 9). The sarcoplasmic reticulum is electrically excited by the muscle action potential to release Ca^{2+} which triggers the contractile event.

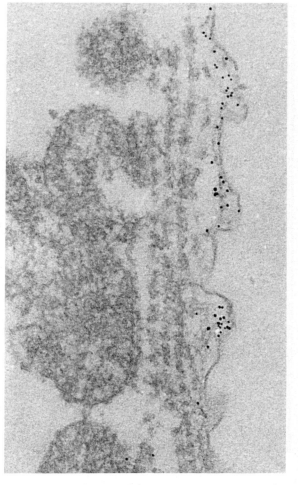

Fig. 10. Colloidal gold particles (black dots) mark the presence of actin at the wall of outer hair cells (Flock et al., 1986).

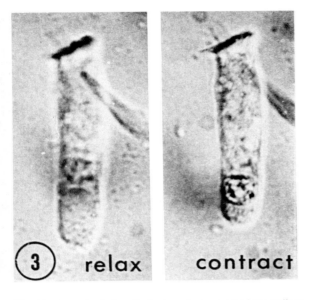

Fig. 11. An outer hair cell shortens in a contraction medium (Flock et al., 1986).

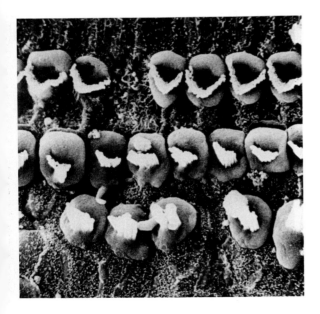

Fig. 12. In waltzing guinea-pigs with hereditary deafness there is a defect in the cytoskeleton.

A deficiency of the actin system in congenital hearing impairment

Ernstson (1972) showed in the late 60s that so-called waltzing guinea-pigs are affected by increasing hearing impairment in parallel with changes of the sensory hair region of the sensory cells. It has been shown that this defect is associated with a deficiency in the formation of actin in the sensory cells during embryological development (Sobin and Flock, 1981). In the hearing organ this is expressed as a swelling of the cell surface as if it loses mechanical stability (Fig. 12). It is therefore of interest to investigate by biochemical methods if these cells lack some cross-linking protein. Here we can, perhaps, see the beginning of clinical relevance.

References

Ashmore, J.F. (1987) A fast motile response in guinea-pig outer hair cells: the cellular basis of the cochlear amplifier. *J. Physiol. (London)*, 388: 323 – 347.

Brownell, W.E., Bader, C.R., Bertrand, D. and de Ribaupierre, Y. (1985) Evoked mechanical responses of isolated cochlear hair cells. *Science*, 227: 194 – 196.

Davis, H. (1983) An active process in cochlear mechanics. *Hear. Res.*, 9: 79 – 90.

Ernstson, S. (1972) Cochlear physiology and hair cell population in a strain of the waltzing guinea pig. *Acta Otolaryngol.*, Suppl., 297: 1 – 24.

Flock, Å., Cheung, H.C., Flock, B. and Utter, G. (1981) Three sets of actin filaments in sensory cells of the inner ear. Identification and functional orientation determined by gel electrophoresis, immunofluorescence and electron microscopy. *J. Neurocytol.*, 10: 133 – 147.

Flock, Å., Flock, B. and Ulfendahl, M. (1986) Mechanisms of movement in outer hair cells and a possible structural basis. *Arch. Otorhinolaryngol.*, 99: 83 – 90.

Kemp, D.T. (1978) Stimulated emissions from within the human auditory system. *J. Acoust. Soc. Am.*, 64: 1386 – 1391.

Orman, S. and Flock, Å. (1983) Active control of sensory hair mechanics implied by susceptibility to media that induce contraction in muscle. *Hear. Res.*, 11: 261 – 266.

Russell, I.J. and Sellick, P.M. (1978) Intracellular studies of hair cells in the guinea pig cochlea. *J. Physiol. (London)*, 284: 261 – 290.

Sellick, P.M., Patuzzi, R. and Johnstone, B.M. (1982) Measurement of basilar membrane motion in the guinea pig

304

using the Mossbauer technique. *J. Acoust. Soc. Am.,* 72: 131 – 141.

Sobin, A. and Flock, Å. (1981) Sensory hairs and filament rods in vestibular hair cells of the waltzing guinea pig. *Acta Otolaryngol.,* 91: 247 – 254.

Strelioff, D. and Flock, Å. (1984) Stiffness of sensory-cell hair bundles in the isolated guinea pig cochlea. *Hear. Res.,* 15: 19 – 28.

Wilson, J.P. and Johnstone, J.R. (1975) Basilar membrane and middle ear vibration in guinea pig measured by capacitive probe. *J. Acoust. Soc. Am.,* 57: 705 – 723.

Zurek, P. (1981) Spontaneous narrowband acoustic signals emitted by human ears. *J. Acoust. Soc. Am.,* 69: 514 – 523.

W. Hamann and A. Iggo (Eds.)
Progress in Brain Research, Vol. 74
© 1988 Elsevier Science Publishers B.V. (Biomedical Division)

CHAPTER 35

Measurement of intracochlear current flow

Toru Hashimoto and Ikuo Taniguchi

Institute for Medical and Dental Engineering, Tokyo Medical and Dental University, Surugadai, Kanda, Chiyoda-ku, Tokyo 101, Japan, and Medical Research Institute, Tokyo Medical and Dental University, Yushima, Bunkyo-ku, Tokyo 113, Japan

Introduction

It was generally believed that the cochlear transduction processes involved a mechanically sensitive process which caused the current flow along the hair cell to be modulated by the acoustic sound input. Since its introduction by Davis, the variable resistance theory (Davis, 1965) has played an important role in cochlear transduction theories. Davis proposed that the cochlear microphonic potential is the result of the modulation process of the intracochlear current flow by the sound-induced conductance change caused by the displacement of the hair cell cilia. The sound-induced electrical impedance change (Johnstone et al., 1966; Strelioff et al., 1972) and the changing resistance synchronized to the acoustic wave form (Geisler et al., 1977; Mountain et al., 1980) were shown to occur when hair cells were mechanically stimulated. Direct measurement of cochlear transduction current in response to hair cell displacement was tried by intracellular recording of the receptor potential (Russell and Sellick, 1978) and by the whole cell voltage clamp study of an isolated hair cell (Lewis and Hudspeth, 1983; Hudspeth, 1985) or patch clamp study (Ohmori, 1984, 1985; Holton and Hudspeth, 1986). Russell suggested the existence of constant current flow along the hair cell from the linear relationship between the resistance change and the associated potential change in response to sound stimulation. But very little is known about the intracochlear current flow

and it should play an important role in cochlear transduction processes.

The present authors attempted to measure the intracochlear current flow by applying the voltage clamp technique to the scala media of the cochlea of a guinea-pig. The cochlear microphonic (CM) current flow, which should be associated with the sound stimulus, was recorded indirectly by the feedback technique. The CM current was modified with command signal for the potential control. The sound-induced conductance change could be estimated by DC command. The sound-induced current should be the spatial summation of the transduction current of ionic channels on the stereocilia of the cochlear hair cell. By a simple electrical circuit model following Thevenin's theorem, the magnitude of the conductance change of the basilar membrane was estimated from the experimental data of the CM potential and current. By AC command signal the sound-induced current was modulated to bring about the distortion product, which was analyzed on the harmonic structure by a sound spectrograph. The sound-induced conductance change was also estimated from the spectral component of the distortion product.

For a simple method of impedance measurement the present authors developed a single electrode technique with the aid of an active bridge circuit. The injection of AC current into the scala media and the CM potential recording could be simultaneously accomplished with a single elec-

306

trode. The frequency spectrum of the CM potential was also analyzed by the sound spectrograph.

Methods

The experiments were done on guinea-pigs (body weight 250 – 350 g) under sodium pentobarbital anesthesia (30 mg/kg). The trachea was cannulated and the animal was artificially respired with a respirator after immobilizing it by an intramuscularly injected neuromuscular blocking agent. A ventral surgical approach was used to

open the bulla and expose the cochlea. A pair of small holes (25 μm in diameter) were drilled in the bony wall overlying the stria vascularis of the basal turn of the cochlea using a sharpened dental burr, ground to a very fine tip. The locations of the holes were chosen in the most accessible part of the bony wall to get into the scala media just near the basilar membrane. A nichrome wire electrode (25 μm in diameter), insulated with globular enamel except at the tip, was inserted tightly into the hole to keep the scala media from endolymph leakage. The wire was fixed to the edge of the bone of the opened

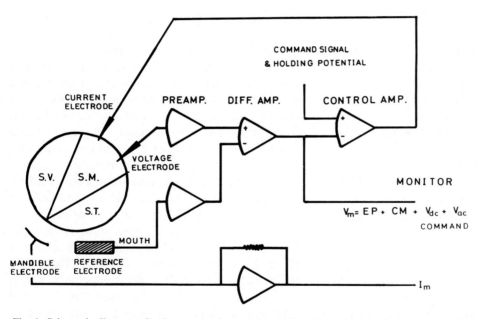

Fig. 1. Schematic diagram of voltage control experiment. The voltage clamp technique was applied to the scala media to measure the intracochlear current flow. A pair of electrodes were inserted into the scala media through small holes drilled in the bony wall overlying the stria vascularis of the basal turn of the guinea-pig cochlea. The holes were adjacent to each other in the spiral direction of the cochlear turn (200 – 300 μm apart). The voltage recording electrode was a nichrome wire electrode (25 μm in diameter) insulated with globular enamel except at the tip. The current injection electrode was a micropipette (4 – 10 μm tip in diameter). The potential of the scala media was differentially measured relative to that of the mouthpiece. The micropipette current electrode was used to supply the feedback current through the control amplifier needed to clamp the scala media potential to a fixed level or to shift the potential and maintain it at any desired level. The injected current should exactly counteract any current flow which might cause the change of the scala media potential. Therefore the intracochlear current flow could be measured indirectly by this feedback technique. On the potential monitor (V_m) the endocochlear DC potential (EP) and the cochlear microphonic (CM) potential were observed when the feedback loop was not closed, that is, in the open loop state. After closing the feedback loop, the command signals ($V_{ac} + V_{dc}$) were observed at the potential monitor. The command signals were applied to shift or control the scala media potential. On the current monitor (I_m) the injected feedback current was observed as a voltage signal through the current to voltage converter connected to the mandible current return electrode in the virtual ground mode of the voltage clamp technique. When the feedback loop was closed, I_m in the resting state was kept null by adjusting the holding potential control. Otherwise the transduction mechanism in the cochlea would be deteriorated by the steady current flow and the experiment would fail.

bulla with cyanoacrylate. The wire electrode was used to record the potential in the scala media. A glass micropipette (3 – 10 μm tip), filled with 3 M KCl, was carefully inserted into the scale media through the other hole drilled as near as possible to the hole for potential recording. The micropipette was used to inject the feedback current into the scala media to clamp the potential to a fixed level through a voltage control amplifier (Dagan: 8500). The schematic diagram of the voltage control experiment is shown in Fig. 1. A stainless steel needle electrode, inserted into the mandibular muscle, was used as the bath ground electrode for current return. The mouthpiece of the headholder of the animal was used as the reference electrode for differential recording of the scala media potential, as shown in Fig. 1. The control amplifier supplies the feedback current needed to shift the scala media potential across the basilar membrane and maintain it at the desired level following the command signal input and the holding potential setting. In response to tonal stimulation, a stimulus-associated current of several hundred nanoamperes was observed at the current monitor, which was a standard current to voltage converter on the virtual ground mode as shown in Fig. 1. This observed current can be a direct measure of ionic movement across the basilar membrane, which would be in-

duced by the conductance change in the transduction process. The feedback current flow would counter exactly any current flowing across the membrane to keep the potential constant. The transduction current could be measured indirectly in response to any sound stimulus at any potential level following the command signal.

A conical earpiece with attached earphone was fitted into the animal's left ear and a tonal stimulus was applied to the ear by the closed system. The frequency spectra of the CM potential and current were analyzed by a sound spectrograph (Bruel and Kjaer: 2010). The frequency response of the measured signal was also analyzed by the spectrograph using the furnished beat frequency oscillator.

General anesthesia was maintained with regular intraperitoneal administration of a small amount of a mixture of pentazocine and droperidol or sodium pentobarbital.

Results

The first object of the experiments was to record intracochlear current flow which would be closely related to the transduction process of sound reception. The conventionally recorded CM potential would be the electrotonic spread of the electrical

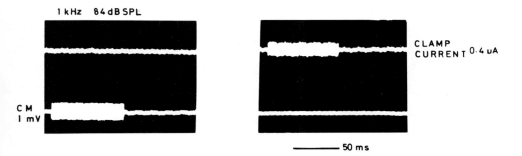

Fig. 2. Voltage clamp of scala media. Upper trace: current monitor. Lower trace: voltage monitor. The left figure is the CM potential record responding to a tone stimulus (1 kHz, 84 dB SPL) before closing the feedback loop of the voltage clamp system. The right figure is the current record corresponding to the CM potential shown in the left figure, after closing the loop of the voltage clamp system. In this situation the potential of the scala media is fixed to a resting level without regard to the tonal stimulus. The sound-induced transduction current was counteracted or compensated exactly by the injected feedback current. The observed current would be a direct measure of the intracochlear current flow which should be associated with the sound reception.

activity of the transduction process. Therefore the location of the CM generating mechanism could not be determined clearly by the potential recording method. Contrary to potential recording, the current recording method would be good for analyzing the local activity just near the recording site. The voltage clamp technique, which was applied to the scala media of the cochlea by the present authors, was developed originally to change the membrane potential in controlled steps and to record the inward or outward current flow across the membrane and analyze ionic conductance or permeability precisely. The accurate measurement of the ionic current through an ionic channel was an important result of the voltage clamp experiment.

Fig. 2 shows a result of the voltage clamp experiment performed at the scala media of the basal turn of a guinea-pig cochlea. The upper right trace was a record of the intracochlear current flow in response to a tonal stimulus (1 kHz, 84 dB sound pressure level (SPL)). The current record corresponds to the CM potential record (as shown at the lower left trace in the figure), which was observed before the feedback loop for the voltage clamp would be closed. After the feedback loop for the scala media was set up, the potential of the scala media was maintained to a fixed level, as shown by the lower right trace in the figure, regardless of the intracochlear transduction of the sound stimulus. The sound-induced intracochlear current flow was indirectly measured by the voltage clamp technique. The fixed potential was the same as that for the resting state, that is, the endocochlear potential. The intracochlear current in response to the tonal stimulus might be named the cochlear microphonic current. The ratio of the CM potential to the CM current should be defined as the impedance of the scala media, which had the value of 2.5 kΩ for the case shown in Fig. 2.

In Fig. 3 the frequency characteristics of the CM potential (upper curve) and the CM current (lower curve) are shown. They were measured by the frequency sweep of the beat frequency oscillator (BFO) synchronized with the frequency analysis of the sound spectrograph. The decline of the frequency response of the CM current at the higher frequency would be caused by the technical limita-

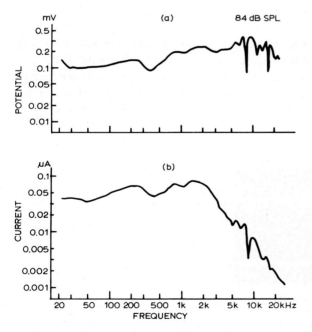

Fig. 3. Frequency response of CM potential (a) and intracochlear current flow (b). At the frequency range above 2 kHz the decline of the frequency response of the current was caused by the frequency characteristic of the loop gain of the voltage clamp system and the electrode impedance.

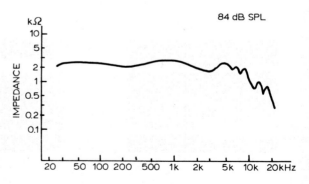

Fig. 4. Frequency characteristic of scala media impedance. The impedance was calculated from the CM potential record and the intracochlear current record shown in Fig. 3. On this calculation the frequency dependence of the loop gain and the electrode impedance were taken into consideration and the frequency characteristic of the current flow was corrected.

tion of the high frequency response of the voltage clamp feedback loop, which should be adjusted to keep the control amplifier from unwanted oscillation.

In Fig. 4 is shown the frequency characteristic of the scala media impedance measured by the voltage clamp technique in response to the sound stimulation with BFO. The impedance value at the higher frequency was appropriately corrected with consideration of the high frequency response of the loop gain of the voltage clamp system.

In Fig. 5 is shown the potential control of the scale media with DC command of positive or negative polarity. The sound-induced intra-cochlear current was increased or decreased by the scala media potential change as shown in the figure. The conductance change of the tranduction process (S_H) in response to the sound stimulus could be estimated by the measured increment or decrement (ΔI_m) of the sound-induced current as follows: $S_H = \Delta I_m / V_{dc}$, where V_{dc} is the scala media potential change following the DC command input. In the left figure S_H was estimated as $S_H = 5.7\ \mu S$. The sound-induced current (I_m) was produced by the conductance change of the transduction process and the resting scala media potential, that is, the endocochlear potential

(V_{EP}), as $I_m = V_{EP} \cdot S_H$. On the left case of the figure V_{EP} was estimated as $V_{EP} = 100$ mV.

In Fig. 6A is shown a simplified method for measurement of the interaction of the injected current with the transduction channel. This method was the improved and simplified form of the impedance measuring method by two micropipettes (Strelioff et al., 1971; Geisler et al., 1977). The constant-amplitude current (1 nA – 1 μA peak) was injected through a 10 MΩ resistor into the scala media and simultaneously the potential was recorded by the same electrode. A severe coupling problem between the recording electrode and the current injecting one in the two-micropipettes method was thoroughly cleared up with aid of the active bridge as shown in the figure. Fig. 6B shows a result of the single electrode experiment. The sound stimulus (7 kHz, 86 dB SPL) and the current injection (1.5 kHz, 0.5 μA peak) were simultaneously applied into the scala media. The interaction of the injected current with the conductance change in the scala media, induced by the sound reception, was clearly observed as the sidebands in the spectrogram of the CM potential recorded in the scala media. The sideband components of the frequencies 7 ± 1.5 kHz were the distortion components produced in the scala media

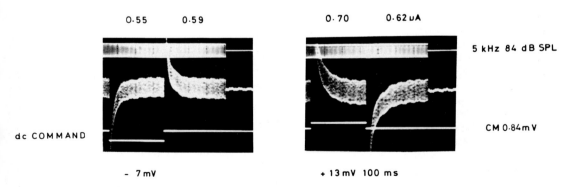

Fig. 5. Voltage clamp of scala media with DC command in response to sound stimulus. Upper trace: monitor of sound stimulus. Middle trace: intracochlear current (AC coupled). Lower trace: scala media potential. The scala media potential was controlled with the DC command of positive or negative step. The CM current was modified by the decrease (in the left figure) or increase (in the right figure) of the scala media potential. The transient rise or fall of the middle trace was brought about by the AC coupling of the oscilloscope amplifier.

of the cochlea. This would be direct evidence of the sound-induced conductance change in the transduction process.

In Fig. 7 is shown the distortion product of the CM spectrum for the sound stimulus (7.4 kHz, 76 dB SPL) and the simultaneously applied current stimulus (1.4 kHz, 0.5 μA peak). Many frequency components of conductance change present in the scala media were measured by the single electrode experiment. Those components should be pro-

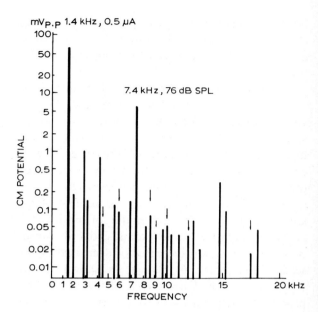

Fig. 7. Distortion products. Many frequency components of the distortion products were produced in the interaction of the CM generating mechanism with the injected current (indicated by arrows over the spectral components). The experimental setup was the same as shown in Fig. 6a. The frequency components indicated by arrows were as follows:

4.6 kHz =   7.4 − 2 × 1.4 kHz,
6   kHz =   7.4 −   1.4 kHz,
8.8 kHz =   7.4 +   1.4 kHz,
9.2 kHz = 2 × 7.4 − 4 × 1.4 kHz,
10.2 kHz =   7.4 + 2 × 1.4 kHz,
12   kHz = 2 × 7.4 − 2 × 1.4 kHz,
17.6 kHz = 2 × 7.4 + 2 × 1.4 kHz.

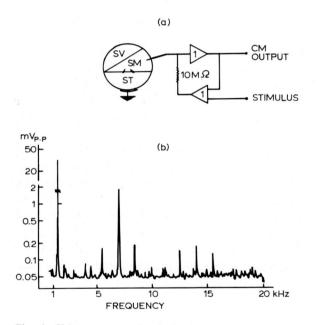

Fig. 6. CM spectrogram in single electrode experiment. (a) Schematic diagram of single electrode experiment. With the aid of the active bridge circuit a constant current was injected through 10 MΩ into the scala media and simultaneously the potential of the scala media was recorded by the same electrode. At the CM output terminal the interaction of the CM potential with the injected current was monitored. (b) Spectrogram of potential record. The frequency spectrum was analyzed by the spectrograph for the sound stimulus of 7 kHz, 86 dB SPL and the injected current stimulus of 1.5 kHz, 0.5 μA peak. At 7 kHz the frequency component of the CM potential was observed and the sideband components observed at both sides (5.5 kHz and 8.5 kHz) would be caused by the interaction of the injected current with the sound-induced conductance change of the transduction channel. Many other small peaks observed in the spectrogram corresponded to the frequency components of the higher harmonics and sidebands. Those components would be produced by the distortion product in the transduction process.

duced in the CM generating mechanism in the cochlea. From the sideband components 7.4 ± 1.4 kHz the sound-induced conductance change was estimated as 18 μS.

Discussion

To analyze the intracochlear current record precisely the present authors would propose a simplified electrical circuit model of the cochlear transduction, as shown in Fig. 8. This model differs from the others in the following points: (1) sound-elicited variable conductance (S_H) shunted with the resting basilar membrane resistance (R_B),

(2) constant current source (I_0). In Davis' original model (Davis, 1965) the primary battery in the hair cell and an accessory battery in series in the stria vascularis were the potential source. The leakage current through the hair cells was assumed to be modulated by an increase or decrease of ohmic resistance due to bending of the cilia or to shearing forces applied to them. The current flow through hair cells should be the essential feature of the transduction. Intracellular studies of hair cells (Russell and Sellick, 1978; Russell, 1983) also sug- gested the existence of the constant current flow through the hair cell in the intact cochlea. The endocochlear potential (EP) would be the voltage drop resulting from the basilar membrane impedance and the intracochlear resting current flow. Therefore the primary source of the steady current flow should be the stria vascularis. The membrane potential of the hair cell could not be a candidate for the source of the steady current flow.

By a simple circuit analysis of the model, the scala media potential can be expressed as follows:

$$V = I_0 \frac{(R_B // R_H)}{1 + j_{\omega f_{bf}} C_B (R_B // R_H)} + I \frac{(R_B // R_H // R_0)}{1 + j_{\omega f_{bf}} C_B (R_B // R_H // R_0)}$$

$$= I_0 R_B - I_0 \frac{R_B^2 S_H}{(1 + j_{\omega f_{bf}} C_B R_B)} + I(R_B // R_0) - I \frac{(R_B // R_0)^2 S_H}{(1 + j_{\omega f_{bf}} C_B (R_B // R_0))}$$

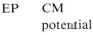

$$\underbrace{\text{EP} \quad \text{CM}}_{\text{potential}} \qquad \left(\underbrace{\begin{array}{c}\text{Command} \\ \text{Current} \\ \text{injection}\end{array}}_{} \quad \underbrace{\begin{array}{c}\text{CM increment} \\ \text{Distortion product}\end{array}}_{} \right)$$

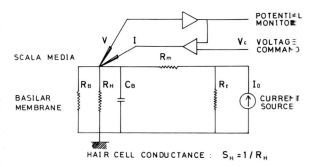

HAIR CELL CONDUCTANCE : $S_H = 1/R_H$

Fig. 8. Simplified electrical circuit model of cochlea and electrode arrangement. V electrode for CM potential recording n scala media and I electrode for current injection into scala media.

R_B: Impedance of basilar membrane in resting state.

R_H: Variable impedance of transduction channels.

C_B: Membrane capacitance.

R_m: Impedance of external tissues which are serially connected to the basilar membrane impedance (R_B).

R_t: Impedance of current source.

I_0: Resting state current source.

V_m: Potential monitor.

V_c: Command signal which controls the injection current.

From this expression the CM potential and the distortion product produced by the current injection could be estimated quantitatively on the circuit parameters.

When the feedback loop for the voltage clamp is closed, the intracochlear current flow would be expressed as follows:

$$I = I_0 \frac{R_B^2 S_H}{(R_B // R_0)} + \frac{V_C}{(R_B // R_0)} + V_C S_H$$

$$\underbrace{}_{\substack{\text{CM} \\ \text{current}}}$$

The first term is the CM current, the second term is the injected current following the command signal and the third term corresponds to the increment of the CM current for the DC command or to the distortion product for the AC command. The scala media impedance ($R_B // R_0$) could be measured by the CM potential and current, DC command or AC command. The sound-induced conductance change (S_H) could be measured by the CM increment for DC command or by the distortion product for AC command.

The single electrode experiment could be analyzed by the simple model of the cochlear transduction shown in Fig. 8. The validity of the model could be confirmed at the lower level of sound stimulation and injected current. Comparison of the spectra of the CM and the CR (sound-elicited changing resistance, Hubbard et al., 1979) should be restricted to the lower sound pressure level and should not be extended to the non-linear region of CM generation, where it would be out of range of the cochlea model.

Acknowledgements

We wish to acknowledge the help and encouragement of Dr. Y. Katsuki, M.J.A. and Dr. S. Yamagishi. This work was supported by a grant from the Japan Academy (for Dr. Katsuki) and by a cooperative program for research project in the National Institute for Physiological Sciences.

References

Davis, H. (1965) A model for transducer action in the cochlea. *Cold Spring Harbor Symposia on Quantitative Biology,* 30: 181 – 189.

Geisler, C.D., Mountain, D.C., Hubbard, A.E., Adrian, H.O. and Ravindran, A. (1977) Alternating electrical-resistance changes in the guinea-pig cochlea caused by acoustic stimuli. *J. Acoust. Soc. Am.,* 61: 1557 – 1566.

Holton, T. and Hudspeth, A.J. (1986) The transduction channel of hair cells from the bull-frog characterized by noise analysis. *J. Physiol. (London),* 375: 195 – 227.

Hubbard, A.E., Geisler, C.D. and Mountain, D.C. (1979) Comparison of the spectra of the cochlear microphonic and of the sound-elicited electrical impedance changes measured in scala media of the guinea pig. *J. Acoust. Soc. Am.,* 66: 431 – 445.

Hudspeth, A.J. (1985) The cellular basis of hearing: the biophysics of hair cells. *Science,* 230: 745 – 752.

Johnstone, B.M., Johnstone, J.R. and Pugsley, I.D. (1966) Membrane resistance in endolymphatic walls of the first turn of the guinea-pig cochlea. *J. Acoust. Soc. Am.,* 40: 1398 – 1404.

Lewis, R.S. and Hudspeth, A.J. (1983) Voltage- and ion-dependent conductances in solitary vertebrate hair cells. *Nature (London),* 304: 538 – 541.

Mountain, D.C., Hubbard, A.E. and Geisler, C.D. (1980) Voltage-dependent elements are involved in the generation of the cochlear microphonic and the sound-induced resistance changes measured in scala media of the guinea pig. *Hear. Res.,* 3: 215 – 229.

Ohmori, H. (1984) Mechanoelectrical transducer has discrete conductances in the chick vestibular hair cell. *Proc. Natl. Acad. Sci. USA,* 81: 1888 – 1891.

Ohmori, H. (1985) Mechano-electrical transduction currents in isolated vestibular hair cells of the chick. *J. Physiol. (London),* 359: 189 – 217.

Russell, I.J. (1983) Origin of the receptor potential in inner hair cells of the mammalian cochlea — evidence for Davis' theory. *Nature (London),* 301: 334 – 336.

Russell, I.J. and Sellick, P.M. (1978) Intracellular studies of hair cells in the mammalian cochlea. *J. Physiol. (London),* 284: 261 – 290.

Strelioff, D., Haas, G. and Honrubia, V. (1972) Sound-induced electrical impedance changes in the guinea pig cochlea. *J. Acoust. Soc. Am.,* 51: 617 – 620.

W. Hamann and A. Iggo (Eds.)
Progress in Brain Research, Vol. 74
© 1988 Elsevier Science Publishers B.V. (Biomedical Division)

CHAPTER 36

Localization of phosphatidylinositol 4,5-diphosphate on the stereocilia of cochlear hair cells

Keiji Yanagisawa[1], Tetsuro Horikoshi[1], Tohru Yoshioka[2] and Masahiro Sokabe[3]

[1] *Department of Physiology, School of Dental Medicine, Tsurumi University, 2-1-3 Tsurumi, Tsurumi-ku, Yokohama 230,*
[2] *Department of Physiology, School of Medicine, Yokohama City University, 2-33 Urafune-cho, Minami-ku, Yokohama 232*
and [3] *Department of Physiology, School of Medicine, Nagoya University, 65 Tsuruma-cho, Showa-ku, Nagoya 466, Japan*

Summary

Antiserum against phosphatidylinositol 4,5-diphosphate ($PI[4,5]P_2$) was obtained from rabbits immunized with $PI[4,5]P_2$ – hapten suspension. To examine the characteristics of this antiserum, cross-reactivities to several phospholipids were tested by liposome lysis assay. The antiserum reacted with $PI[4,5]P_2$ and phosphatidylinositol 4-monophosphate ($PI[4]P$), but not with other lipids. The possibility that the antiserum bound to negatively charged materials was excluded histochemically. Further reactivity of the antiserum was tested electrically in lysophosphatidylinositol 4,5-diphosphate (lyso-$PI[4,5]P_2$) channels formed in artificial membrane. The antiserum decreased K^+ conductance of lyso-$PI[4,5]P_2$ channels. From these data, we concluded that this antiserum reacts with $PI[4,5]P_2$ and $PI[4]P$. Using this antiserum the stereocilia of both inner and outer hair cells in the organ of Corti were stained immunohistochemically. Therefore, $PI[4,5]P_2$ and/or $PI[4]P$ may be localized on the stereociliary membrane of hair cells.

Introduction

Aminoglycosides are known to be ototoxic, and they compete with Ca^{2+} which is indispensable for mechanoelectrical transduction of hair cells (Wersäll and Flock, 1964; Yanagisawa et al., 1984). Phosphatidylinositol 4,5-diphosphate ($PI[4,5]P_2$, triphosphoinositide) has been proposed as a candidate for the binding site of aminoglycoside, since metabolic turnover of $PI[4,5]P_2$ appears to be inhibited by binding of aminoglycosides to this lipid in the organ of Corti (Schacht, 1976), and since direct interaction between aminoglycosides and $PI[4,5]P_2$ was observed in monomolecular films of $PI[4,5]P_2$ (Lodhi et al., 1979) and in a neomycin affinity column for purifying $PI[4,5]P_2$ (Schacht, 1978). To identify the sites of $PI[4,5]P_2$, we attempted to make antiserum against $PI[4,5]P_2$, and succeeded in staining the stereocilia of both inner and outer hair cells in the organ of Corti immunohistochemically (Horikoshi et al., 1984, 1985).

In immunohistochemistry, it is important to identify the characteristics of antibody such as its cross-reactivity to several molecules and its reactivity in tissue (Landis, 1985). In order to examine the characteristics, we report here (1) the cross-reactivities of the antiserum to other lipids by liposome lysis assay, (2) the cross-reactivity of the antiserum to negatively charged materials other than lipids histochemically, (3) the direct binding of antibodies to $PI[4,5]P_2$ by electrical assay, which measures the effect of the antiserum on the

314

electric conductance of monovalent cations in lyso-PI[4,5]P$_2$ channels formed in artificial lipid membrane. All results show that the antiserum reacts highly with PI[4,5]P$_2$ and phosphatidylinositol 4-monophosphate (PI[4]P) but not with other lipids nor with negatively charged materials. From these results we conclude that PI[4,5]P$_2$ and/or PI[4]P are localized on the stereocilia of hair cells.

Materials and methods

Immunization

New Zealand White rabbits were immunized with PI[4,5]P$_2$ complexed with methylated bovine serum albumin as described by Inoue and Nojima (1967). Each rabbit received the immunogen every other day for 3 weeks by intravenous injection. Sera were obtained 3 weeks after the last injection.

Liposome lysis assay

Multilamellar liposomes were prepared as described by Inoue (1974). The dried lipid film (2.5 μmol of lipids) was swollen in 0.25 ml of marker solution containing 20 mM 4-methylumbelliferyl phosphate (UmP) and 240 mM glucose. Complement-dependent immune damage to liposomes was assayed by release of trapped UmP according to the method of Six et al. (1974). The quantity of UmP released from the liposomes was determined using an RF-501 spectrophotometer (Simadzu Seisakusho Co., Kyoto, Japan) with excitation at 340 nm and emission at 448 nm.

Assay of the antiserum on lysophosphatidylinositol 4,5-diphosphate (lyso-PI[4,5]P$_2$) channels

Preparation of lyso-PI[4,5]P$_2$, the channel forming technique in the membrane and the method of electrical conductance measurements were the same as previously reported (Hayashi et al., 1978; Sokabe et al., 1982). Potassium conductance of the membrane modified with lyso-PI[4,5]P$_2$ was measured by applying 15-mV square pulses and measuring the corresponding currents.

Preparation of tissue and immunohistochemical processing

Guinea-pigs were decapitated and the temporal bone was removed from the skull. The organ of Corti was fixed by local perfusion with fixative containing 3% paraformaldehyde and 1% glutaraldehyde in 0.1 M phosphate buffer at pH 7.4 for 2 h at room temperature. Segments of the organ of Corti were cut loose from the modiolus with some spiral osseous lamina attached. Processing for immunohistochemistry was carried out according to the procedure of Sternberger et al. (1970). The tissue was incubated with the diluted antiserum (1:1000) for 24 h at 4°C. Goat anti-rabbit immunoglobulin G (IgG) (Miles-Yeda, Israel) and rabbit peroxidase-antiperoxidase (PAP, Miles-Yeda) were used. The tissue was stained with diaminobenzidine tetrahydrochloride (Sigma) solution containing H$_2$O$_2$ (Horikoshi et al., 1984).

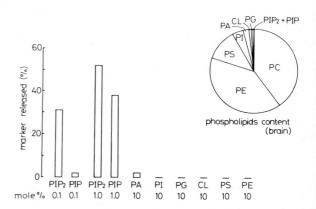

Fig. 1. Reactivity of the antiserum to various phospholipids by liposome lysis assay. PIP$_2$, phosphatidylinositol 4,5-diphosphate; PIP, phosphatidylinositol 4-monophosphate; PA, phosphatidic acid; PI, phosphatidylinositol; PG, phosphatidylglycerol; CL, cardiolipin; PS, phosphatidylserine; PE, phosphatidylethanolamine. Ordinate: marker (UmP) released (%). Inset: typical constitution of phospholipids of brain tissue.

Results and discussion

Eight acidic phospholipids incorporated into liposomal membrane were used as test antigens to examine the binding specificity of the antiserum. As shown in Fig. 1, the serum showed strong reactivity against liposomes containing 1 mol% PI[4,5]P$_2$ as well as 1 mol% PI[4]P, whereas no appreciable reaction was observed with liposomes containing the other acidic phospholipids even at a content of 10 mol%. And also, the serum showed certain marker release against liposomes containing 0.1 mol% PI[4,5]P$_2$, but the reaction against liposomes containing 0.1 mol% PI[4]P was slight. Although PI[4,5]P$_2$ and PI[4]P together constitute only about 1% of the plasma membrane phospholipids (inset of Fig. 1), the reactivity of the antiserum to PI[4,5]P$_2$ and PI[4]P may be enough to recognize these phospholipids from other plasma membrane lipids. Details of these experiments will be reported in a separate paper (Horikoshi et al., in preparation).

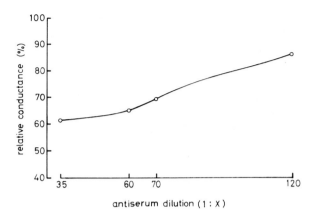

Fig. 3. Relative K$^+$ conductance in various dilutions of antiserum added to one side of the lyso-PI[4,5]P$_2$ channel. No antiserum indicated as 100%.

Results of antiserum assay of the lyso-PI[4,5]P$_2$ channel in the lipid bilayer membrane are shown in Fig. 2. The antiserum diluted 60 times decreased membrane K$^+$ conductance to as low as 65% of the original value. Application of 1 mM neomycin to the antiserum containing solution further reduced the membrane conductance (Sokabe et al., 1982). Relative K$^+$ conductance of the lyso-PI[4,5]P$_2$ channel was plotted as a function of dilution of the antiserum (Fig. 3). The membrane conductance reduction was consistently decreased with the dilution of the antiserum. It is not clear from the present experiment if more concentrated antiserum would block the lyso-PI[4,5]P$_2$ channel completely or not, because the artificial membrane tended to be destroyed by the too high concentration of antiserum. This membrane break was also observed at high concentrations of normal rabbit serum. The conductance inhibition of the lyso-PI[4,5]P$_2$ channel by the antiserum indicates a direct interaction of the antibody with lyso-PI[4,5]P$_2$.

Fig. 4 shows a surface preparation of guinea-pig organ of Corti stained by the PAP method using the antiserum described above as a primary antiserum. Stereocilia of both inner and outer hair cells are stained clearly, but the cell bodies of the hair cells and supporting cells are not stained. The

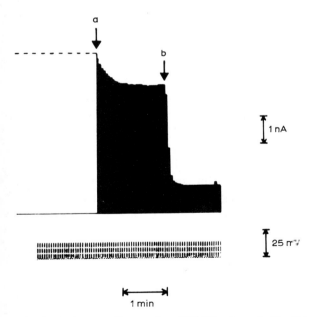

Fig. 2. Antiserum effect on lyso-PI[4,5]P$_2$ channel. The K$^+$ current was measured by 15-mV electrical pulses. At a, 60 times diluted antiserum was added to one side of the membrane. At b, 1 mM neomycin was added to the same side.

stereocilia were found to be stained uniformly. No specific staining of stereocilia was observed when normal rabbit serum, which did not react with PI[4,5]P$_2$ or PI[4]P, was applied. After antiserum was absorbed by incubation with excess PI[4,5]P$_2$, this antiserum stained the stereocilia weakly. When the antiserum was applied in the presence of neomycin ($10^{-4} - 10^{-3}$ M), PAP staining intensity was somewhat reduced. Staining of the tectorial membrane and the stria vascularis was concluded to be non-specific, since they were also stained by normal rabbit serum.

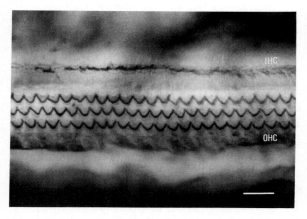

Fig. 4. Surface preparation of guinea-pig organ of Corti stained by the PAP method using the antiserum. Stereocilia of both inner hair cells (IHC) and outer hair cells (OHC) are stained clearly. Bar = 20 μm. (Horikoshi et al., 1984.)

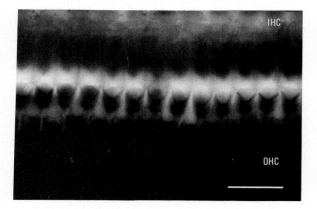

Fig. 5. Surface preparation of guinea-pig organ of Corti stained by ruthenium red. Inner hair cells (IHC), outer hair cells (OHC) and supporting cells similarly stained. Bar = 10 μm.

In cochlear tissue, it is known that the apical surface of both sensory hair cells and supporting cells are coated by negatively charged materials such as acidic mucopolysaccharides (AMPS) and glycoproteins (Flock et al., 1977; Hama, 1978; Slepecky and Chamberlain, 1985). To exclude the possibility that negatively charged materials were stained by this antiserum, we applied ruthenium red (RR) to cochlear tissue, prepared as described above, for detection of negatively charged materials in the organ of Corti. RR stained the tectorial membrane and the cell bodies of sensory and supporting cells as well as stereocilia of both inner and outer hair cells, but their staining intensity of the stereocilia was the same as that of the cell bodies (Fig. 5). The staining patterns of alcian blue and toluidine blue which stain AMPS were quite similar to that of RR (data not shown). If the antiserum can bind negatively charged materials, the staining patterns of the antiserum and RR must be the same in cochlear tissue. Comparing Fig. 4 and Fig. 5, we concluded that the antiserum does not react with negatively charged materials in a non-specific manner.

From these results, we conclude that the antiserum reacts with PI[4,5]P$_2$ and PI[4]P, but not with other acidic phospholipids or negatively charged materials. Since the reactivity of the antiserum to PI[4,5]P$_2$ and PI[4]P is enough to recognize these lipids in the cellular membrane, PI[4,5]P$_2$ and/or PI[4]P are localized on the stereocilia of hair cells in the organ of Corti.

The role of PI[4,5]P$_2$ in hair cells is unclear at present. A possible explanation is as follows. In hair cell mechanoelectrical transduction, it is known that extracellular calcium ions are important. In the lateral line organ, synchronization of afferent nerve firing with mechanical stimulation was enhanced by calcium ion application and depressed by EGTA application (Sand, 1975). In mammalian cochlear endolymph the concentration of calcium ions is low (Bosher and Warren, 1978), but iontophoretic injection of EDTA into the scala media reduced cochlear microphonics, and this effect was weakened by injection of calcium ions prior to the EDTA application (Tanaka et al., 1979). The minimal concentration of calcium ions required for transduction is estimated to be 10–100 μM (Sand, 1975; Corey and Hudspeth, 1979). Since the apical surface of hair cells is covered by the tectorial membrane which restricts ion movement, it is a convenient way to maintain the concentration of calcium ions that PI[4,5]P$_2$ works as sites on the stereocilia which regulate calcium concentration. Really PI[4,5]P$_2$ is known to have high affinity for binding calcium ions (Michell, 1975).

Acknowledgements

We wish to express our thanks to Dr. Y. Katsuki and Dr. A. Asanuma for their valuable suggestions and encouragement. This work was supported by Grants-in-Aid for Special Research on Molecular Mechanism of Bioelectrical Response (59123005, 60123006, 61107006) from the Japanese Ministry of Education, Science and Culture and by a grant from the Japan Academy to Dr. Y. Katsuki.

References

Bosher, S.K. and Warren, R.L. (1978) Very low calcium content of cochlear endolymph, and extracellular fluid. Nature (London), 273: 377–378.

Corey, D.P. and Hudspeth, A.J. (1979) Ionic basis of the receptor potential in a vertebrate hair cell. Nature (London), 281: 675–677.

Flock, Å., Flock, B. and Murray, E. (1977) Studies on the sensory hairs of receptor cells in the inner ear. Acta Otolaryngol., 83: 85–91.

Hama, K. (1978) A study of the fine structure of the pit organ of the common Japanese sea eel Conger myriaster. Cell Tissue Res., 189: 375–388.

Hayashi, F., Sokabe, M., Takagi, M., Hayashi, K. and Kishimoto, U. (1978) Calcium-sensitive univalent cation channel formed by lysotriphosphoinositide in bilayer lipid membrane. Biochim. Biophys. Acta, 510: 305–315.

Horikoshi, T., Yanagisawa, K. and Yoshioka, T. (1984) A highly specific staining of cochlear hair cells by TPI (triphosphoinositide) antibody. Proc. Japan Acad., 60B: 157–160.

Horikoshi, T., Yanagisawa, K. and Yoshioka, T. (1985) Staining of cochlear hair cells by triphosphoinositide (TPI) antiserum. Neurosci. Res., Suppl., 1: S1.

Inoue, K. (1974) Permeability properties of liposomes prepared from dipalmitoyllecithin, dimirystoyllecithin, egg lecithin, rat liver lecithin and beef brain sphingomyelin. Biochim. Biophys. Acta, 339: 390–402.

Inoue, K. and Nojima, S. (1967) Immunochemical studies of phospholipids, III. Production of antibody to cardiolipin. Biochim. Biophys. Acta, 144: 409–414.

Landis, D.M.D. (1985) Promise and pitfalls in immunocytochemistry. Trends Neurosci., 8: 312–317.

Lodhi, S., Weiner, N.D. and Schacht, J. (1979) Interaction of neomycin with monomolecular films of polyphosphoinositides and other lipids. Biochim. Biophys. Acta, 557: 1–8.

Michell, R.H. (1975) Inositol phospholipids and cell surface receptor function. Biochim. Biophys. Acta, 415: 81–147.

Sand, O. (1975) Effects of different ionic environments on the mechano-sensitivity of lateral line organs in the mudpuppy. J. Comp. Physiol. A, 102: 27–42.

Schacht, J. (1976) Biochemistry of neomycin ototoxicity. J. Acoust. Soc. Am., 59: 940–944.

Schacht, J. (1978) Purification of polyphosphoinositides by chromatography on immobilized neomycin. J. Lipid Res., 19: 1063–1067.

Six, H.R., Young, Jr., W.W., Uemura, K. and Kinsky, S.C. (1974) Effect of antibody-complement on multiple vs. single compartment liposomes. Application of a fluorometric assay for following changes in liposomal permeability. Biochemistry, 13: 4050–4058.

Slepecky, N. and Chamberlain, S.C. (1985) The cell coat of inner ear sensory and supporting cells as demonstrated by ruthenium red. Hear. Res., 17: 281–288.

Sokabe, M., Hayase, J. and Miyamoto, K. (1982) Neomycin effect on lysotriphosphoinositide channel as a model for an acute ototoxicity. Proc. Japan Acad., 58B: 177–180.

Sternberger, L.A., Hardy, Jr., P.H., Cuculis, J.J. and Meyer, H.G. (1970) The unlabeled antibody enzyme method of immunohistochemistry. Preparation and properties of soluble antigen-antibody complex (horseradish peroxidase-antihorseradish peroxidase) and its use in identification of spirochetes. J. Histochem. Cytochem., 18: 315–333.

Tanaka, Y., Asanuma, A. and Yanagisawa, K. (1979) Effect of EDTA in the scala media on cochlear potentials. Proc. Japan Acad., 55B: 31–36.

Wersäll, J. and Flock, Å. (1964) Suppression and restoration of the microphonic output from the lateral line organ after local application of streptomycin. Life Sci., 3: 1151–1155.

Yanagisawa, K., Yoshioka, T. and Katsuki, Y. (1984) Sound transducer mechanism and phospholipids in the hair cell of the ear. In: W. Hamann and A. Iggo (Eds.), Sensory Receptor Mechanisms. World Scientific Publ. Co., Singapore, pp. 109–116.

W. Hamann and A. Iggo (Eds.)
Progress in Brain Research, Vol. 74
© 1988 Elsevier Science Publishers B.V. (Biomedical Division)

CHAPTER 37

Efferent modulation of penile mechanoreceptor activity

Richard D. Johnson

Department of Physiological Sciences, College of Veterinary Medicine, University of Florida, Gainesville, FL 32610, USA

Introduction

The mammalian penis is richly innervated by sensory receptors. The mechanoreceptors, responsible for tactile sensation and the afferent limb of the spinal sexual reflexes, have been studied physiologically in several species using computer controlled mechanostimulators (Cottrell et al., 1978; Kitchell et al., 1982; Johnson et al., 1986; Johnson and Kitchell, 1987). These studies have demonstrated the presence of rapidly adapting and slowly adapting mechanoreceptors capable of responding, albeit in a manner somewhat different from receptors found in the digits, to a wide variety of indentations. However, those investigations dealt only with response characteristics and neural codes of mechanoreceptors in the flaccid, non-erect penis. Because the penis is subject to efferent control, namely a tumescence of the penile tissue following activation of a set of autonomic and somatic nerves, the following study was undertaken to determine if modulation of penile mechanoreceptor activity could be detected following efferent stimulation.

Methods

Mature male Sprague – Dawley rats with body weights between 300 and 500 g were anesthetized with an intraperitoneal injection of pentobarbital sodium (50 mg/kg), maintained at a deep surgical plane of anesthesia throughout the duration of the experiment (via a cannula in the external jugular

vein) and then given an anesthetic overdose. Penile erection in the rat is a complicated neurovascular event (Benson, 1981; Hart and Leedy, 1985) requiring the activation of parasympathetic and sympathetic nerve fibers (causing the relaxation of cavernosal blood vessels and smooth muscle) along with the activation of skeletal motor fibers in the somatic pudendal nerve (causing the contraction of the bulbocavernosus muscle which forces blood rapidly into the erectile spaces). Each animal was placed on its back and two incisions were made, one on the ventral midline from the umbilicus to the prepuce and a second one along the ventral midline of the scrotum. Following surgical exposure via the abdominal cavity, bipolar platinum stimulating electrodes were placed around the right cavernous nerves, a bundle of unmyelinated autonomic (parasympathetic and sympathetic) postganglionic nerve fibers travelling on the lateral aspect of the pelvic urethra. At the scrotal site, the large bulbocavernosus muscle was exposed after removal of the testes. A pair of fine gauge nickel wire stimulating electrodes (uninsulated at the tip) were placed bilaterally into the muscle bellies so that electrical stimulation produced a simultaneous bilateral contraction of the muscle. The wire leads were exteriorized and the wound closed.

The free edges of skin resulting from the abdominal incision were sutured onto a metal ring to make a mineral oil pool. The right dorsal nerve of the penis was severed along the penile body and the desheathed distal end placed over 30 gauge bipolar recording electrodes. Whole fascicle and teased

320

single fiber neural activity was obtained using conventional dissection and recording procedures as described previously (Kitchell et al., 1982; Johnson et al., 1986). The flaccid, non-erect glans penis was directed caudally and adhered, on its left lateral aspect, to the surface of a warm plate (38°C) with a drop of cyanoacrylate glue thereby providing mechanical and thermal stabilization. Various combinations of stimulation paradigms were tried on the cavernous nerves and the bulbocavernosus muscle until a reproducible and reversible erection of the penile body and glans was produced.

An electromagnetic mechanostimulator/transducer (Chubbuck, 1966) was employed for discrete punctate stimulation of the receptive field of single mechanoreceptors as described previously (Johnson and Kitchell, 1987). All mechanical stimulations were given in the displacement feedback control mode while monitoring both skin displacement and reactive force with an oscilloscope and voltmeter. Before each stimulus, the stimulator probe tip (0.5 mm diameter) was placed on the skin surface with a resting force of 10 mg. Sustained stimulus commands (long duration square waves) were delivered with a Grass stimulator and variable velocity commands (short duration, half cycle triangle waves) delivered with a function generator. Single unit response patterns to controlled stimulation were recorded before and after efferent stimulation of the cavernous nerves and/or bulbocavernosus muscle.

Results

Penile responses

Electrical stimulation of the cavernous nerves (CN) produced a slowly developing (time course 5 s) erection of the penile body (corpus cavernosum) but only a slight tumescence of the glans. Optimal stimulation parameters were as follows: pulse rate 20 Hz, pulse duration 0.75 – 0.85 ms and intensity 10 – 18 V. Isolated stimulation of the bulbocavernosus muscle (BCM) did not give rise to any penile tumescence regardless of the stimulation

parameters. However, when preceded by 5 s of CN stimulation, a 500 ms long train of high frequency stimulus pulses (0.25 ms duration) to the BCM produced a rapid engorgement of the glans which appeared to be identical to the 'flared cup' erection seen during sexual reflex testing in awake rats. A pulse frequency range of 60 – 160 Hz to the BCM was effective in generating an erection of the glans, however, the upper range was typically used to produce a fused tetanus of the BCM to prevent possible movement artifact during recording sessions. At cessation of BCM stimulation (or BCM fatigue) the erection of the glans would rapidly subside (detumescence). Because of the need to record neural responses to static erect and non-erect states, sustained glans erection was produced by CN and BCM stimulation combined with temporary occlusion of the large and superficial dorsal penile vein in the body of the penis. This was achieved by touching, and therefore collapsing, the vein with a tapered glass probe having a balled tip diameter of 1 mm. A glans erection was therefore maintained as long as the venous occlusion

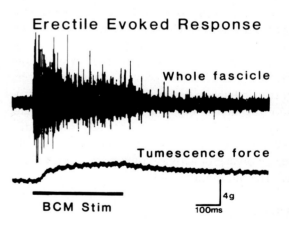

Fig. 1. Evoked burst of neural activity in a large fascicle of the dorsal nerve of the penis in response to a brief erection of the glans. The cavernous nerves were stimulated throughout the entire period shown and the bulbocavernosus muscle (BCM) was stimulated during the period indicated by the bar. Tumescence of the glans was monitored by the mechanostimulator (reaction force against the probe) placed on the penile surface in a region not supplied by this fascicle.

prevented the blood (driven into the glans by BCM contraction) from returning to the general circulation.

Neural responses

Erection of the glans elicited by simultaneous CN and BCM stimulation produced a large burst of activity in desheathed whole fascicles of the dorsal nerve of the penis (Fig. 1). These bursts were never seen following isolated CN or BCM stimulation indicating that the rapid tumescence of the glans provided the stimulus to the receptors. Only some of the receptors activated during the elicited flared cup erection have been identified with single unit recording. Slowly adapting (SA) glans mechanoreceptors responded to BCM induced tumescence of the glans with a slowly adapting discharge correlated with the magnitude of the erection. Some of the more sensitive SA units developed a slow, regular discharge in response to the slight and slowly developing glans engorgement induced by isolated CN stimulation. Only a few rapidly adapting (RA) glans mechanoreceptors were found that fired impulses in response to rapid tumescence. The identity of many of the fibers firing during the initial erectile response has yet to be determined.

Three SA units were driven with rectangular mechanical pulses of 400 ms duration during periods when the penis was either erect or flaccid in order to determine if there was a change in response. In all cases, an equal amplitude static displacement produced a greater response in the erect state compared with the non-erect state. A stimulus–response sequence in a representative SA unit is shown in Fig. 2. However, as seen in this

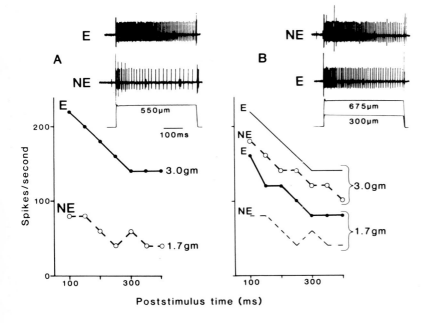

Fig. 2. Response of one SA unit to static indentation with controlled displacement rectangular pulses given when the penis was erect (E) and non-erect (NE). (A) A displacement of 550 μm (indicated by the displacement output trace) during each penile configuration produced a different neural response of which the static response is plotted below as mean firing frequencies of 50 ms bins. The reaction force against the probe, however, was not the same in each configuration as indicated by the force measurement in grams (though not shown, stress relaxation was not significant during this short stimulus). (B) The displacement was increased to 675 μm in the NE state and decreased to 300 μm in the E state in order to give the same respective force of stimulation generated in A. The neural response was subsequently increased in NE and decreased in E and more closely correlated with the responses generated in A (responses in A are replotted without data points in B).

figure, a given displacement amplitude produced more static stimulus force (measured as reaction force by the mechanostimulator system) in the erect state relative to the non-erect. If the displacement amplitude was then decreased for stimulation of the erect penis and increased in the non-erect state, thereby creating an equal force stimulation, the neural response differential was reduced, suggesting these receptors were encoding mechanical force amplitude more accurately than displacement amplitude. Despite the balanced stimulus force, however, the neural response in the erect state was always greater than in the non-erect state (Fig. 2B).

To determine the effect of efferent stimulation and erection on the single unit response to changing stimulus velocity, stimulus – response curves were compiled for two RA units and two SA units. Sustained electrical stimulation of the CN did not by itself produce a change in response. When coupled with BCM stimulation and venous occlusion, however, the resultant glans erection changed the stimulus – response curves. The stimulus – response curves for one RA unit are shown in Fig. 3. The upward shift of the curve without a significant change in slope seen during erection was evident in

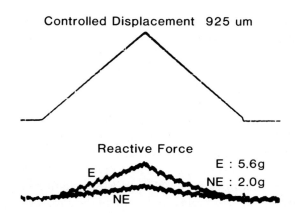

Fig. 4. Change in reactive force of the penile tissue against the mechanostimulator probe during a constant displacement ramp stimulus generated from the penile surface. The reactive force (dynamic force) is greater in the erect (E) penis when compared to the non-erect (NE). The indentation velocity was 2.5 μm/ms.

all four units and suggested that a change in stimulus intensity rather than a change in receptor sensitivity was responsible for the response differential. Although the displacement amplitude during the variable velocity stimulus regimen was the same in both the erect and non-erect states, the dynamic stimulus force (measured as reaction force against the probe) was not the same. As shown in Fig. 4, the dynamic stimulus force on erect penile tissue was greater than on the non-erect penis, despite an equal displacement.

Discussion

The results of this preliminary study demonstrate that a group of receptors in the penis of the rat are affected by the efferent stimulation of elements involved in the generation of erection of the glans. The receptors responding to the dynamic period of tumescence were only partially identified, those being slowly adapting mechanoreceptors. These mechanoreceptors are therefore functioning as exteroceptors, responding to external stimuli, and as interoceptors, responding to internal mechanical stimuli. The identity of other receptors transiently responding to the erection is still to be determined

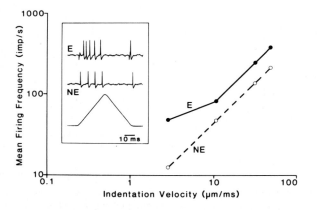

Fig. 3. Response of one RA unit to variable velocity ramp stimulation while the penis was erect (E) or non-erect (NE). The displacement throughout the two series remained constant at 800 μm. The inset shows the evoked neural responses at one point in the series (stimulus is indicated by the displacement output trace).

as only a few of the rapidly adapting mechanoreceptors discharged during this period.

Analysis of discharge patterns of single mechanoreceptors demonstrated that isolated autonomic nerve stimulation did not appear to change mechanical sensitivity, unlike the effect observed in mechanoreceptors of the hairy skin by a number of investigators (see Roberts et al., 1985), and therefore does not provide an explanation for the small unmyelinated neurites seen entering the genital corpuscles of the rat penis (Patrizi and Munger, 1965). When the glans penis enlarges during flared cup erection, however, the response characteristics do change most likely due to the change in skin compliance, that is, the erect penis is less compliant. This would appear to particularly apply to the static response pattern of the SA units. A given displacement in compliant skin produces less reaction force when compared to firmer skin (Pubols, 1982; Pubols and Benkich, 1986) and when coupled with the greatly increased response of penile SA units in the erect state, a suggestion that these units encode the force of stimulation can be made. Recent evidence from other laboratories studying given SA mechanoreceptor populations in rats suggests that when the viscoelastic properties of the surrounding tissue are changed due to aging (Baumann et al., 1986) and arthritis (Guilbaud et al., 1985), the neural code for force is more accurate than the code for displacement. In the present report, where the same SA unit could be studied before and after a natural change in tissue compliance, the response to stimulus force appeared to be the more sensitive neural signal. The fact that the static response to constant force was always greater in the erect state might be explained on the basis of an increased temperature at the receptor loci resulting from the increase in blood flow into the erectile tissue. Most penile mechanoreceptors in the ram (Cottrell et al., 1978) and the dog (Johnson and Kitchell, 1987) are more sensitive at temperatures near body temperature.

The upward shift in the indentation velocity coding curves described in this study is again probably due to the decrease in penile compliance during a state of erection. The observed phenomenon of greater force stimuli (dynamic force) generated on firmer skin has been described previously in the hand (Pubols and Maliniak, 1984) and along with a possible thermal effect (Johnson and Kitchell, 1987), the modulation of the velocity coding curves is probably not due to a direct change in mechanoreceptor sensitivity. The higher dynamic burst frequencies and shorter adapting responses seen in SA mechanoreceptors during erection (shown but not plotted in Fig. 2) are again undoubtedly caused by an increase in dynamic force, an effect reported in the glabrous skin of the squirrel monkey (Pubols and Pubols, 1976).

In summary, the results of this preliminary study demonstrate that many of the mechanoreceptors in the penis of the rat can respond to internal as well as external stimuli to the penis and their stimulus – response characteristics can be modulated with efferent stimulation of the autonomic and somatic components of erection.

Acknowledgements

The author is grateful to Dr. Paul Davenport for the use of equipment and facilities for some of the experiments and to Victoria Dugan for technical support. This study was funded in part by a grant from the Division of Sponsored Research, University of Florida.

References

Baumann, K.I., Hamann, W. and Leung, M.S. (1986) Mechanical properties of skin and responsiveness of slowly adapting type I mechanoreceptors in rats at different ages. *J. Physiol. (London)*, 371: 329 – 337.

Benson, G.S. (1981) Mechanisms of penile erection. *Invest. Urol.*, 19: 65 – 69.

Chubbuck, J.G. (1966) Small motion biological stimulator. *APL Tech. Dig.*, 5: 18 – 23.

Cottrell, D.F., Iggo, A. and Kitchell, R.L. (1978) Electrophysiology of the afferent innervation of the penis of the domestic ram. *J. Physiol. (London)*, 283: 347 – 367.

Guilbaud, G., Iggo, A. and Tegner, R. (1985) Sensory receptors in ankle joint capsules of normal and arthritic rats. *Exp. Brain Res.*, 58: 29 – 40.

324

Hart, B.L. and Leedy, M.G. (1985) Neurological bases of male sexual behavior. In: N. Adler, D. Pfaff and R.W. Goy (Eds.), *Handbook of Behavioral Neurobiology, Vol. 7, Reproduction.* Plenum, New York, pp. 373 – 422.

Johnson, R.D. and Kitchell, R.L. (1987) Mechanoreceptor response to mechanical and thermal stimuli in the glans penis of the dog. *J. Neurophysiol.,* 57: 1813 – 1836.

Johnson, R.D., Kitchell, R.L. and Gilanpour, H. (1986) Rapidly and slowly adapting mechanoreceptors in the glans penis of the cat. *Physiol. Behav.,* 37: 69 – 78.

Kitchell, R.L., Gilanpour, H. and Johnson, R.D. (1982) Electrophysiologic studies of penile mechanoreceptors in the rat. *Exp. Neurol.,* 75: 229 – 244.

Patrizi, G. and Munger, B.L. (1965) The cytology of encapsulated nerve endings in the rat penis. *J. Ultrastruct. Res.,* 13: 500 – 515.

Pubols, B.H. (1982) Factors affecting cutaneous mechanoreceptor response. I. Constant-force versus constant-displacement stimulation. *J. Neurophysiol.,* 47: 515 – 529.

Pubols, B.H. and Pubols, L.M. (1976) Coding of mechanical stimulus velocity and indentation depth by squirrel monkey and raccoon glabrous skin mechanoreceptors. *J. Neurophysiol.,* 39: 773 – 787.

Pubols, B.H. and Maliniak, C.H. (1984) The role of skin mechanics in tactile receptor discharge. In: W. Hamann and A. Iggo (Eds.), *Sensory Receptor Mechanisms.* World Scientific Publ. Co., Singapore, pp. 152 – 166.

Pubols, B.H. and Benkich, M.E. (1986) Relations between stimulus force, skin displacement, and discharge characteristics of slowly adapting type I cutaneous mechanoreceptors in glabrous skin of squirrel monkey hand. *Somatosens. Res.,* 4: 111 – 125.

Roberts, W.J., Elardo, S.M. and King, K.A. (1985) Sympathetically induced changes in the responses of slowly adapting type I receptors in cat skin. *Somatosens. Res.,* 2: 223 – 236.

W. Hamann and A. Iggo (Eds.)
Progress in Brain Research, Vol. 74
© 1988 Elsevier Science Publishers B.V. (Biomedical Division)

CHAPTER 38

Modulation of testicular polymodal receptor activities

T. Kumazawa, K. Mizumura and J. Sato

Department of Nervous and Sensory Functions, Research Institute of Environmental Medicine, Nagoya University, Nagoya, 464 Japan

Introduction

The difficulty encountered in investigations of polymodal receptors is the limited reproducibility of responses, like well-known 'heat sensitization' (Bessou and Perl, 1966; Kumazawa and Perl, 1977; Kumazawa and Mizumura, 1977, 1980). Such behavior of the receptor might be expected, however, considering the role of this receptor in signalling the changes in tissues caused by noxious, tissue damaging, stimuli. The activities of the receptor should be easily modulated by various processes presumed to occur in the microenvironment of the receptor site.

Recently we have developed an in vitro testis – spermatic nerve preparation, which is quite suitable for systematically studying chemical and thermal modulations of this visceral nociceptor activity (Kumazawa et al., 1987b).

This report summarizes modifying effects on the unitary activity of polymodal receptors caused by (1) putative chemical mediators and related substances, (2) temperature elevation both supra- and sub-threshold for receptor activation, and (3) changes in the ionic concentration of the Krebs solution bathing their receptive fields.

Methods

The experimental methods are basically the same as reported previously (Kumazawa et al., 1987a). The testis and epididymis with the spermatic cord attached were excised from dogs that were deeply anesthetized with pentobarbital sodium and kept in an areflexic state. Single- or multi-fiber activity was recorded from the superior spermatic nerve placed in an oil pool, while the testis and epididymis, exposed at the tunica vaginalis visceralis, were immersed in a test pool of Krebs – Henseleit solution (Krebs solution) equilibrated with a gas mixture of 5% CO_2 and 95% O_2. The composition of the solution normally used was (in mM): NaCl 110.9; KCl 4.8; $CaCl_2$ 2.5; $MgSO_4$ 1.2; KH_2PO_4 1.2; $NaHCO_3$ 24.4; glucose 20. The temperature of the solution bathing the scrotal contents was adjusted by regulating the water temperature circulating in the trough surrounding the test pool. After the temperature of the receptive field reached a pre-set level, chemical stimulation was applied by replacing the Krebs solution with a stimulus solution of the same temperature: hypertonic saline and high K^+ solution for 30 s, or bradykinin (BK) for 1 min with an interval of 10 min between trials. Heat stimulation was carried out by replacing the Krebs solution of base temperature with that of a set temperature for 30 s.

Modulations by chemical mediators and related substances

Various substances are known to appear in damaged or inflamed tissues (Johansson, 1960; Ohuchi et al., 1976; Barbieri et al., 1977; Essman, 1978;

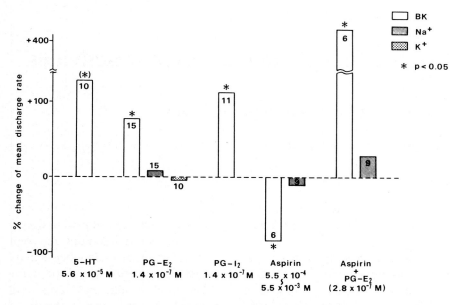

Fig. 1. Effects of 5-HT, PGE$_2$, PGI$_2$ and aspirin on the discharges of polymodal receptors to algesic substances. Modulation effects are expressed as percentage changes against the responses before application of the modifying substances indicated at the bottom. Bar numerals indicate number of units tested.

Higgs et al., 1983), some of them are implicated in the alarm signals, or 'dolor' from these tissues.

Fig. 1 summarizes the changes in discharge rate of polymodal receptor units to algesic substances by adding serotonin (5-HT), prostaglandin E$_2$, I$_2$ (PGE$_2$, PGI$_2$), and acetylsalicylic acid (aspirin). These values are expressed as percentage change induced by these substances. Responses to BK were significantly augmented after application of 5-HT and PGs. 5-HT was also effective in augmenting responses to hypertonic saline, although this is not shown in the figure because of differences in the method of application. When PGE$_2$ (1.4 × 10^{-7} M) was applied simultaneously with hypertonic saline and a high K$^+$ solution, its effect was unclear, but pretreatment or a higher concentration of PGE$_2$ significantly augmented the responses to these algesic substances as well (Mizumura et al., 1987). 5-HT and PGs per se seldom caused excitation of these receptors at these concentrations, while BK, a known pain producing substance at this concentration, consistently caused

a clear excitation of the receptor. 5-HT and PGs are thus considered to sensitize the responses of the receptor to algesic substances.

Although BK induces excitation at a very low concentration, the excitation process involves interactive effects of PGs induced by BK in the tissue. Aspirin, an inhibitor of cyclo-oxygenase (Ferreira et al., 1971), suppressed BK responses while adding PGE$_2$ restored it, and aspirin did not alter responses to hypertonic saline.

As shown in Table 1, substance P and calcitonin gene-related peptide (CGRP), neuropeptides released from the nociceptor terminal, and combination of both peptides caused only a slight excitatory and modifying effect, if any. Des-Arg^9-BK and des-Arg^9-[Leu^8]-BK, which are a putative agonist and antagonist of the B$_1$ receptor respectively (Marceau et al., 1980), did not cause any effect. 6-Keto PGF$_{1\alpha}$, a degradation product of PGI$_2$, and leukotriene D$_4$, a lipoxygenase product of arachidonate, did not cause any excitatory and sensitizing effects on the recep-

TABLE 1

Stimulation and modulation effects of various substances on polymodal receptors

Substance	Character	Concentration tested (M)	Direct excitatory effect	Modifying effect Sensitizing	Suppressing
Substance P	Neuropeptide from nociceptor	$6 \times 10^{-8} - 6 \times 10^{-5}$	±	−	−
CGRP	Neuropeptide from nociceptor	$10^{-10} - 10^{-8}$	−	−	−
Des-Arg^9-BK	B$_1$ receptor agonist	10^{-5}	−	−	−
Des-Arg^9-[Leu^8]-BK	B$_1$ antagonist	10^{-5}	−	−	−
6-Keto-PGF$_{1\alpha}$	PGI$_2$ degraded	1.4×10^{-7}	−	−	−
Leukotriene D$_4$	Lipoxygenase product	10^{-5}	−	−	−
Morphine	Opioid μ agonist	$10^{-5} - 10^{-4}$	+ (10^{-5} M : 12/31)	−	−
DADLE	Opioid δ agonist	10^{-5}	+ (7/29)		
Dynorphin	Opioid $\varkappa$ agonist	10^{-5}	+ (7/17)		

tor. Analgesic effects of opioids on peripheral nociceptors have been reported (Ferreira and Nakamura, 1979). However, morphine did not reveal suppressive effects on polymodal receptor activity but morphine as well as D-Ala^2,D-Leu^5-enkephalin (DADLE) and dynorphin frequently caused excitation.

Modulation by temperature elevation

It is well known that heat stimulation sensitizes subsequent responses to the same heat stimulus: 'heat sensitization'. Sensitizing effects of a heat stimulus of 55°C were tested on two groups of units: with heat thresholds above and below 45°C. A conditioning stimulus of 55°C itself evoked a larger response in units with lower thresholds, but larger augmentation effects were observed in units with higher thresholds (Fig. 2). In previous investigations on polymodal receptors of skin (Kumazawa and Perl, 1977), of muscle (Kumazawa and Mizumura, 1977), and of testis (Kumazawa and Mizumura, 1980; Kumazawa et al., 1987b) using ramp heat stimulation, a reduction of the subsequent heat response was noted. This deactivation tended to be observed when units were stimulated far in excess of their thresholds.

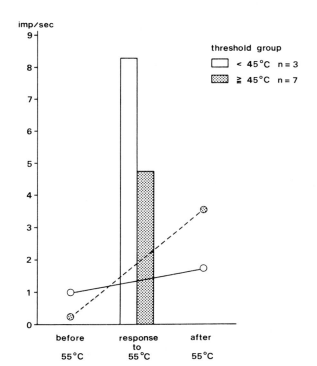

Fig. 2. Effects of 55°C heat stimulation on units with high and low heat threshold. Averaged mean discharge rate induced by heat stimulation on units with heat thresholds below 45°C (white) and above 45°C (dotted). Columns indicate responses to 55°C heating, circles indicate responses to heating close to the threshold temperature before and after 55°C heating.

The present results provided evidence supporting these previous observations.

After supra-threshold heat stimulation, responses to hypertonic saline were also sensitized (Kumazawa et al., 1987a). As shown in Fig. 3, after 55°C heat stimulation, the response to 10^{-7} M BK was augmented to 150% of the control responses, while the response to moderate heat stimulation was augmented to 350% after 55°C heat stimulation. In both groups of units, the discharge rate evoked by either BK or heat before conditioning heat stimulation was similar. Although supra-threshold heat stimulation sensitizes responses of polymodal receptors to both heat and algesic substances, the sensitizing effect on heat responses was stronger and lasted longer than on algesic substances.

Under the influence of aspirin, 55°C heating clearly sensitized responses to BK as well as to heat. Furthermore, PGE_2 at concentrations causing a definite enhancement of the BK response augmented heat responses only inconsistently or slightly. Thus, participation of prostaglandins in heat sensitization phenomena appears to be minimal or absent.

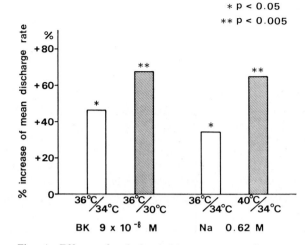

Fig. 4. Effects of sub-threshold temperature rise on the responses to bradykinin and hypertonic saline. Increase of responses at higher temperature is expressed as percentage of the response at base temperature.

A temperature rise of 6°C from the base temperature that itself did not induce excitation also enhanced the response to various concentrations of BK and hypertonic saline (Kumazawa et al., 1987a). A temperature increase of 2°C caused a significant enhancement of the response to algesic substances, although the degree of enhancement was less than that obtained by a 6°C rise (Fig. 4). This indicates that responses to algesic substances would be enhanced by temperature rise observable in inflamed tissues.

Modulations related to ionic changes

When responses to hypertonic saline and high K^+ solutions were tested in a Ca-free state, the responses were significantly increased as compared with that in normal Krebs solution. This enhancing effect of a Ca-free solution was restored by adding Mg ions. In high Ca Krebs solution, the response to high K^+ solution was significantly suppressed (Fig. 5). These results suggest that the effect is not Ca ion specific but may be due to the change in ionic charge at the membrane. When the concentration of K^+ in the Krebs solution was reduced to

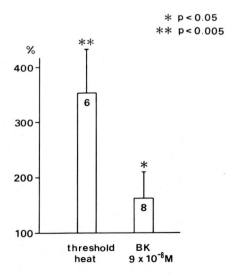

Fig. 3. Sensitizing effects of 55°C heat stimulation on the responses to threshold heat and bradykinin. Sensitizing effects are expressed as percentage of the control response before application of the 55°C heat stimulus.

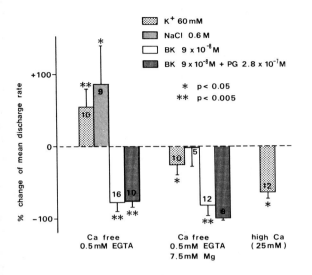

Fig. 5. Effects of changes in Ca^{2+} concentration of Krebs solution on the responses to algesic substances. Comparison of the response to algesic substances in control, Ca-free (with or without Mg^{2+}) and high Ca expressed as percentage change for each Ca condition vs. control.

half (3 mM) or doubled (12 mM), the responses to hypertonic saline as well as BK decreased and increased, respectively, as compared to the control (6 mM) K^+ concentration, thus indicating the influence of membrane depolarization on the response to both BK and hypertonic saline.

However, as shown in Fig. 5, the BK response was suppressed in a Ca-free solution, and the addition of neither PGE_2 nor Mg ions restored it. The BK response in the absence of Ca may be interpreted as the membrane depolarization being overcome by the lack of the Ca-dependent facilitatory processes involved in the BK response. As mentioned above, PGs triggered by BK participate in the BK response. In this process, Ca-dependent activation of phospholipase A_2 is known to be implicated. This may be one of the Ca-dependent facilitatory processes, but this would not be the sole mechanism involved, since exogenously applied PGE_2 did not effectively restore the decreased response of BK in the Ca-free state. Ca-dependent processes in nociceptor activity remain an interesting problem to be clarified.

As mentioned above, a reduced K^+ concentration of Krebs solution suppressed responses to algesic substances, but if the concentration of K^+ is reduced to zero resting discharges and response tend to increase with some time lag. This might be caused by suppression of electrogenic $Na^+ - K^+$ pump activity due to the elimination of K ions from the outside of the membrane, since similar phenomena were observed by application of ouabain. In both the K^+-free and ouabain-treated condition, (1) spontaneous discharges increased, (2) response to hypertonic saline augmented, and (3) cold temperatures suppressed, and warming increased the discharges. The appearance of thermosensitivity of this receptor in these two conditions may be interpreted as follows: temperature-dependent membrane depolarization as caused by a larger temperature coefficient for P_{Na} than P_K (Carpenter, 1981) may be unmasked by eliminating another temperature-dependent activation of the $Na^+ - K^+$ pump, which acts in the opposite direction.

In summary, noxious stimuli act on nociceptors to elicit impulse discharges for an alarm signal on the one hand, and on the surrounding tissues to produce various cell reactions for defense on the other. The reaction in the surrounding tissues involves production of pain producing substances like BK and sensitizing substances like PGs derived from lipoproteins of the cell membrane, as well as release of sensitizing substances like histamine or 5-HT, resulting in inflammatory changes including vascular reactions causing rubor, tumor and calor. All of these factors influence nociceptor activity. Nociceptor activation accompanies release of neuropeptides from the endings and these act on various cell components and blood vessels to modify the tissue reactions. A full understanding of these mutual interrelations of the tissue microenvironment is needed to understand the function of nociceptors and indeed is a quite interesting and fundamental problem for further exploration.

References

Barbieri, E.J., Orzechowski, R.F. and Rossi, G.V. (1977) Measurement of prostaglandin E_2 in an inflammatory exudate: effects of nonsteroidal anti-inflammatory agents. *J. Pharmacol. Exp. Ther.,* 201: 769 – 777.

Bessou, P. and Perl, E.R. (1966) A movement receptor of the small intestine. *J. Physiol. (London),* 182: 404 – 426.

Carpenter, D.O. (1981) Ionic and metabolic bases of neuronal thermosensitivity. *Fed. Proc.,* 40: 2808 – 2813.

Essman, W.B. (1978) Serotonin distribution in tissues and fluids. In: W.B. Essman (Ed.), *Availability, Localization and Disposition, Vol. 1.* Spectrum, New York, pp. 132 – 181.

Ferreira, S.H. and Nakamura, M. (1979) II. Prostaglandin hyperalgesia: the peripheral analgesic activity of morphine, enkephalins and opioid antagonists. *Prostaglandins,* 18: 191 – 200.

Ferreira, S.H., Moncada, S. and Vane, J.R. (1971) Indomethacin and aspirin abolish prostaglandin release from the spleen. *Nature New Biol.,* 231: 237 – 239.

Higgs, G.A., Moncada, S., Salmon, J.A. and Seager, K. (1983) The source of thromboxane and prostaglandins in experimental inflammation. *Br. J. Pharmacol.,* 79: 863 – 868.

Johansson, S.-A. (1960) 5-Hydroxytryptamine in burns. *Acta Physiol. Scand.,* 48: 126 – 132.

Kumazawa, T. and Mizumura, K. (1977) Thin-fibre receptors responding to mechanical, chemical and thermal stimulation in the skeletal muscle of the dog. *J. Physiol. (London),* 273: 179 – 194.

Kumazawa, T. and Perl, E.R. (1977) Primate cutaneous sensory units with unmyelinated (C) afferent fibers. *J. Neurophysiol.,* 40: 1325 – 1338.

Kumazawa, T. and Mizumura, K. (1980) Mechanical and thermal responses of polymodal receptors recorded from the superior spermatic nerve of dogs. *J. Physiol. (London),* 299: 233 – 245.

Kumazawa, T., Mizumura, K. and Sato, J. (1987a) Thermally potentiated responses to algesic substances of visceral nociceptors. *Pain,* 28: 255 – 264.

Kumazawa, T., Mizumura, K. and Sato, J. (1987b) Response properties of polymodal receptors studied using in vitro testis spermatic nerve preparation of dogs. *J. Neurophysiol.,* 57: 702 – 711.

Marceau, F., Barabe, J., St-Pierre, S. and Regoli, D. (1980) Kinin receptors in experimental inflammation. *Can. J. Physiol. Pharmacol.,* 58: 536 – 542.

Mizumura, K., Sato, J. and Kumazawa, T. (1987) Effects of prostaglandins and other putative chemical intermediaries on the activity of canine testicular polymodal receptors studied in vitro. *Pflugers Arch.,* 408: 565 – 572.

Ohuchi, K., Sato, H. and Tsurufuji, S. (1976) The content of prostaglandin E and prostaglandin $F_{2\alpha}$ in the exudate of carrageenin granuloma of rats. *Biochim. Biophys. Acta,* 424: 439 – 448.

W. Hamann and A. Iggo (Eds.)
Progress in Brain Research, Vol. 74
© 1988 Elsevier Science Publishers B.V. (Biomedical Division)

CHAPTER 39

Psychophysical and neurophysiological studies of chemically induced cutaneous pain and itch

The case of the missing nociceptor

Robert H. LaMotte

Department of Anesthesiology, Yale University School of Medicine, 333 Cedar Street, New Haven, CT 06510, USA

Introduction

Algesic or pruritic chemicals may contact the skin from the outside or be endogenously released, either from non-neural tissue, or from the endings of certain peripheral nerve fibers. Certain cutaneous nociceptors, such as the C fiber polymodal nociceptor, may be directly excited and/or sensitized by such chemicals (Beck and Handwerker, 1974; Handwerker, 1976). There have been few, if any, direct attempts to quantitate the relationships among the types and concentrations of chemicals, the graded discharges of evoked responses in cutaneous sensory receptors and psychophysical measurements of evoked sensations. Toward this goal, we designed three sets of experiments.[a] (1) We measured, psychophysically in humans, the sensation of pain or itch produced by an intradermal injection of capsaicin or histamine dihydrochloride respectively. (2) We characterized the two different types of mechanical hyperesthesia to lightly stroking the skin around the injection site: tenderness (allodynia) after cap-

saicin and itch ('alloknesis'[b]) after histamine. (3) We searched for the cutaneous receptors contributing to these chemically induced sensations and hyperesthesias by recording from single peripheral nerve fibers in both monkeys and humans. Surprisingly, none of the known types of cutaneous receptors studied could account for the observed sensory events, hence the subtitle of this paper and our hypothesis for the existence of a class of 'missing' nociceptors.

Methods

Human subjects ($n = 10 - 15$) were injected intradermally with 10 μl of either capsaicin or histamine into the volar forearm in doses of 0.01, 0.1, 1, 10, or 100 μg. The vehicles were Tween – saline for capsaicin, and normal saline alone for histamine. The subjects were instructed to judge the magnitude of pain (after capsaicin) or itch (after histamine) by calling out a number every 15 s that was proportional to the magnitude of sen-

---

[a] As some of this work is to be published in full-length manuscripts or has been previously described in abstracts, only a brief summary is provided here. The author gratefully acknowledges collaboration with many colleagues including Drs. M. Alreja, T.K. Baumann, C.N. Shain, and D.A. Simone.

---

[b] The term 'alloknesis' is suggested for mechanically evoked itch, since light stroking is 'other than' ('allo' in Greek) a normal itch-provoking stimulus and 'knesis' is the ancient Greek word for 'itching'.

sation (the method of magnitude estimation, see Stevens, 1975). Once the magnitude estimates had fallen to zero, the skin surrounding the injection site was mapped by lightly stroking the skin with a cotton swab in order to define the area of abnormal sensation, i.e., allodynia (tenderness or pain) that occurred after a sufficiently high dose of capsaicin or alloknesis (itch) after a sufficiently high dose of histamine.

In neurophysiological experiments, evoked responses in single nociceptive afferent fibers innervating the hairy skin of the arm or leg were recorded electrophysiologically from anesthetized monkey using conventional methods (LaMotte et al., 1983). Receptive fields of these fibers were typically searched for and mapped using mechanical stimuli, such as lightly pinching the skin with the experimenter's fingers or poking the skin with von Frey filaments. In a small number of experiments, heat or cold stimuli were used instead of the mechanical stimuli. These search stimuli were faintly or moderately painful but did not pro-

duce hyperalgesia, when applied to human skin. In a collaborative study with Drs. Torebjörk and Lundberg in Uppsala, similar experiments were conducted in awake humans while recording percutaneously from single nociceptive afferent fibers from the common peroneal nerve.

Results and discussion

Psychophysical measurements of chemogenic pain and itch

Capsaicin produced pain (and never itch) that reached a peak magnitude immediately after injection, and then usually decreased to zero within 15 min (for a dose of 100 μg). The peak magnitude of pain from 100 μg was typically judged as 3 – 5 times greater than the pain from a 5-s heat stimulus of 51°C (given during a previous test without chemical stimuli). Both the peak magnitude and the duration of pain increased with the dose of capsaicin from 0.01 to 100 μg (Simone et al.,

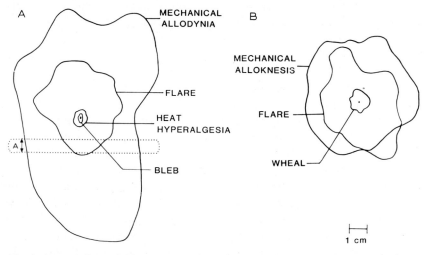

Fig. 1. A comparison of skin reactions and areas of altered sensation produced by an intradermal injection of capsaicin vs. histamine dihydrochloride into the human volar forearm. One subject was given 10 μl of 100 μg of capsaicin and another subject 10 μl of 10 μg of histamine. The injection site is marked by a dot. Top to bottom is proximal to distal. (A) Capsaicin produced a small, raised area (bleb), a local region of heat hyperalgesia, an area of reddening (flare), and an area of mechanical hyperalgesia (allodynia) that encompassed the above areas and within which a light cutaneous stroke elicited pain or tenderness. (B) Histamine produced a local edema (wheal), a flare and an area of mechanical alloknesis (typically including the area within the flare) within which a light cutaneous stroke evoked itch. If a strip of skin 1 cm away from the injection site was anesthetized with lidocaine (e.g., the dashed region marked by an 'A'), allodynia or alloknesis was prevented from occurring on the side of the strip away from the injection site.

1987a). In contrast, histamine produced itch (and not pain) that reached a peak magnitude within a minute and decreased gradually to zero within 30 min (for a dose of 100 μg). The peak magnitude and the duration of itch increased with the dose from 0.01 to 100 μg (Simone et al., 1987c). We interpret these results as follows. (1) The intradermal injection technique was successful in delivering a quantitated continuum of stimulus intensities (chemical concentrations). (2) The evoked sensation could be measured psychophysically and was dose-related in magnitude and duration. (3) Since capsaicin and histamine each elicited a singular and different quality of sensation, namely pain and itch, these two types of sensation are probably served by different sensory receptors.

Psychophysical studies of neurogenic hyperesthesia

Capsaicin and histamine each produced, at the higher doses, a different quality of mechanical hyperesthesia to lightly stroking the skin around the injection site (Simone et al., 1985; LaMotte et al., 1987a). This is illustrated in Fig. 1 for an intradermal injection of each chemical in two different subjects. Capsaicin produced a small bleb at the injection site without a wheal. There was a small area of heat hyperalgesia close to the bleb, wherein thresholds for heat pain were typically about 32°C (Simone et al., 1987b). Surrounding this region was a much larger area, greater than the area of erythema, i.e., flare, within which light stroking with a cotton swab evoked pain or tenderness and von Frey filaments elicited a greater than normal magnitude of pain ('allodynia'). In contrast, histamine (10 μg) elicited a wheal, a flare and a surrounding area that was typically the same size or slightly larger than the flare within which light stroking elicited itch ('alloknesis') and not tenderness or pain. The phenomenon of 'itchy skin' surrounding a histamine injection was studied by Bickford (1938) and Graham et al. (1951).

Neural mechanisms underlying chemogenic pain, itch and hyperalgesia

Experiments were conducted to determine whether the allodynia from capsaicin was controlled neurogenically, and if so, whether the mechanism was in the peripheral or the central nervous system. An injection of lidocaine into the capsaicin bleb greatly reduced and typically eliminated the pain and hyperalgesia. This resulted in normal cutaneous sensation around the injection site. Similarly, placing a cold thermode (1 cm diameter, 5°C) over the bleb for several minutes eliminated or reduced the area of tenderness to a diameter of about 1 – 1.5 cm while rewarming brought it back. In other experiments, the area of tenderness was eliminated distal but not proximal to a thin medialateral strip of lidocaine injected intradermally 1 cm distal to the injection site (Fig. 1, left panel). We therefore conclude that peripheral neural activity at the injection site continuously maintained the surrounding mechanical tenderness and did so by a peripheral neuronal pathway such as an axon reflex (Lewis, 1937) and not by a central facilitatory neuronal mechanism (e.g., Hardy et al., 1950). The results of experiments in which conduction was selectively blocked in A fibers by either ischemia or nerve compression or in C fibers by local anesthetization indicated that both the injection pain and the subsequent allodynia were mediated primarily by A-δ and/or C fibers (Simone et al., 1985).

The same experiments are currently being carried out to determine the underlying mechanism of alloknesis after histamine. Preliminary results exactly parallel those described for allodynia after capsaicin.

In single fiber recordings from the anesthetized monkey, 40 C fiber and 30 A fiber mechano-heat ('polymodal') nociceptors (CMHs and AMHs, respectively) were studied (Simone et al., 1986; LaMotte et al., 1987a). Each fiber received an injection of 100 μg of capsaicin inside, adjacent to or outside (5 – 7 mm) its cutaneous receptive field (RF). Only about half of the CMHs and one of the

AMHs responded to any of these injections and then usually did so weakly and transiently (e.g., less than 3 min) and responded with a discharge rate typically much less than that evoked by a 5-s heat stimulus of 51°C. Six C fiber 'heat nociceptors' were discovered that responded weakly or not at all to noxious mechanical stimulation but responded readily to heat stimuli that were painful to human observers. These nociceptors all responded better than CMHs to capsaicin and several gave a much greater peak discharge rate to capsaicin than to a 51°C heat stimulus. One 'cold nociceptor' that responded well to cold stimuli (< 10°C), but not at all to noxious mechanical or heat stimuli, did not respond to capsaicin. None of the fibers tested became sensitized to mechanical stimulation and only a few were sensitized to heat. In fact, most became desensitized after an injection inside their receptive fields and often ceased responding to any natural stimulation.

In single unit recordings from peripheral nerves in awake humans, the responses of 11 CMH nociceptive afferents were studied after injection of capsaicin (100 μg, 10 μl) outside, adjacent to or inside their RFs on the dorsum of the foot (LaMotte et al., 1987b). Each injection produced the usual pain and an area of mechanical hyperalgesia that enveloped the fiber's RF. Only those injections that were inside or close (< 8 mm) to the receptive field evoked responses and then only a weak and transient response in about half of those tested. None of the fibers tested became significantly sensitized to mechanical stimulation. Thus, we found no evidence that CMHs in humans were different from those in monkeys, i.e., their responses could not account for the pain or hyperalgesia from capsaicin.

We conclude the following. (1) Activity in mechano-heat (polymodal) nociceptors contribute little to the capsaicin injection pain produced by the 100-μg dose and does not account for the greater pain to capsaicin than to heat of 51°C. Whether C heat nociceptors or other (unknown) nociceptors make the major contribution to capsaicin pain awaits further investigation. (2) Only a few of the fibers responsive to capsaicin could provide a candidate mechanism for maintaining allodynia around the injection site since most ceased responding within 3 min of the injection while allodynia in humans typically persisted for an hour or more. (3) There was no evidence that any of these fibers contributed significantly to the mechanical or heat hyperalgesia from capsaicin.

In neurophysiological studies of itch in the monkey, none of the 21 CMHs tested and none of six AMHs responded to an intradermal injection of 0.1 (or 1) μg of histamine given adjacent to or inside their RFs (LaMotte et al., 1987a). Since these doses always produced itch in humans either there is a species difference as to fiber sensitivity between monkey and man or the CMH and AMH nociceptive afferents do not play a major role in histamine induced itch.

In some of our fiber recording experiments in monkeys or humans, one or more fibers that were previously silent and unresponsive to mechanical or thermal stimuli prior to chemical injection began responding after an injection of capsaicin or histamine. These observations, however, are still anecdotal and further investigation is needed. But such findings and, more importantly, our psychophysical observations lead me to postulate the existence of a new class of nociceptors in humans which I term chemical nociceptors or 'chemonociceptors'. Most of these would have C fibers and be relatively insensitive to noxious mechanical or thermal stimuli but respond readily to specific exogenous and/or endogenous chemical substances. I predict that there are at least four subcategories of fiber types. The first type (call it 'A1') would respond best to algesic chemicals and release from its widely arborizing terminal endings a chemical ('X') that mechanically sensitizes another subclass of chemonociceptors (A2) – those mediating allodynia. A third subclass (P1) responds best to pruritic chemicals, and releases a chemical ('Y') that mechanically sensitizes the fourth subclass of fibers (P2) – those that mediate alloknesis.

The hypothetical fibers A1 and 2 are

physiologically coupled as are P1 and 2. There is recent evidence for physiological coupling in the periphery between certain afferent C fibers in the monkey (Meyer et al., 1985). The majority of these coupled C fibers do not have mechanical receptive fields and some of these respond to algesic or pruritic chemicals injected into a local region of the skin (Meyer and Campbell, 1987).

Why have somatic chemonociceptors not been found in earlier studies? The answer may be that there has been little motivation to search for them. Since our observations now provide such a motive, it is hoped that a concerted effort will eventually be successful and solve the case of the 'missing nociceptor'.

Acknowledgement

This research was supported by a grant from the USPHS (14624).

References

Beck, P.W. and Handwerker, P.O. (1974) Bradykinin and serotonin effects on various types of cutaneous nerve fibres. *Pflüger's Arch.,* 347: 209 – 222.

Bickford, R.G. (1938) Experiments relating to the itch sensation, its peripheral mechanism and central pathways. *Clin. Sci.,* 3: 377 – 386.

Graham, D.T., Goodell, H. and Wolff, H.G. (1951) Neural mechanisms involved in itch, 'itchy skin', and tickle sensations. *J. Clin. Invest.,* 30: 37 – 49.

Handwerker, H.O. (1976) Pharmacological modulation of the discharge of nociceptive C-fibers. In: Y. Zotterman (Ed.), *Sensory Functions of the Skin in Primates,* Pergamon Press, Oxford, pp. 427 – 439.

Hardy, J.D., Wolff, H.G. and Goodell, H. (1950) Experimental evidence on the nature of cutaneous hyperalgesia. *J. Clin. Invest.,* 29: 115 – 140.

LaMotte, R.H., Thalhammer, J.G. and Robinson, C.J. (1983) Peripheral neural correlates of magnitude of cutaneous pain and hyperalgesia: a comparison of neural events in monkey with sensory judgments in human. *J. Neurophysiol.,* 50: 1 – 26.

LaMotte, R.H., Simone, D.A., Baumann, T.K., Shain, C.N. and Alreja, M. (1987a) Hypothesis for novel classes of chemoreceptors mediating chemogenic pain and itch. *Pain,* Suppl. 4: S15.

LaMotte, R.H., Torebjörk, E. and Lundberg, L. (1987b) Neural mechanisms of cutaneous hyperalgesia in humans: peripheral or central? *Neurosci. Abstr.,* 13: 189.

Lewis, T. (1937) The nocifensor system of nerves and its reactions. I and II. *Br. Med. J.,* 1: 431 – 437, 491 – 494.

Meyer, R.A. and Campbell, J.N. (1987) A novel electrophysiological technique for locating cutaneous nociceptors and chemospecific receptors. *Brain Res.,* in press.

Meyer, R.A., Raja, S.N. and Campbell, J.N. (1985) Coupling of action potentials between unmyelinated fibers in the peripheral nerve of the monkey. *Science,* 227: 184 – 187.

Simone, D.A., Ngeow, J.Y.F. and LaMotte, R.H. (1985) Neurogenic spread of hyperalgesia after intracutaneous injection of capsaicin in humans. *Soc. Neurosci. Abstr.,* 11: 123.

Simone, D.A., Baumann, T.K., Shain, C.N. and LaMotte, R.H. (1986) The common polymodal nociceptor does not contribute to hyperalgesia produced by intracutaneous injection of capsaicin. *Soc. Neurosci. Abstr.,* 12: 331.

Simone, D.A., Baumann, T.K., Shain, C.N. and LaMotte, R.H. (1987a) Magnitude scaling of chemogenic pain and hyperalgesia in humans. *Soc. Neurosci. Abstr.,* 13: 109.

Simone, D.A., Ngeow, J.Y.F., Putterman, G.J. and LaMotte, R.H. (1987b) Hyperalgesia to heat after intradermal injection of capsaicin. *Brain Res.,* 418: 201 – 203.

Simone, D.A., Ngeow, J.Y.F., Whitehouse, J., Becerra-Cabal, L., Putterman, G.J. and LaMotte, R.H. (1987c) The magnitude and duration of itch produced by intracutaneous injections of histamine. *Somatosens. Res.,* 5: 81 – 92.

Stevens, S.S. (1975) *Psychophysics.* John Wiley and Sons, New York.

W. Hamann and A. Iggo (Eds.)
Progress in Brain Research, Vol. 74
© 1988 Elsevier Science Publishers B.V. (Biomedical Division)

CHAPTER 40

Possible role of capillary permeability in the excitation of sensory receptors by chemical substances

Ashima Anand and A.S. Paintal

DST Centre for Visceral Mechanisms, V.P. Chest Institute, University of Delhi, Delhi-110 007, India

Introduction

At the first Hong Kong symposium on sensory receptor mechanisms held in 1983, Paintal and Anand (1984) concluded that histamine might reveal the presence of sub-threshold activity in certain sensory receptors. This conclusion was based on observations made on type J receptors, pulmonary stretch receptors and the slowly adapting type 1 cutaneous receptor (SA1) following intravenous injections of histamine. In all three receptors the stimulus was adjusted such that the receptor gave an occasional response of one impulse or did not respond at all following most repeated mechanical stimuli. After the injection of histamine a clear response appeared following each stimulus. This effect of histamine is shown in Fig. 1. In the case of type J receptors a paranatural stimulus was used while in the case of the pulmonary stretch receptor the natural stimulus, i.e., inflation of the lungs, was used. In both cases the stimulus was adjusted such that it was below threshold for the receptor.

From observations such as those shown in Fig. 1 it followed that histamine revealed the presence of sub-threshold activity. It was concluded that this effect of histamine could not be due to an enhancement of the generator potential as the effects of chemical substances on the generator potential were known to be very small when compared to their effects on the regenerative region (Paintal, 1964). It was also felt that vascular changes were unlikely as the effect on the SA1 receptor occurred only briefly after a long delay. However, recent experiments suggest that the effect of histamine could be due to an increase in permeability of the capillaries in the vicinity of the receptor leading to an increase in tissue fluid which through a mechanical effect lowers the threshold of the receptor to the fixed stimulus. We give here a preliminary report of some initial observations on type J receptors.

Methods

Adult cats were anaesthetised either with chloralose 75 mg/kg (i.v.) after induction with trichlorethylene or with 35 mg/kg sodium pentobarbital (i.p.).

The vagus nerve near the nodose ganglion was separated from the surrounding tissues and placed on a glass plate for dissecting filaments containing afferent fibres from type J receptors. Type J receptors were identified by the fact that an injection of phenyldiguanide into the right atrium produced a discharge of impulses within 2.5 s in them, that no

338

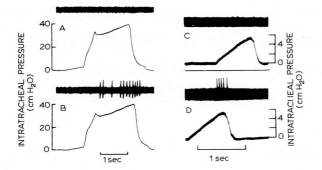

Fig. 1. Reduction in the threshold of type J (A, B) and pulmonary stretch receptors (C, D) by histamine. The stimulus used for stimulating the J receptor was hyperinflation which was just sub-threshold in A. After injecting histamine (i.v.) the same stimulus produced a clear burst of impulses in B. C and D are records from a pulmonary stretch receptor before and after histamine (i.v.) respectively; note the clear reduction and sensitisation after histamine as in the J receptor (A, B). (Adapted from Paintal and Anand, 1984.)

activity followed a similar injection into the left atrium and that they yielded a burst of impulses following sudden inflation with air bubbled through halothane kept at 4°C within 0.3 s (see Paintal, 1969).

A catheter was inserted into the femoral artery for recording arterial blood pressure with a Statham type P 23 Gb pressure transducer. A second catheter was inserted into the external jugular vein such that its tip lay in the right atrium or right ventricle. A third catheter was inserted into the left atrium after opening the chest. The cats were ventilated with a Palmer respiratory pump (Ideal).

Histamine (Fluka) in a concentration of 100 μg/m was used. Phenyldiguanide (Light Co.) was also used in the same concentration.

Results and discussion

The main results are shown in Figs. 2 and 3. Samples of records relating to one J fibre are shown in Fig. 2. Fig. 2A shows the response of the receptor to an injection of 150 μg phenyldiguanide into the right ventricle. Thereafter histamine 150 μg was injected and about 2 min later the same

dose of phenyldiguanide was injected again; the effect is shown in Fig. 2B; clearly the response is much greater than before injection of histamine. Fig. 3 shows the responses in another receptor; note the duration of stimulation, peak frequency of discharge and the total number of impulses produced by phenyldiguanide is clearly greater after a previous injection of histamine. The responses obtained in 12 other receptors were similar, i.e., in nearly all of them the discharge produced by the same dose of phenyldiguanide was much greater after histamine. Since there is no evidence to suggest that histamine directly potentiates the effect of phenyldiguanide, the results of Figs. 2 and 3 (and other receptors) suggest that the greater effect after histamine (Figs. 2B and 3B) could be due to a greater concentration of phenyldiguanide reaching the site of the J receptors after histamine injection and thus the greater response to the same dose of phenyldiguanide. This could happen if histamine increased the permeability of the pulmonary capillaries particularly in view of the fact that it is now well recognised, following the observations of Meyrick and Reid (1971) and Hung et al. (1972), that the type J receptors are located in the interstitium close to the pulmonary capillaries (see Paintal, 1983; Coleridge and Coleridge, 1984). However, the observations of Pietra et al. (1971) with colloidal carbon particles and their subsequent observations using haemoglobin (Pietra et al., 1979) indicate that the pulmonary capillaries do not show obvious evidence of leakiness follow-

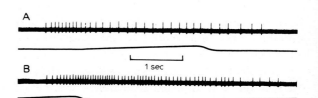

Fig. 2. Potentiation of the excitatory effect of phenyldiguanide on a J receptor by histamine. A shows the impulses produced following an injection of 150 μg phenyldiguanide into the right ventricle. B shows the response following a similar injection about 2 min after an injection of histamine (150 μg, i.v.); note that the effect of phenyldiguanide is much greater.

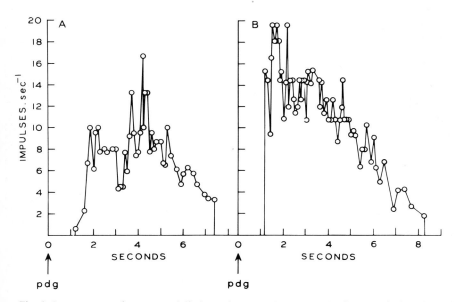

Fig. 3. Instantaneous frequency of discharge in a type J receptor. At time zero in both A and B 150 μg phenyldiguanide (pdg) was injected. B shows the response after a prior intravenous injection of histamine; note the obviously greater effect of phenyldiguanide.

ing histamine. Their observations were made in dogs and it is possible that the pulmonary capillaries of cats may be affected differently by histamine although the haemodynamic effects of histamine on the pulmonary circulation of cats (Colebatch, 1970) and dogs (Pietra et al., 1971) seem to be qualitatively the same.

If it is assumed that histamine does indeed increase the permeability of the pulmonary capillaries (in the vicinity of the J receptors), as the observations shown in Figs. 2 and 3 would in-

dicate, then fluid would increase temporarily in the collagen tissue surrounding the J receptor (see Paintal, 1969, 1983). This would alter the response of the receptor to mechanical stimulation. In the case of the pulmonary stretch receptors which are located in the airways (see Paintal, 1983) the position is more certain because here Pietra et al. (1971, 1979) found clear evidence of leaky bronchial vessels after histamine. Thus in the case of the pulmonary stretch receptors the reduction in the threshold of the receptor to the same

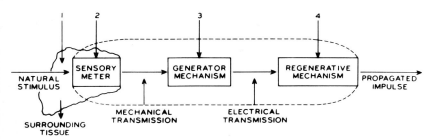

Fig. 4. Possible sites of action of histamine at the sensory receptor complex enclosed by the dotted line. In the case of the type J and pulmonary stretch receptors (Fig. 1) it is suggested that histamine increases the permeability of capillaries thereby leading to the presence of a greater amount of fluid in the tissue surrounding the receptor, i.e., at site 1. This then lowers the threshold of the receptor to the natural stimulus revealing the presence of sub-threshold activity as shown in Fig. 1.

mechanical stimulus could certainly be due to the temporary increase in tissue fluid near the receptor and this makes the mechanical stimulus more effective. This is how histamine reveals the presence of sub-threshold activity in this receptor.

In conclusion at present one can explain the results of Fig. 1 on the assumption that histamine increases the permeability of the capillaries close to the sensory receptors leading to the accumulation of fluid at point 1 of Fig. 4. It is through an action at this point that histamine is able to reveal the presence of sub-threshold activity at certain receptors as shown at the first symposium held in Hong Kong in 1983 (Paintal and Anand, 1984). Histamine could, like other substances, also act at site 4 (Fig. 4) by lowering the threshold of the regenerative region to the unchanged generator potential. Indeed this has to be kept in mind in the case of J receptors because larger doses produce a clear excitatory effect (Armstrong and Luck, 1984) presumably by an action at the regenerative region (site 4). Chemical substances have a much weaker effect on the generator region, i.e., site 3 (Paintal, 1964, 1971). Action at site 2 (Fig. 4), i.e., the sensory meter which filters the mechanical stimulus (e.g., the capsule of the Pacinian corpuscle) (see Paintal, 1971, 1976) has so far not been suggested by any investigator.

References

Armstrong, D.J. and Luck, J.C. (1974) A comparative study of irritant and type J receptors in the cat. *Respir. Physiol., 21:* 47 – 60.

Colebatch, H.J.H. (1970) Adrenergic mechanisms in the effects of histamine in the pulmonary circulation of the cat. *Circulat. Res.,* 26: 379 – 396.

Coleridge, J.C.G. and Coleridge, H.M. (1984) Afferent vagal C fibre innervation of the lungs and airways and its functional significance. *Rev. Physiol. Biochem. Pharmacol.,* 99: 1 – 110.

Hung, K.-S., Hertweck, M.S., Hardy, J.D. and Loosli, C.G. (1972) Innervation of pulmonary alveoli of the mouse lung: an electron microscopic study. *Am. J. Anat.,* 135: 477 – 495.

Meyrick, B. and Reid, L. (1971) Intra-alveolar wall nerve in rat lung: an electron-microscopic study. *J. Physiol. (London),* 214: 6P – 7P.

Paintal, A.S. (1964) Effects of drugs on vertebrate mechanoreceptors. *Pharmacol. Rev.,* 16: 341 – 380.

Paintal, A.S. (1969) Mechanism of stimulation of type J pulmonary receptors. *J. Physiol. (London),* 203: 511 – 532.

Paintal, A.S. (1971) Action of drugs on sensory nerve endings. *Annu. Rev. Pharmacol.,* 11, 231 – 240.

Paintal, A.S. (1976). Natural and paranatural stimulation of sensory receptors. In: Y. Zotterman (Ed.), *Sensory Functions of the Skin.* Pergamon Press, Oxford, pp. 3 – 12.

Paintal, A.S. (1983) Lung and airway receptors. In: D.J. Pallot (Ed.), *Control of Respiration.* Croom Helm, London, pp. 78 – 107.

Paintal, A.S. and Anand, A. (1984) The detection of subthreshold activity of J and other receptors. In: W. Hamann and A. Iggo (Eds.), *Sensory Receptor Mechanisms.* World Scientific Publ. Co., Singapore, pp. 207 – 218.

Pietra, G.G., Szidon, J.P., Leventhal, M.M. and Fishman, A.P. (1971) Histamine and interstitial pulmonary edema in the dog. *Circulat. Res.,* 29: 323 – 337.

Pietra, G.G., Magno, M., Johns, L. and Fishman, A.P. (1979) Bronchial veins and pulmonary edema. In: A.P. Fishman and E.M. Renkin (Eds.), *Pulmonary Edema.* American Physiological Society, Bethesda, MD, pp. 195 – 206.

W. Hamann and A. Iggo (Eds.)
Progress in Brain Research, Vol. 74
© 1988 Elsevier Science Publishers B.V. (Biomedical Division)

CHAPTER 41

The expression of sensory receptors on regenerating and regenerated cutaneous C fibres

John Leah, Gabriele-Monika Koschorke, Eckhard Welk and Manfred Zimmermann

II. Physiologisches Institut, Universität Heidelberg, Im Neuenheimer Feld, Heidelberg, D-6900, FRG

Introduction

Afferent cutaneous C fibres are grouped into several subclasses based on the combinations of the types of sensory receptors at their endings. The different types of mechanical or thermal stimuli or chemical ligands to which the individual receptor moieties react have been delineated in a number of species. A minority of C fibres have receptors responding to light mechanical pressure, or to cooling or warming. The endings of the majority of cutaneous C fibres, however, are polymodal nociceptive in that they possess sensory receptors activated by intense mechanical pressure, by high temperatures, or by a variety of chemical agents (Perl, 1984). There is also increasing evidence that there exist on C fibre endings receptor moieties sensitive to other types of stimuli, and that the types of afferent C fibre endings might yet be further subdivided (LaMotte et al., 1987; Meyer et al., 1987).

A characteristic of cutaneous C fibre sensory receptors, and probably also of those on C fibres innervating deeper structures, is their propensity to undergo long-term changes in sensitivity to these various stimuli following a variety of perturbations to the nerve or its endings. This can give rise to sensory disturbances, such as the pain consequent on peripheral nerve injury in humans, and those which result in the autotomy seen in many species of animals after peripheral nerve transection.

Many studies have been made of the types and characteristics of receptors present on the endings of regenerating A fibres (Devor, 1984). The more important problem of changes in the functioning of the different types of sensory receptors at regenerating C fibre endings, which could underlie painful sensory abnormalities, is now increasingly the subject of investigation (see Pubols and Sessle, 1987; Cervero and Morrison, 1986). Here we survey the accumulating findings, including recent results from our own laboratory (Koschorke and Zimmermann, in preparation; Leah and Zimmermann, in preparation; Welk and Zimmermann, in preparation). We do so in the context of considering that each of the receptors specific for the different types of stimuli are separate molecular ensembles whose syntheses in the soma are under separate control mechanisms and which are transported axonally to be inserted into the membranes of the fibre endings. This view of an independent expression of sensory receptor types is evidenced, for example, by the finding that one day after treating a cutaneous nerve with capsaicin there is a selective loss of the mechanoreceptors which are normally present on the same C fibre endings as the thermoreceptors (Welk et al., 1983).

Sensory receptors on C fibre endings in neuromas

Most of the information concerning the functioning of sensory receptors on regenerating peripheral nerve endings is derived from studies where peripheral nerves in animals have been ligated and transected distally. This results in the formation of a nerve end neuroma which contains regenerating nerve sprouts (Devor, 1984). Although in the majority of these studies it has been the sensory receptors of the A fibre endings that have been examined (Devor, 1984), many results have now also been obtained from the C fibre endings.

Spontaneous activity

While the spontaneous activity observed in regenerating nerves is probably generated solely by alterations in their membrane ion channels (Devor, 1983, 1984; Gallego et al., 1987; Lisney and Devor, 1987; Kelly et al., 1986; Lipton, 1987) and not via any sensory receptors per se, the degree of spontaneous activity in damaged afferent nerves is likely to be a measure of the excitability of their membranes. Should these generators of spontaneous activity reside only along the axons then the effects of stimuli applied at the nerve endings are likely to remain the same. However, if the nerve ending membranes themselves are nearer threshold and more excitable, then some alteration of the responsiveness of the endings to stimulation of their receptors might be expected. Spontaneous activity in the regenerating nerves is therefore an important parameter to be considered when evaluating sensory receptor functions in these nerves, especially considering that in intact cutaneous afferents spontaneous activity in C fibres is rare.

Recording from electrically identified fibres, most of which were C fibres, Blumberg and Jänig (1984, 1987) have shown that 4–14% of C fibres ending in neuromas of the cutaneous superficial peroneal nerves in the cat are spontaneously active. The peak incidence of activity occurs about 100 days after formation of the neuroma and maximal discharge frequencies are rarely above 1 Hz. A similar percentage of A and also of apparent C fibres has been reported to be spontaneously active

in sciatic (mixed nerve) neuromas in mice (Scadding, 1981). Spontaneously active C fibres are also recordable from peroneal and median nerve neuromas in humans (Nystrom and Hagbarth, 1981) but the percentage of C fibres which are spontaneously active in these cases is not known. In Sabra strain rats the incidence of spontaneous activity seen in A fibres of sciatic nerve neuromas is also high (Govrin-Lippmann and Devor, 1978; Devor and Govrin-Lippmann, 1983; Lisney and Devor, 1987; Matzner and Devor, 1987) but for C fibres it is usually less than 2% in neuromas up to several weeks old (Devor and Govrin-Lippmann, 1983; Devor and Raber, 1983).

Some caution is warranted in interpreting these findings, as well as those relating to the degree of sensory receptor sensitivity of regenerating nerve endings (see below). Recent reports (Burchiel and Russell, 1985, 1987) have shown that gallamine, used as a muscular paralysing agent in many in vivo experiments, itself causes a more than eight-fold increase in the number of spontaneously active A fibres ending in neuromas. In the absence of this compound few spontaneously active A fibres, and no spontaneously active C fibres, were seen. Gallamine is a potassium channel blocking agent and most likely acts on such channels in the endings of damaged A and C fibre afferents and alters their excitability since it has been found that another potassium channel blocker, 4-aminopyridine, excites normal cutaneous C fibre endings (Kirchof et al., 1988). Gallamine has also been found to enhance the release of noradrenaline from sympathetic nerves (Kobayashi et al., 1987) and this may further influence the excitability of regenerating C fibre endings (see below). Thus the experimental protocol in some in vivo experiments may have rendered the membranes of the nerve sprouts of both the A and C fibres in the neuromas more depolarised than usual, and thus perhaps more likely to be excited by any stimulation of their sensory receptors.

In our laboratory we also see spontaneous C fibre (but not A fibre) discharge at less than 1 Hz in approximately 26% of identified C fibres ending in 3-week-old sural nerve neuromas in the cat. In saphenous nerve neuromas up to 2 months old in Sprague–Dawley rats we find that approximately 6% of C fibres (but rarely A fibres) are active when recordings are made in vivo; and that in this and tibial nerve neuromas up to 1 month old in Sprague–Dawley rats or in guinea-pigs, approximately 3% of C fibres (but virtually no A fibres) are active when the recordings are made from these neuroma nerves in an in vitro chamber.

Chemosensory receptors

Although it is commonly reported that both adrenergic compounds acting at α-receptors, as well as activation of the sympathetic supply, can excite A fibre endings in neuromas (Wall and Gutnick, 1974; Devor and Jänig, 1981; Scadding, 1981; Blumberg and Jänig, 1984; Devor, 1984), the degree to which C fibres are so excitable is less well defined. A study of those fibres which already had on-going activity in the cat superficial peroneal nerve neuroma, most of which were C fibres, showed that 26% could be weakly excited by sympathetic stimulation and 39% could be excited by intravenous injection of adrenaline or noradrenaline (Blumberg and Jänig, 1984). In marked contrast, only one of a total of 815 electrically identifiable but silent C fibres could thus be excited.

This latter finding accords with the results from this laboratory that adrenaline (at concentrations up to 100 μg/ml) excites only 3% of all the C fibre endings in cat sural nerve neuromas, and at most 2% of those in rat or guinea-pig saphenous nerve neuromas (Welk et al., 1987).

The study of the mechanism of action of adrenergic compounds on C fibre endings in neuromas is complicated by the recent evidence that they do not act directly on the afferent endings themselves but rather presynaptically on the sympathetic efferent terminals, possibly releasing prostaglandins (Levine et al., 1986). Since the effects of axotomy on sympathetic efferent functioning are largely unknown, elucidating the details of adrenergic actions on C fibre endings in regenerating nerves and neuromas, which is of clinical relevance, will certainly require further study.

A consistent finding in this laboratory is that C fibre endings in neuromas can be excited by some of the chemical compounds known to act at receptors on normal cutaneous C fibres. Thus the peptide bradykinin (at concentrations up to 100 μg/ml) excites 26% of C fibre endings in 3-week-old sural nerve neuromas in cats (Koschorke and Zimmermann, 1984a,b; Koschorke et al., 1985a; Zimmerman et al., 1987). In contrast, in rat or guinea-pig saphenous nerve neuromas up to 2 months old only 4% or less of C fibre endings are excited by similar concentrations of bradykinin when studied either in vivo or in vitro (Welk et al., 1987). In rat saphenous nerves with 3- to 7-month-old neuromas, studied in vitro, this percentage increases to about 10% of the C fibres.

We have found that there are chemoreceptors for histamine on C fibre endings in neuromas. In the cat sural nerve neuroma 16% of the C fibres can be excited by histamine at 1–100 μg/ml (Koschorke et al., 1985b), but in rat or guinea-pig saphenous nerve neuromas only about 3% of the endings are excitable by such concentrations of this compound (Welk et al., 1987). We have also found that some chemoreceptors on normal cutaneous C fibre endings appear not to be expressed by C fibres ending in neuromas. Thus we have been unable to excite C fibre endings in neuromas in cats by serotonin (Koschorke and Zimmermann, 1984a). In addition to physiological methods, study of the altered expression of chemosensory receptors on regenerating nerve endings would be facilitated by including ligand binding autoradiographic techniques (Ninkovic et al., 1983).

At normal cutaneous C fibre endings some of the sensory receptor types can be sensitised by chemical and other stimuli. Thus prostaglandin E_2 can potentiate the excitation produced by heat and bradykinin (Handwerker, 1976) and serotonin can potentiate the responses to bradykinin (Mizumura et al., 1987). Although Blumberg and Jänig (1987) report that responses to mechanical stimuli are not enhanced by adrenaline in cat superficial peroneal nerve neuromas, we do observe some interactive effects at the sensory receptors on C fibre endings in neuromas. Thus in cat sural nerve neuromas, prior exposure to either adrenaline or noradrenaline potentiates the excitation produced by bradykinin (Koschorke and Zimmermann, 1984a,b). We have not, however, seen such an effect with C fibre endings in rat saphenous nerve neuromas. Substance P has also been seen to suppress C fibre responses to both bradykinin and to heat in cat sural nerve neuromas (Koschorke et al., 1985a). It will be of interest to investigate whether there exist other modulatory events at regenerating C fibre endings, particularly in relation to the prostaglandins.

Mechanosensory receptors

C fibre endings in neuromas express mechanosensitive receptors. Blumberg and Jänig (1984) have found that the percent of fibres (mostly C fibres) whose endings could be excited by 'light' to 'strong' pressure from small-tipped glass rods increased with the age of the neuroma; from 20% in neuromas 6 – 27 days old to 33% in those 53 – 222 days old. All afferents which were spontaneously active were also mechanosensitive. Mechanical stimulation of median and peroneal nerve neuromas in humans also excites the C fibre endings (Nystrom and Hagbarth, 1981).

In saphenous nerve neuromas in Sprague – Dawley rats we have found that, when studied in vivo, an average of 13% of C fibre endings can be excited by probing with von Frey hairs of 0.8 to 160 mN, but this percentage does not increase with neuroma age up to 2 months. When these neuroma nerves are examined in vitro with blunt probes there does seem to be an increase in mechanosensitivity: from 7% of the C fibre endings in neuromas up to 1 month old to 20% in those 3 months old. However, quantification of the presence of, and thresholds for, mechanosensitivity in all of these studies is made difficult by the susceptibility of the neuroma tissue to damage, especially by von Frey hairs used in the manner to examine receptors in skin.

Thermosensory receptors

Few studies have been made of whether C fibre endings in neuromas have receptors sensitive to thermal stimuli. Matzner and Devor (1987) have found that, in sciatic nerve neuromas of Sabra strain rats, cooling the neuroma by an average of 10°C from an original pool temperature of 33 – 34°C excites 1.2% of silent C fibres; and over 50% of those C fibres which are already spontaneously active (about 4% of the total C fibres in these neuromas) at least double their firing rate. The remainder of the spontaneously active C fibres were neither excited nor depressed by cooling. Warming the neuroma by 3 – 4°C decreased the firing rate of the three spontaneously active C fibres examined.

Such results agree with our findings that, in Sprague – Dawley rats, neither cooling the saphenous nerve neuromas by 10°C or more from 32 – 34°C, nor heating to noxious temperatures (50 – 52°C) ever excited more than 2% of the C fibres (Welk et al., 1987). This result in rat neuromas is somewhat surprising and the responsiveness of C fibre endings in neuromas to thermal stimuli warrants further investigation and clarification. In contrast, we find that heating of sural nerve neuromas in cats to 50°C does excite many of the C fibres (Koschorke et al., 1985a).

The nerve endings in the neuromas that form after transecting and ligating cutaneous nerves may not be an entirely appropriate model with which to study the sensory receptors expressed by regenerating C fibres. In such neuromas, the forward growth of the nerve sprouts is physically impeded and there is an accumulation of neurofilaments and membranous organelles in the terminal regions (Liuzzi and Lasek, 1987). Moreover, such enveloped nerve sprouts are less likely to be influenced by any trophic signals released from distal glial cells or denervated tissue, or by signals resulting from the contact of the growing sprouts with membranes of distal glial cells (Carlstedt, 1985; Windebank and Poduslo, 1986; Daniloff et al., 1986). Thus gene expression in such regenerating nerves may be influenced differently to that in freely regenerating C fibres and the types of sensory receptors that they express may be different. In addition, after neuroma formation approximately 50% of C fibres die (Lisney, 1987; Leah and Zimmermann, in preparation) and it may be that those having particular receptor types are lost selectively.

Regenerating cutaneous C fibre endings

Few studies have been made of the sensory receptors expressed by afferent C fibres which have been damaged or sectioned and then allowed to regenerate freely (Lisney, 1987). Diamond (1959) found that many nerve endings in regenerating sural nerves in the rabbit, some of which seem to have been those of C fibres, are excited by acetylcholine. Regenerating sprouts of C fibres in the rabbit auricular nerve trunk are commonly sensitive to mechanical stimuli (Shea and Perl, 1985). Beyond these results, however, nothing is yet known of the sensory receptors of regenerating afferent C fibres.

Regenerated cutaneous C fibre endings

As with regenerating C fibres, there have been few studies specifically of the sensory receptors on previously damaged cutaneous C fibres which have subsequently regenerated into the skin. The results do show, however, that the types of sensory receptors expressed by regenerated cutaneous C fibres are quite similar, but not identical, to those of normal cutaneous C fibre endings. The proportion of regenerated C fibres with the different types of receptors is also similar to that of the normal nerves.

After regeneration of transected auricular nerves in the rabbit the relative proportion of C fibres ex-

pressing each of the different types of receptors, and the characteristics of these receptors are also nearly identical to those in normal skin. However, the mean threshold for those responding to noxious heating is lower by about 3.8°C (Shea and Perl, 1985). Similar results have been found in this laboratory. Thus, after crushing the plantar nerves in the cat the regenerated C fibre endings in the skin have receptors responding to both low and high threshold mechanical stimuli, and to noxious heating of the skin (Dickhaus et al., 1976). The mean threshold for the latter stimulus is again lower by about 3.7°C compared to that in normal nerves.

Discussion

The above results illustrate how the types of sensory receptors found at regenerating cutaneous C fibre endings may differ, depending on both the species of animal considered and the time after the initial damage at which the nerve endings are studied. Generally, for example, most C fibre endings in neuromas less than 1 month old in cats have many of the receptors of normal endings in skin. In contrast, those in rats are initially more quiescent, with only a few expressing some receptor types after several months. These differences are likely to be, in part, a consequence of genetic differences in the requirement of the regenerating nerves for trophic influences from distal glial and target cells (or perhaps from central sources) to initiate receptor expression. The expression of some types of receptors in a few of the C fibre endings in neuromas in rats after several months may be because they have made contact with epithelial tissue or blood vessels of sufficient efficacy to initiate expression of some receptors (Russell and Burchiel, 1987).

Although the results at this stage are somewhat disparate (for example, there are no detailed studies of all the possible types of receptors on single regenerating C fibre endings), this review does seem to support our initial consideration and an emerging general principle: the different molecular ensembles that constitute each of the different sensory receptor types may be expressed independently, and that spectrum of sensory receptors expressed during the course of regeneration of C fibres is different from that of normal and regenerated C fibres. Thus, for example, many normal cutaneous C fibres have receptors for mechanical pressure, high temperatures and bradykinin present on the same endings, whereas with regenerating endings in neuromas it may be that only the receptors for bradykinin are expressed. Indeed, receptors for high temperatures, and for serotonin and histamine have thus far rarely been encountered on regenerating nerve endings, whereas those for bradykinin and mechanical stimuli appear to be common.

This differential expression of sensory receptor types in regenerating nerves is analogous to the differential changes in the synthesis of neuropeptides also seen following peripheral nerve transection. Here, for example, the synthesis of substance P and of somatostatin is decreased but that of vasoactive intestinal peptide and galanin is increased (Shehab and Atkinson, 1986; Hökfelt et al., 1987). Thus, this differential expression of sensory receptor types in regenerating C fibres should be seen in the broader context of a generalised alteration in gene expression (or post-transcriptional processing) by the nerves following damage to their peripheral axons. Although the functional significance of these alterations is difficult to envisage, since the spectrum of receptors present on regenerated cutaneous C fibres is essentially the same as that on such normal C fibre endings, it would appear that the alterations are under some controlling influence from the skin.

Clearly much remains to be learnt about the nature of sensory receptors of regenerating C fibres, not only those of cutaneous afferents but also those with muscle and visceral projections.

References

Blumberg, H. and Jänig, W. (1984) Discharge pattern of afferent fibres from a neuroma. *Pain,* 20: 335–353.

Blumberg, H. and Jänig, W. (1987) Changes in primary afferent neurons following lesions of their axons. In: L.M. Pubols and B.J. Sessle (Eds.), *Effects of Injury on Trigeminal and Spinal Somatosensory Systems. Neurology and Neurobiology, Vol. 30.* Alan R. Liss, New York, pp. 85–92.

Burchiel, K.J. and Russell, L.C. (1985) Effects of potassium channel-blocking agents on spontaneous discharges from neuromas in rats. *J. Neurosurg.,* 63: 246–249.

Burchiel, K.J. and Russell, L.C. (1987) Has the amount of spontaneous electrical activity in experimental neuromas been overestimated?. In: L.M. Pubols and B.J. Sessle (Eds.), *Effects of Injury on Trigeminal and Spinal Somatosensory Systems. Neurology and Neurobiology, Vol. 30.* Alan R. Liss, New York, pp. 77–83.

Carlstedt, T. (1985) Regenerating axons form nerve terminals at astrocytes. *Brain Res.,* 347: 188–191.

Cervero, F. and Morrison, J.F.B. (Eds.) (1986) *Visceral Sensation, Progress in Brain Research, Vol. 67.* Elsevier, Amsterdam.

Daniloff, J.K., Levi, G., Grumet, M., Rieger, F. and Edelman, G.M. (1986) Altered expression of neuronal cell adhesion molecules induced by nerve injury and repair. *J. Cell Biol.,* 103: 929–945.

Devor, M. (1983) Potassium channels moderate ectopic excitability of nerve-end neuromas in rats. *Neurosci. Lett.,* 40: 181–186.

Devor, M. (1984) The pathophysiology and anatomy of damaged nerve. In: P. Wall and R. Melzack (Eds.), *Textbook of Pain.* Churchill-Livingstone, London, pp. 49–64.

Devor, M. and Jänig, W. (1981) Activation of myelinated afferents ending in a neuroma by stimulation of the sympathetic supply in the rat. *Neurosci. Lett.,* 24: 43–47.

Devor, M. and Govrin-Lippman, R. (1983) Axoplasmic transport block reduces ectopic impulse generation in injured peripheral nerves. *Pain,* 16: 73–85.

Devor, M. and Raber, P. (1983) Autotomy after nerve injury and its relation to spontaneous discharge originating in nerve-end neuroma. *Behav. Neural Biol.,* 37: 276–283.

Diamond, J. (1959) The effects of injecting acetylcholine into normal and regenerating nerves. *J. Physiol. (London),* 145: 611–629.

Dickhaus, H., Zimmermann, M. and Zotterman, Y. (1976) The development in regenerating cutaneous nerves of C-fibre receptors responding to noxious heating of the skin. In: Y. Zotterman (Ed.), *Sensory Functions of the Skin in Primates.* Pergamon Press, Oxford, pp. 415–425.

Gallego, R., Ivorra, I. and Morales, A. (1987) Effects of central or peripheral axotomy on membrane properties of sensory neurones in the petrosal ganglion of the cat. *J. Physiol. (London),* 391: 39–56.

Govrin-Lippmann, R. and Devor, M. (1978) Ongoing activity in severed nerves: source and variation with time. *Brain Res.,* 159: 406–410.

Handwerker, H.O. (1976) Influences of algogenic substances and prostaglandins on the discharges of unmyelinated cutaneous nerve fibres identified as nociceptors. In: J.J. Bonica and D.G. Albe-Fessard (Eds.), *Advances in Pain Research and Therapy*. Raven Press, New York, pp. 41 – 51.

Hökfelt, T., Wiesenfeld-Hallin, S., Villar, M. and Melander, T. (1987) Increase of galanin-like immunoreactivity in dorsal root ganglion cells after peripheral axotomy. *Neurosci. Lett.*, 83: 217 – 220.

Kelly, M.E.M., Gordon, T., Shapiro, J. and Smith, P.A. (1986) Axotomy affects calcium-sensitivity potassium conductance in sympathetic neurones. *Neurosci. Lett.*, 67: 163 – 168.

Kirchoff, C., Leah, J., Jung, S. and Reeh, P.W. (1988) That cutaneous nerve endings within homogenous sensory categories show different sensitivity to 4-AP and TEA. *Eur. J. Physiol.*, in press.

Kobayashi, O., Nagashima, H., Duncalf, D., Chaudhry, I.A., Harsing, G.J., Foldes, F.F., Goldiner, P.L. and Vizi, E.S. (1987) Direct evidence that pancuronium and gallamine enhance the release of norepinephrine from the atrial sympathetic nerve by inhibition of prejunctional muscarinic receptors. *J. Autonom. Nerv. Syst.*, 18: 55 – 60.

Koschorke, G.M. and Zimmermann, M. (1984a) Response to algesic substances of non-myelinated fibres in normal and chronically damaged cutaneous nerves of the cat. *Pain*, Suppl., 2: S6.

Koschorke, G.M. and Zimmermann, M. (1984b) Responses to bradykinin of non-myelinated fibres in chronically damaged cutaneous nerves of the cat. *Eur. J. Physiol.*, Suppl., 400: S15.

Koschorke, G.M., Helme, R.D. and Zimmermann, M. (1985a) Substance P suppresses the response to bradykinin and to heat of non-myelinated fibres in experimental neuroma of the cat's sural nerve. *Soc. Neurosci. Abstr.*, 11: 118.

Koschorke, G.M., Westerman, R.A. and Zimmermann, M. (1985b) Histamine excites non-myelinated fibres in experimental neuroma of the cat's sural nerve. *Neurosci. Lett.*, Suppl., 22: S32.

LaMotte, R.H., Simone, D.A., Baumann, T.K., Shain, C.N. and Alreja, M. (1987) Hypothesis for novel classes of chemoreceptors mediating chemogenic pain and itch. *Pain*, Suppl. 4: S15.

Levine, J.D., Taiwo, Y.O., Collins, S.D. and Tam, J.K. (1986) Noradrenaline hyperalgesia is mediated through interaction with sympathetic postganglionic neurone terminals rather than activation of primary afferent nociceptors. *Nature (London)*, 323: 158 – 160.

Lipton, S.A. (1987) Bursting of calcium-activated cation-selective channels is associated with neurite regeneration in a mammalian central neuron. *Neurosci. Lett.*, in press.

Lisney, S.J.W. (1987) Studies on unmyelinated fibre regeneration in rat peripheral nerve. In: L.M. Pubols and B.J. Sessle (Eds.), *Effects of Injury on Trigeminal and Spinal Somatosensory Systems. Neurology and Neurobiology, Vol. 30*. Alan R. Liss, New York, pp. 107 – 114.

Lisney, S.J.W. and Devor, M. (1987) Afterdischarge and interactions among fibers in damaged peripheral nerve in the rat. *Brain Res.*, 415: 122 – 136.

Liuzzi, F.J. and Lasek, R.J. (1987) Astrocytes block axonal regeneration in mammals by activating the physiological stop pathway. *Science*, 237: 642 – 645.

Matzner, O. and Devor, M. (1987) Contrasting thermal sensitivity of spontaneously active A- and C-fibers in experimental nerve-end neuromas. *Pain*, 30: 373 – 384.

Meyer, R.A., Campbell, J.N. and Hartke, T.V. (1987) A novel technique to search for nociceptors. *Pain*, Suppl. 4: S16.

Mizumura, K., Sato, J. and Kumazawa, T. (1987) Effects of prostaglandins and other putative chemical intermediaries on the activity of canine testicular polymodal receptors studied in vitro. *Eur. J. Physiol.*, 408: 565 – 572.

Ninkovic, M., Hunt, S.P., Gleave, J.R.W., Iversen, S.D. and Iversen, L.L. (1983) Autoradiographic localization of neurotransmitter receptors on sensory neurons. In: H.L. Fields, R. Dubner and F. Cervero (Eds.), *Advances in Pain Research and Therapy*. Raven Press, New York, pp. 257 – 263.

Nystrom, B. and Hagbarth, K.E. (1981) Microelectrode recordings from transected nerves in amputees with phantom limb pain. *Neurosci. Lett.*, 27: 211 – 216.

Perl, E.R. (1984) Pain and nociception. In: I. Darian-Smith (Ed.), *Handbook of Physiology*. American Physiological Society, Bethesda, MD, pp. 915 – 975.

Pubols, L.M. and Sessle, B.J. (Eds.) (1987) *Effects of Injury on Trigeminal and Spinal Somatosensory Systems. Neurology and Neurobiology, Vol. 30*. Alan R. Liss, New York.

Russell, L.C. and Burchiel, K.J. (1987) Chronic pain from the periphery: the role of neuroma. In: L.M. Pubols and B.J. Sessle (Eds.), *Effects of Injury on Trigeminal and Spinal Somatosensory Systems. Neurology and Neurobiology, Vol. 30*. Alan R. Liss, New York, p. 485.

Scadding J.W. (1981) Development of ongoing activity, mechanosensitivity, and adrenaline sensitivity in severed peripheral nerve axons. *Exp. Neurol.*, 73: 345 – 364.

Shea, V.K. and Perl, E.R. (1985) Regeneration of cutaneous afferent unmyelinated (C) fibres after transection. *J. Neurophysiol.*, 54: 502 – 512.

Shebab, S.A.S. and Atkinson, M.E. (1986) Vasoactive intestinal polypeptide (VIP) increases in the spinal cord after peripheral axotomy of sciatic nerve originate from primary afferent neurons. *Brain Res.*, 372: 37 – 44.

Wall, P.D. and Gutnick, M. (1974) Properties of afferent nerve impulses originating from a neuroma. *Nature (London)*, 248: 740 – 743.

Welk, E., Petsche, U., Fleischer, E. and Handwerker, H.O. (1983) Altered excitability of afferent C-fibres of the rat distal to a nerve site exposed to capsaicin. *Neurosci. Lett.,* 38: 245 – 250.

Welk, E., Leah, J., Hauch, A. and Zimmermann, M. (1987) Differential expression of sensory functions in regenerating cutaneous C-fibres in rats. *Pain,* Suppl. 4: S200.

Windebank, A.J. and Poduslo, J.F. (1986) Neuronal growth factors produced by adult peripheral nerve injury. *Brain Res.,* 385: 197 – 200.

Zimmermann, M., Koschorke, G.M. and Sanders, K. (1987) Response characteristics of fibers in regenerating and regenerated cutaneous nerves in cat and rat. In: L.M. Pubols and B.J. Sessle (Eds.), *Effects of Injury on Trigeminal and Spinal Somatosensory Systems. Neurology and Neurobiology, Vol. 30.* Alan R. Liss, New York, pp. 93 – 106.

W. Hamann and A. Iggo (Eds.)
Progress in Brain Research, Vol. 74
© 1988 Elsevier Science Publishers B.V. (Biomedical Division)

Modulation and Efferent Control of Transduction: Summary

E.R. Perl

These presentations were an eclectic mixture dealing with excitation and modulation of sensory apparatus of the ear, viscera and skin. The common message was that sense organ responsiveness is, if anything, plastic. Sensitivity may be modified by neural efferent control and possibly in some instances by local neural networks, by changes in the physical environment, and by chemical agents produced by the surrounding tissue. None of this should be surprising given what has been learned from 20th century work on sensory transduction although the session served up new concepts about sense organ modulation as well as offering evidence on older suggestions.

Three of the talks dealt with processes in the inner ear. Å. Flock's evidence for movement of the outer hair cells by a contraction-like action which in turn would modify transduction at the inner hair cells elicited a considerable reaction. Other presentations of the session by T. Hashimoto on current flow within the cochlea and by K. Yanagisawa on the localization of triphosphoinositide on the surface membrane of the stereocilia, while not directly addressing the issue, could relate to an induced motility of the outer hair cells. Voltage-dependent calcium fluxes are established as part of the molecular reconfigurations of contraction and triphosphoinositide's known interactions with calcium fit with a role in contraction. The discussion of Flock's paper emphasized the evidence for at least two kinds of movement, one an overall displacement of the outer hair cells and the second a motion or fixation of the stereocilia. In answer to a query, Dr. Flock suggested that the movements of the cells and of the stereocilia might be independent, the latter being more rapid and phasic with the slower movement of the hair cells serving as a background modulation. Background modulation could conceivably serve to alter sensitivity of specific subsets of hair cells and thereby faces maximum sensitivity on particular parts of the frequency spectrum. The discussion also brought out that a possible contractile material, myosin, has not yet been specifically localized in the hair cells or stereocilia. Another point made was that since the stereocilia can move rapidly, their induced movements could flex the tectorial membrane and thereby actually excite eighth nerve fibers at the base of hair cells. In this context Flock mentioned objective tinnitus, noises produced in the ear and heard by others as well as the subject.

Another three of the presentations were concerned with chemical initiation or modification of the responsiveness or excitability of sensory terminals (Paintal, Kumazawa et al., LaMotte). The sense organs in question were both visceral and cutaneous. This set of discussions made it clear that chemical agents produced or released in the vicinity of certain sensory fibers can substantially, if not profoundly, modify responsiveness. They emphasized a point made earlier in this symposium: chemical responsiveness by specific sense organs may be quite selective. There was discussion only of A. Anand's description of the possible part played by capillary permeability changes in the responsiveness of bronchial receptive elements.

Questions were raised about the directness of the effects of histamine in the reported enhancement of responsiveness of the pulmonary sense organs. A possible relationship between bronchial constriction produced by histamine and the increased reactivity was suggested; Dr. Anand countered that the J receptors are not activated by bronchial constriction. She also argued that histamine was not directly excitatory to these sensory units since the effects took 60 s to develop, a timing more in keeping with a secondary effect such as alteration of capillary permeability. Part of her argument for increased interstitial fluid as the basis of the changes in receptor responsiveness was the production of a similar increased responsiveness by other agents which caused edema without a direct excitatory effect upon the sense organs.

The remaining two presentations of this session described work on mechanoreceptors in what was labelled by discussors as exotic preparations: J. Diamond's Merkel cell sense organs of the salamander skin and R.D. Johnson's cutaneous mechanoreceptors of the penis. Dr. Diamond's conclusion that the Merkel cell is not a crucial link in the excitation of the sensory nerve terminals through a synaptic linkage evoked considerable debate. While there was no substantive disagreement over the proposal that in the absence of Merkel cells, the nerve receptive terminals are still mechanically excitable, there were objections to the implication that the Merkel cell was not involved in providing the special reaction of the complex to mechanical distortion. The comments suggested that after dissociation of the nerve terminal from the Merkel cell definitive tests on alterations of responsiveness of the terminal, rather than solely trials on complete inactivation, are needed to help settle the issue of the importance of the Merkel cell to afferent function.

Modification of responses of penile receptors under conditions controlled by efferent activity sparked discussion on the possible functional significance of such changes in responsiveness, particularly of the velocity or dynamic components of the response. Some comments appeared to reflect introspectively generated viewpoints, a source which other participants were quick to point out did not necessarily apply to the species used for the experiment. It was emphasized that while the penis has a common reproductive function in mammals, details of intercourse and the timing of the male ejaculation vary from one species to another. Therefore alterations in movement detection capacity by the sensory elements of contact surface could have major importance for successful mating in certain species.

In the general discussion, the definition of transduction was debated at some length. Where and when should it be considered that the stimulus is transduced? Is the process of transduction the production of a generator potential in the primary afferent nerve terminal? Is it proper to consider transduction as the production of a 'receptor' potential in elements such as hair cells? Even among this gathering of active workers of the field, the place or process of transduction appeared in dispute. One argument put forth, transduction occurs when the stimulus initiates opening of ionic channels, would imply that transduction is the process of converting a stimulus into charge separation. The idea behind this view argues that conversion of the energy of the stimulus to another form represents the essential feature of transduction. If charge separation and current flow are to be taken as the mark of transduction by organs of sensory signalling, that event may occur in afferent nerve terminals in some cases to produce the current flow causing a 'generator potential' while in others it may occur as a 'receptor potential' in cells associated with the terminals. Obviously, the issue is not easy to decide until we know the nature of the intimate molecular changes. Meanwhile any decision on the point seems arbitrary.

Subject Index